Global Perspectives in Professional Reasoning

Global
Perspectives
in Professional
Reasoning

Global Perspectives in Professional Reasoning

Edited by

Marilyn B. Cole, MS, OTR/L, FAOTA
Professor Emerita of Occupational Therapy
Quinnipiac University
Hamden, Connecticut, United States

Jennifer Creek, PhD
Freelance Occupational Therapist
North Yorkshire, United Kingdom

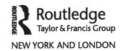

Routledge
Taylor & Francis Group

NEW YORK AND LONDON

Instructors: *Global Perspectives in Professional Reasoning, Instructor's Manual,* is also available from SLACK Incorporated. Don't miss this important companion to *Global Perspectives in Professional Reasoning.* To obtain the *Instructor's Manual,* please visit www.routledge.com/9781617116353

First published 2016 by SLACK Incorporated

Published 2024 by Routledge
605 Third Avenue, New York, NY 10158

and by Routledge
4 Park Square, Milton Park, Abingdon, Oxon OX14 4RN

Routledge is an imprint of the Taylor & Francis Group, an informa business

Names: Cole, Marilyn B., 1945- , editor. | Creek, Jennifer, editor.
Title: Global perspectives in professional reasoning / [edited by] Marilyn B.
  Cole, Jennifer Creek.
Description: Thorofare, NJ : Slack Incorporated, [2016] | Includes
  bibliographical references and index.
Identifiers: LCCN 2016003214 (print) | ISBN
  9781617116353 (hardback) | ISBN 9781630913458 (web)
Subjects: | MESH: Occupational Therapy | Thinking | Professional Competence |
  Cultural Competency | Internationality
Classification: LCC RM735 (print) | NLM WB 555 | DDC
  615.8/515--dc23
LC record available at http://lccn.loc.gov/2016003214

ISBN: 9781617116353 (hbk)
ISBN: 9781003524373 (ebk)

DOI: 10.4324/9781003524373

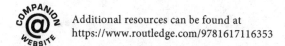

Additional resources can be found at
https://www.routledge.com/9781617116353

CONTENTS

Instructors: *Global Perspectives in Professional Reasoning, Instructor's Manual,* is also available from SLACK Incorporated. Don't miss this important companion to *Global Perspectives in Professional Reasoning.* To obtain the *Instructor's Manual,* please visit www.routledge.com/9781617116353

ABOUT THE EDITORS

Jennifer and Marli first met at the World Federation of Occupational Therapists (WFOT) Congress in Stockholm, Sweden, in 2002. At the Congress banquet, planners had randomly arranged the seating so that delegates were placed at tables with people they did not know. We found ourselves sitting directly across from each other at the long banquet table, with everyone discussing the keynote talks of the day. Jennifer contends that it was a completely random meeting, but Marli thinks that some of our colleagues got to the planners and intentionally put us together, knowing that we were both writers of textbooks who loved to talk theory. Perhaps the others were expecting to be entertained at dinner by a lively argument, but to our mutual delight, we ended up feeling we had each found a kindred spirit. Before leaving, we exchanged addresses and agreed to send each other our latest publications—Marli's *Group Dynamics in Occupational Therapy* and Jennifer's *Occupational Therapy and Mental Health*—and we continued to discuss interesting questions about occupational therapy theory via email.

A year or so later, Jennifer invited Marli to write a chapter for the Fourth Edition of the *Occupational Therapy and Mental Health* textbook, an offer Marli accepted, as the only author from the United States to be included. One of our points of agreement is that the occupational therapy literature has been too isolationistic, each country developing and publishing its own theories and research without looking to what is happening outside its borders. This is something we hope this textbook will help to change.

The next time we met was again at a WFOT Congress, this time in Sydney, Australia, in the summer of 2006. By the time of the Congress, Marli had already spent 3 months traveling in Australia with two other professors and 14 occupational therapy students from Quinnipiac University, for whom they had arranged a series of international fieldwork experiences. (Marli had done this previously in London, England, and in San Jose, Costa Rica.) In Sydney, we frequently found ourselves attending the same lectures and workshops, where we met each other's international colleagues and conversed over tea during breaks. We continued to be amazed at how much we had in common, including a mutual love of world travel.

In 2009, a good friend offered Marli a prepaid trip for two for an African Safari, which she had won in a raffle but could not use. Her husband, not an adventurer, did not want to go, nor were any of her friends free to go. So she emailed Jennifer, who loves Africa and readily agreed to accompany her. Among the zebras, giraffes, elephants, and baboons, we managed to talk about occupational therapy and our current projects. Marli was working on a textbook called *Social Participation* with coauthor Mary Donohue, and Jennifer was working on her PhD project about occupational therapy on the margins (a study of therapists practicing in nontraditional settings). We compared publishers, Jennifer unhappy with hers, and Marli very enthusiastic about SLACK Incorporated. Jennifer had previously published an edited book about clinical reasoning (*Contemporary Issues in Occupational Therapy*) with a coeditor and was looking for a new publisher for a similar, updated text. Marli suggested SLACK Incorporated.

Back home, we collaborated via email on a proposal for *Global Perspectives in Professional Reasoning*, which we would coedit. We were delighted to receive a contract from SLACK Incorporated on November 19, 2012, and both began to contact potential contributors. The process took about 2 years, with authors coming from Europe, Africa, and the United States. We agreed to meet at Marli's vacation home in Freeport, Bahamas, to complete our final edits, which, after two deadline extensions, turned out to be in January 2015. Both of us were grateful to be away from unusually cold winters (New England in the United States and North Yorkshire in the United Kingdom).

As soon as Jennifer arrived in Freeport, we went right to work. Although Marli had previously published four textbooks with SLACK Incorporated, she had never attempted an edited text, whereas Jennifer has extensive experience in the art of editing. Marli was grateful to have her mentorship during our January meeting, even though she arose 2 hours before dawn and presented a "to-do" list before morning coffee! Jennifer appreciated Marli's extensive knowledge of occupational therapy theory and beautiful writing style. Jennifer had done most of the rewriting and reorganizing of her chapters before our meeting, so Marli had the lion's share to do during the week. It turned out we keyed off each other in collaborative reasoning and even produced a cowritten chapter within the week (Chapter 1).

This collaboration has been a great joy to both of us. We have shared our knowledge, skills, and experiences; learned from each other; delighted in the quality of the chapters submitted; and reconfirmed our commitment to the global profession of occupational therapy.

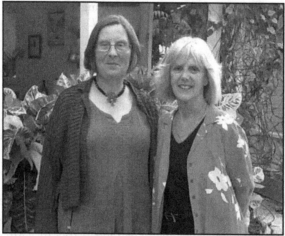

Figure A-1. Jennifer and Marli in Freeport, Bahamas, January 2015.

CONTRIBUTING AUTHORS

Angela Birleson, Dip COT, MSc, PhD (Chapter 4)
Specialist Neurological Occupational Therapist
Let's Accomplish Change Ltd.
Darlington, Co Durham, United Kingdom

Estelle B. Breines, PhD, OTR, FAOTA (Chapter 10)
President, Geri-Rehab, Inc., Retired
Lebanon, New Jersey, United States

E. Madeleine Duncan, BAOT, BA Hon (Psych), MScOT, DPhil (Psychology) (Chapter 12)
Associate Professor
Division of Occupational Therapy
Department of Health and Rehabilitation Sciences
University of Cape Town
South Africa

Ivelisse Lazzarini, OTD, OTR/L (Chapter 11)
Professor and Chair
Le Moyne College
Syracuse, New York, United States

Theresa Lorenzo, BSc (Occupational Therapy) (Wits), HDipEdAd (Wits),
MSc (Community Disability Studies) (University of London), PhD in Public Health (UCT),
PgDip (Higher Education Studies) (UCT) (Chapters 6 and 7)
Professor in Disability Studies and Occupational Therapy
Faculty of Health Sciences
University of Cape Town
South Africa

Sílvia Martins, MS, OT (Chapter 5)
Adjunct Professor
Escola Superior de Saúde do Alcoitão
Alcabideche, Portugal

Anne Hiller Scott, PhD, FAOTA, OTR/L (Chapter 8)
Occupational Therapy Program Founder, Long Island University
Associate Professor, Retired
Brooklyn, New York, United States

Richard Scott (Chapter 8)
Special Education Grant Program Coordinator, NYC Department of Education
Creative Director, Independent Artists Company
Music and Film Studies, Brooklyn College
Brooklyn, New York, United States

Hanneke van Bruggen, Bsc OT, Hon.Dscie, FWFOT (Chapter 3)
Director of Facilitation and Participation of Disadvantaged Groups (FAPADAG)
Netherlands

PREFACE

Jennifer and Marli have in common a love of theory. In our conversations about occupational therapy, we take great pleasure in analyzing our own thinking processes and challenging one another to try out alternate approaches to the problems we have encountered in our professional lives. As world travelers, we have met many original thinkers among our professional colleagues across the globe, and in this book we wanted to create a venue for them to express their unique reasoning processes. The idea for the book was born at an Occupational Therapy Africa Regional Group congress in Zambia, when a number of therapists from around the world discussed the need for a new, more comprehensive text explaining the many and varied modes of thinking used by occupational therapists in different situations. Several of these people have contributed chapters to the book.

The styles in which the chapters are presented vary greatly, as do the people, situations, and environments they address. As editors, we did not aim for consistency of style; rather, we opted to embrace diversity. Therefore, Chapter 3 (van Bruggen) uses complex and cerebral language to describe a multifaceted, strategic type of reasoning, while Martins, in Chapter 5, expresses herself in a very personal way as she takes the reader through her own ethical and spiritual processes in grappling with a very different culture.

Variations also exist with respect to the applications of professional reasoning. We chose some authors who applied previously known thought processes to new areas of occupational therapy practice. For example, Chapter 8 (Scott and Scott) shows how narrative reasoning influences our understanding of disability as portrayed in films, enriching our appreciation of clients' illness experiences. Chapter 10 (Breines) demonstrates the creative aspects of professional thinking in current occupational therapy practice and how they have evolved over time. Chapter 11 (Lazzarini) applies concepts from nonlinear science in occupational therapy approaches with cognition and for clients with cognitive issues. Other authors have derived theories of reasoning inductively from their own professional experience. For example, Chapter 4 (Birleson) unpacks and analyzes the tangle of issues influencing the development of a collaborative partnership between the National Health Service and a third sector organization in the Prof. Adjunto do Departamento de Terapia Ocupacional, Escola Superior de Saúde do Alcoitão. Chapter 5 (Martins) describes the interplay of the personal and the professional identified in the process of establishing a new occupational therapy program in a foreign country. From whichever direction the authors have approached professional reasoning, all the chapters include descriptions of theory and how it can be applied in practice.

Although each chapter represents, as one of the text's reviewers noted, a "unique experience of a therapist overcoming challenges to implement occupational therapy" (SLACK Incorporated Reviewer B, 2015), many of the situations described will remind readers of similar dilemmas in their own lives and professional roles. Coping with new problems often requires new ways of conceptualizing the problem itself. We need to take a fresh look and to acknowledge the many layers that influence both problem creation and problem solution. That is what these authors help us do.

An accompanying *Instructor's Manual* is available on the SLACK website containing brief outlines for lecture planning as well as additional learning activities.

In economically and politically uncertain times, occupational therapy can no longer rely on tradition to secure its place in the changing systems of health care. The profession must "acknowledge and embrace changes in health care provision and how political and environmental issues impact occupation. Many occupational therapists are struggling to understand or advocate for our place in the changing landscape of health care. This manuscript is an excellent roadmap for change" (SLACK Incorporated Reviewer B, 2015). Together, the original reasoning strategies described in the book offer some much-needed guidelines for moving the occupational therapy profession forward and establishing it more firmly in emerging health care models, while keeping intact the value of occupation for personal meaning, identity, health, and well-being.

For both the editors, it has been exciting to recruit both new and established authors, to help them develop their ideas and to see the book come to fruition as a coherent, scholarly whole. Each author has contributed a unique perspective on professional reasoning, and some of them have found ways to articulate aspects of reasoning that have not appeared previously in the literature. As part of the editing process, we collaborated with them to identify appropriate titles for the particular modes of reasoning described, such as strategic reasoning (Chapter 3), political reasoning (Chapter 6), and development reasoning (Chapter 12).

The book represents a future-oriented approach to professional reasoning, moving occupational therapy well beyond the clinic. It transcends national and continental borders in its pursuit of occupational justice for all nations and populations. We hope that readers will learn from the book and try out some of the reasoning strategies in practice. But we also hope they will be inspired to pay more attention to their own thinking skills and to value them as an essential component of occupational therapy.

FOREWORD

This new addition to the professional reasoning literature provides an excellent opportunity for health care professionals to reflect on their own reasoning skills and offers a foundation for exploration of broader concepts and contexts in reasoning in the local and global health care arenas. The added value of this book on professional reasoning is in facilitating occupational therapists to take a broader view, to think differently and creatively, and to step outside the box.

Health care professionals need to rethink situations and plan strategically for change, as noted in the many case studies throughout *Global Perspectives in Professional Reasoning*. This book is about change—in thinking, in practice, in ways we consider our own work contexts and the broader social and environmental contexts—taking professional reasoning outside of the clinical setting and into society, taking it to the next level. Change can be as basic as facilitating students to understand and develop creativity and creative thinking, as particularly noted by Breines in Chapter 10. Or it can be as complex as working at an international level with governments, as noted by van Bruggen in Chapter 3.

As the socially connected world evolves, there are increasing opportunities to test directions, explore solutions, and use theory and evidence in practice. As shown throughout this book, occupational therapists are using their professional skills to meet challenges in varying situations and are creating new perspectives by thinking outside the box and opening their minds to all possibilities. These situations can be client related or community or political in nature. *Global Perspectives in Professional Reasoning* facilitates the exploration of perspectives through examples offered by some of the occupational therapists who actually practice what they propose, thus allowing for the exploration of professional reasoning beyond the clinical encounter.

These perspectives have broad implications for sustainability in our rapidly changing society. For many occupational therapists, these are uncharted waters. We often remain in our clinical situations, becoming experts at what we do, which can be a good thing, but do we really become the experts we want to be by remaining only in our clinical situations and not taking up opportunities to expand our horizons? *Global Perspectives in Professional Reasoning* challenges occupational therapists to do just that.

The United Nations (UN), in March 2015, held a major conference on disaster risk reduction (DRR) directed toward reducing the impact of natural disasters and helping to prevent man-made disasters. The World Federation of Occupational Therapists (WFOT) contributed a position statement to the session on inclusion, noting that the post-2015 Framework for DRR should be rights based, equity oriented, people centered, and environmentally sustainable. To fulfill the requirement for inclusiveness, a disability-inclusive, gender-sensitive, community-driven approach should be adopted. The Framework should be designed to build on and strengthen local resilience capabilities (WFOT, 2015). Where are occupational therapists in the mix? How can we use these concepts in our practice? Lorenzo, in Chapter 6, offers perspectives on getting involved.

The UN Millennium Development Goals, which ended in 2015, were a call for action to countries and organizations around the world, and the post-2015 Sustainable Development Goals (SDGs) are taking the quest to the next level. The SDGs are intended to be universal in the sense of embodying a "universally shared common global vision of progress toward a safe, just and sustainable space for all human beings to thrive on the planet" (UN, 2015). The goals were identified to promote global action toward ending poverty, promoting prosperity and well-being for all, protecting the environment, and addressing climate change. They reflect the moral principles that no one and no country should be left behind and that everyone and every country should be regarded as having a common responsibility for playing their part in delivering the global vision. In general terms, all of the goals have therefore been conceived both as ambitions and as challenges to all countries. The UN requires regular reports on actions from member countries. With the increasing pressure for improved ecological systems, improved human rights, and reduced poverty, this book identifies where occupational therapists fit in the mix.

This book challenges assumptions about clinical and professional reasoning and promotes broader perspectives. *Global Perspectives in Professional Reasoning* will encourage occupational therapists to consider the examples shared here and to think outside the box. As noted by Creek in Chapter 2, it is important to recognize that the language we use when working with clients, teaching students, developing existing services, and establishing new services, and in many other ways, is culture bound and influences our thinking skills and cognitive processes, as well as the way we explain our practice to colleagues, clients, and the wider community. It is also important to consider the social context of our practice and work with clients and others, as noted by Cole in Chapter 9.

Occupational therapists thinking outside the box with nonlinear (creative) reasoning and who are open to alternative ways of thinking are more likely to challenge personal preconceptions, develop toward leadership in sustainable practices, and advocate for social change and healthy communities. It is a broad-ranging, evolving process as occupational therapists find their skills applicable not only in direct client therapy but at the level of populations and governments, using a wide range of professional reasoning. It is a process toward sustainable practice in which we challenge barriers and constraints. The chapters in this book highlight themes of partnership and collaboration, openness, social networking, and the use of personal relationships, as well as occupational therapy's identity in the broader social and political arenas. With these concepts in place, we can anticipate a changed future where occupational therapists are well positioned and well prepared to meet the future needs of society.

—*Kit Sinclair, PhD*
Fellow, World Federation of Occupational Therapists

References

United Nations. (2015). *Universal sustainable development goals stakeholder forum 2015.* Retrieved from https://sustainabledevelopment.un.org

World Federation of Occupational Therapists. (2015). *Position statement on disaster risk reduction.* Retrieved from http://www.wfot.org/Practice/DisasterPreparednessandResponseDPR.aspx

1

Introduction to the Book

Jennifer Creek, PhD and Marilyn B. Cole, MS, OTR/L, FAOTA

Professional reasoning takes the reader beyond the boundaries of the clinic and into a wider world of practice. We looked to therapists, educators, and scholars who have explored new areas of professional practice, such as the humanities, social networks, underserved populations, and underserved communities, and asked them to write about their thought processes in accomplishing their visions for practice. Some types of reasoning have clinical applications, while others serve to guide therapists in establishing occupational therapy educational and community programs where the profession has never been before. Our contributors come from around the world, providing a global perspective while demonstrating that occupational therapists within vastly different cultures serve remarkably similar human needs: to be included in their communities, to have occupational choices, and to determine their own life course. The stories told are inspiring as well as enlightening. They serve as examples of what occupational therapists can accomplish when they expand their professional reasoning.

WHAT IS PROFESSIONAL REASONING?

Professional reasoning has been defined as the full range of thinking skills and "cognitive processes used to guide professional actions" (Schell & Schell, 2008, p. 447). The professional reasoning used by occupational therapists has a broad range of applications, including clinical practice, the development of services, expanding occupational therapy's role in community practice, teaching students, and creating social and political change. All of these applications can be found within this book.

The term *clinical reasoning* is used to refer more narrowly to the modes of thinking that the therapist uses when trying to understand people's needs and what to do about them, such as defining problems, making judgments, and reaching clinical decisions (Schell & Schell, 2008; Sinclair, 2007).

At the outset, clinical reasoning had to be differentiated from theoretical reasoning. Whereas therapists often use theories within their practice, clinical reasoning refers to their practical

Cole, M. B., & Creek, J. (Eds.).
Global Perspectives in Professional Reasoning (pp. 1-6).
© 2016 Taylor & Francis Group.

application in therapy and in everyday life. Although clinical reasoning came to the forefront of occupational therapy practice during the 1980s, the now-classic research study by Mattingly and Fleming (1994) identified the first evidence-based categories of reasoning demonstrated by master occupational therapy clinicians: procedural, interactive, and conditional. Procedural reasoning is similar to medical problem solving, relative to the client's physical and mental health conditions, symptoms, and the functional consequences of these for everyday occupations. Interactive reasoning refers to the therapist's encounters with clients as people, as social beings, considering their subjective illness and wellness experiences. Conditional reasoning applies to the impact of contexts and environments, as well as timing, including clients' life stage, their past, present, and future. Because occupational therapy practitioners appear to think in all three of these modes, simultaneously applying them to different aspects of the same problem, Mattingly and Fleming dubbed occupational therapy practitioners "therapists with the three track mind" (1994, p. 119). Subsequently, Schell and Schell (2008) identified and defined a wider range of clinical reasoning categories: scientific, narrative, pragmatic, ethical, interactive, and conditional reasoning. Definitions of these terms may be found in the Glossary at the end of this book.

Some of the chapters in this book cover aspects of clinical reasoning (e.g., Chapter 2 presents findings from clinical reasoning research), but all of them go far beyond the confines of the clinical encounter. This book expands our understanding of the term professional reasoning, a broader term encompassing all of our professional activities, from past and present to future.

The contributors to this book are all experienced occupational therapists, demonstrating expertise in a range of professional reasoning skills.

THE AUTHORS

The chapters in this book encompass a wide range of thinking skills and cognitive processes, from reflecting on practice to solving problems, and from clinical reasoning to strategic reasoning. Most authors focus their attention on the process of reasoning rather than on the specific types of reasoning they are employing, or on desired outcomes. This may be because they all found themselves in situations that demanded new ways of thinking and working—for example, helping to develop a new occupational therapy program in an unfamiliar country (Chapters 3 and 5) or carrying out research in collaboration with people with disabilities (Chapters 6 and 10). All the authors were willing to travel outside the boundaries of what was familiar to them, into situations that drove the development of new forms of reasoning or forms that were new to them. The chapters chart the learning process that authors went through as they extended their thinking skills and processes to meet the challenges they encountered.

The authors come from a wide range of nationalities and backgrounds. Countries represented include the United States (5), United Kingdom (2), South Africa (2), Portugal, and the Netherlands. The topics, however, represent both developed and developing nations worldwide. Because of the complexity of the subject, authors approach professional reasoning from a variety of perspectives that take us into unfamiliar worlds (disability film, evolution of creativity) and unexpected levels of professional leadership (establishing educational programs in third-world countries, partnerships with disability organizations, creating an occupational therapy network across all of Europe). Their work challenges readers to expand their views of where occupational therapy may be applicable and relevant and what social changes it might accomplish. They do so in a variety of writing styles, each appropriate to the chosen topic. Some are scholarly, referring to many researchers and experts, and others are highly personal and reflective. Yet despite these differences, their themes and the lessons they have to teach are surprisingly similar. A brief review of some of these themes follows.

THEMES FLOWING THROUGH THE BOOK

The 10 themes described here are representative of the content of this text: collaboration, learning through reflection, aligning occupational therapy with the principles of humanity, openness, the power of personal relationships and social networks, modeling, pragmatism, complexity, occupational therapy's identity in the larger social arena, and, finally, creating social change.

The theme of collaboration comes through in nearly every chapter. By that we mean working in partnership with others, whether the client–therapist relationship, occupational therapists working with other professionals, or therapists within service provision entities collaborating with other organizations to achieve mutual goals. For example, Birleson describes the process and benefits of collaborating with community organizations representing consumers with head injuries (Chapter 4). Van Bruggen demonstrates strategic thinking in the creation of the European Network of Occupational Therapy in Higher Education, through involving both regulatory and funding organizations with a common interest in providing inclusion for persons with disabilities in their respective countries (Chapter 3). Cole stresses the importance of collaboration with social connections and networks to achieve individual occupational goals (Chapter 9).

This collection of writings charts the journeys the authors took toward developing expert professional reasoning for particular applications. For example, Chapter 4 describes the learning process that an experienced practitioner went through as she worked in partnership with a third sector organization to develop new services. Acquiring new skills through experience did not happen automatically, but as the authors of each chapter explain, they learned from reflecting deeply on their experiences and testing that learning against new challenges. Individual authors each had their own preferred style of reflective learning, which included both personal and cultural aspects. Birleson (Chapter 4), employed within statutory neurological health services in the United Kingdom, thought about her investment of time in a head injury charity in terms of the potential benefits to her service. Lorenzo (Chapter 6), working in rural South Africa, measured the efficacy of her reasoning by the range and quality of the people and organizations with whom she was able to collaborate.

The philosophy of occupational therapy from the outset has included the belief that occupations provide meaning in people's lives. That value continues to guide occupational therapists' reasoning—not only in the therapy we provide but in the way that we make professional decisions and in the projects we choose to undertake. For example, in Chapter 5, Martins describes using reflection to better understand her own reasoning with respect to taking on a challenging project, the establishment of an occupational therapy educational program in Mozambique. This includes moral and ethical thinking as well as the human attributes of empathy and compassion. Duncan articulates this question best (Chapter 12): "How may the profession align itself with a human development agenda?" In other words, how can we find ways to improve conditions within which people can engage in occupations that will improve their lives, such as gaining employment or establishing food security—projects with broader social impact?

The practice and thinking of the authors is characterized by openness to alternative ways of working, to the possibility of change and to other people's points of view. In Chapter 2, Creek demonstrates how changing the words we use can change how we think, whereas in Chapter 5, Martins describes being willing to abandon or adapt her carefully prepared teaching materials when she discovered that they were not appropriate for her students. All the authors demonstrate a willingness to learn and develop, both as people and as therapists. Martins expresses her gratitude for having been given the opportunity to work in a foreign country and for the intense learning experiences it offered. In Chapter 12, Duncan writes about the risks and rewards of employing a participatory methodology. Without this openness to new experiences and willingness to challenge personal assumptions and preconceptions, none of these authors would have made the decision to become involved in the projects described in this book.

Several authors acknowledge that the bonds established between people in various decision-making positions can make or break the success of a program or the achievement of a vision or a desired goal. For example, Martins (Chapter 5) identifies that the bonds developed between individuals while establishing an occupational therapy program in Mozambique kept participants from abandoning the project in its beginning stages. Cole (Chapter 9) shows how social relationships provide support and meaning, motivating people to continue their occupational engagements. Van Bruggen (Chapter 3) calls on her personal contacts to help her navigate difficult political situations, acknowledging the effectiveness of the strategic mention of an influential personal connection when applying for a grant.

Another theme that can be traced through many of the chapters is that of modeling. For example, authors often describe modeling appropriate professional behavior to their students and colleagues. In Chapter 4, Birleson describes working in partnership with her mentee, who learned in turn to work as an equal partner with her service users. In Chapter 7, Lorenzo describes mutual learning as a way of modeling person-centered practice to her students. Some chapters discuss how therapists model ways in which people can take control of their own lives, by working in partnership rather than taking the lead. In Chapter 6, Lorenzo highlights the need to involve local people in making decisions about projects that will affect them so that development is owned and, hence, more likely to be sustainable. In Chapter 5, Martins emphasizes the importance of engaging students as active partners in the process of program development and delivery so that they will feel committed to establishing the new profession in their country.

Throughout history, occupational therapists have favored action and doing over thinking and reflection. This practical aspect of our profession makes us especially useful in situations where action is needed, such as reducing the negative effects of poverty or facilitating the inclusion of children with disabilities in schools and communities. In Chapter 10, Breines articulates the connection between creativity and pragmatism as ancient cultures attempted to solve the problems of their day. This same resourcefulness can help today's occupational therapists find creative solutions to problems with funding or overcome barriers to participation in wellness and primary care. In Chapter 6, Lorenzo demonstrates some practical projects to raise community awareness of the need for inclusion among citizens with disabilities in South Africa, and in Chapter 7, she describes concrete activities to encourage occupational therapy students to become effective leaders.

Complexity is a theme that runs through most of the chapters, from the more reflective to the more theoretical. Creek introduces the European Conceptual Framework for Occupational Therapy, a theory that is organized as a complex system (Chapter 2). Duncan discusses the complexity involved in attempting to align the different values by which people live through a process of axiological reasoning (Chapter 12). Self-organization is a key feature of nonlinear cognition, which requires occupational therapists to make a fundamental shift in thinking (Lazzarini, Chapter 11). Complex systems are self-organizing, and the challenge of promoting self-organization in communities is another theme that several authors address. Duncan writes about the role of the occupational therapist in developing healthy societies that meet the needs of their members, rather than working with individuals. In Chapter 10, Breines describes people as self-organizing systems, developing through interaction with their environments.

Many authors discuss practice areas that are outside the traditional or established systems. In the United States, these might be called *emerging practice areas* or *emerging niches*. In the United Kingdom, they are often called *role emerging areas* or working *"on the margins"* (Creek, 2014). They include community development (Chapters 6 and 12), participating in political and organizational efforts to comply with global health and human rights standards (Chapter 6), and establishing occupational therapy education and services where they have never been before (Chapters 3, 4, 5, and 12).

One of the themes of this book echoes the social activism of early occupational therapists. Authors are less concerned with clinical interventions than with bringing about social change to create healthier communities. Duncan, in Chapter 12, describes a development role for occupational therapists in which they work to create the conditions for people to live dignified and meaningful lives. In Chapter 4, Birleson recognizes that involving people with head injuries in developing services for themselves will reduce their dependence on statutory services. In Chapter 6, Lorenzo demonstrates how occupational therapists can interpret public policies in ways that encourage groups of disadvantaged persons to advocate for needed social change.

How the Book Is Organized

The title of each chapter includes the specific type of professional reasoning addressed within it, often followed by the pertinent application areas. Just scanning the titles can therefore give the reader an overview of the broad range of reasoning from which he or she might learn. The applications, in turn, model the ways in which different types of reasoning can be useful, and we hope, will help the reader to see possible parallels with his or her own dilemmas or opportunities.

Each of the chapters in this book covers a number of the themes identified in the last section, so it was not possible to organize the book thematically. Instead, the editors identified a continuum of approaches along which the chapters can be organized. Some authors describe finding themselves in unfamiliar and challenging situations in which they begin by observing what is going on, try to make sense of it, and then work out what to do. Other authors are fascinated by, and see potential in, a theory, a policy, or an approach; study it; and then look for ways to utilize it in practice. We have called these the *bottom-up* and the *top-down* approaches. Both approaches use theory, and both describe reasoning in practice; the difference is in the direction of travel.

Chapters in the first half of the book (with the exception of Chapter 2) describe the bottom-up approach. For example, in Chapter 5, Martins is offered an opportunity to help set up a new occupational therapy program in an unfamiliar country. This is the starting point for a complex process of professional reasoning through which she learns the thinking skills needed for such a project.

Chapters in the second half of the book describe the top-down approach. For example, in Chapter 11, Lazzarini recognizes that nonlinear cognition could enhance occupational therapists' professional reasoning, making it more flexible, open, and dynamic. Scott and Scott, in Chapter 8, explore the nature of narrative reasoning and then illustrate how it can be used to analyze the illness narratives in disability-themed films as a way of teaching this mode of reasoning to students and deepening its meaning for practitioners.

Chapter 2 discusses the language of professional reasoning and provides the reader with a vocabulary for thinking about the themes and issues covered in the rest of the book.

How to Use the Book

How many occupational therapy practitioners find themselves wishing to be free of the many constraints that limit today's practice? Yet most of us continue in our current positions, unsure of how to do otherwise. The professional reasoning put forth in this book can help occupational therapy professionals understand how they can rethink their situations; consider the social, political, and economic dimensions of their practice; and think and plan strategically to take steps to change the conditions that currently constrain us.

The people invited to contribute to this book are already leaders in their fields who have pioneered projects or engaged in opportunities that were often well outside the normal scope of occupational therapy practice. Because of this, their modes of thinking are original, created as part of their own response to the situations they encountered. Each has outlined some of the lessons they learned, and their ways of thinking have much to teach us all about how we can bring about the kinds of change that are needed in our respective societies. These accounts of professional reasoning may represent the professional thinking of the future, helping us to position occupational therapy to become well recognized and well prepared to meet future occupational needs.

We suggest that therapists, educators, and students use this book to broaden their range of professional reasoning as it might apply to the problems they see in their own situations. For example, thinking in clinical practice can be greatly enhanced by considering the narrative reasoning made apparent in disability films, teaching us to appreciate the emotional and spiritual dimensions of the illness experience. Through nonlinear cognition, therapists can appreciate the need to step back and allow clients the opportunity to self-organize or find ways to guide them through this process. Educators can learn to appreciate the need to model true collaboration and partnership with their students and thus to prepare them to become more effective therapists and leaders. Those of us who are already experienced might take courage from the examples described here to seize opportunities to lead the profession into uncharted waters within larger social and political contexts.

There are many ways in which you, the reader, might decide to use the wealth of information and experience represented by the following chapters. You may decide to read the book from start to finish, or to begin with the chapter that looks most interesting or most relevant to your own situation. Or you may wish to think about a problem you have encountered in your own position as an occupational therapist, or a position you might aspire to. What barriers and constraints do you see? Chances are, one or more of these chapters describes a situation with similar characteristics, and the authors' experience and reflections can serve as models for the reasoning required to begin to make some changes.

CONCLUSION

The different types of professional reasoning are evident from the titles of the chapters. This collection of alternative ways of thinking can guide both students and professionals in becoming more thoughtful and effective clinicians, establishing programs that serve their communities, operating in nontraditional settings, partnering with community organizations, initiating educational programs, and sharing knowledge and evidence with each other and with other professionals. Our international authors have much to teach us about how occupational therapists can create visions of a better health care system, establish strategic social connections, advocate for inclusiveness, and lead the way in effecting needed policy changes. Much of the reasoning described here could be essential knowledge for occupational therapy leaders, educators, and scholars to effect the social and political change that is needed to move the profession forward toward broader and more inclusive roles and recognition.

REFERENCES

Creek, J. (2014). *Transformative occupational therapy practice: Learning from the margins*. Unpublished PhD thesis. University of Sheffield, United Kingdom.

Mattingly, C., & Fleming, M. (1994). *Clinical reasoning: Forms of inquiry in a therapeutic practice*. Philadelphia, PA: F. A. Davis.

Schell, B., & Schell, J. (2008). *Clinical and professional reasoning in occupational therapy*. Philadelphia, PA: Wolters Kluwer/Lippincott Williams & Wilkins.

Sinclair, K. (2007). Exploring the facets of clinical reasoning. In J. Creek & A. Lawson-Porter (Eds.), *Contemporary issues in occupational therapy: Reasoning and reflection* (pp. 143-160). Chichester, England: Wiley.

2

The Language of
Professional Reasoning

Jennifer Creek, PhD

During a training session on outcome measurement for staff working in a National Health Service trust, one of the participants expressed concern that a particular client's score on an anxiety scale had not gone down after occupational therapy intervention. I suggested that occupational therapy is not so much concerned with levels of anxiety as with what people do, and asked whether the client was able to engage in more activities or be active for longer periods after the intervention program. The occupational therapist paused for a few moments and then said, in a surprised voice, "I thought occupational therapy hadn't worked for this woman, but she started shopping on her own and going out for coffee with friends. It was a success; she was doing the things she wanted to do, even though she was still anxious!"

To measure the effectiveness of occupational therapy, we have to be able to say what we are trying to achieve and how our goals differ from those of other professions. For this, we need a professional vocabulary that makes clear the difference between, for example, reducing anxiety and improving occupational performance.

This chapter is concerned with the language of occupational therapy and with the relationship between the words we use and how we think. *Language* is commonly understood as "a system of human communication using words, written and spoken, and particular ways of combining them" (*Shorter Oxford English Dictionary*, 2002). But language is also an important tool for making sense of the world and of our own interactions with it. In fact, the words we use to refer to things and events have a strong influence on how we perceive and react to them: Describing the glass as half full feels more positive than saying it is half empty.

To think is to "exercise the mind . . . in a positive, active way, [to] form connected ideas, meditate, cogitate" (*Shorter Oxford English Dictionary*, 2002). Thinking "includes such mental actions as applying rules, choosing, conceptualising, evaluating, judging, justifying, knowing, perceiving and understanding" (Creek, 2007b, p. 9). Some types of thinking do not require language and are

Cole, M. B., & Creek, J. (Eds.).
Global Perspectives in Professional Reasoning (pp. 7-23).
© 2016 Taylor & Francis Group.

difficult to express in words, such as the thinking involved in playing tennis: A player coordinates his or her responses to everything that is happening on the court without having to put his or her thinking processes into words. Indeed, he or she would probably not be able to do so. Expert practice in any field tends to be largely nonlinguistic, or tacit, making it difficult to explain in words (Fleming, 1994).

In contrast to nonlinguistic thinking, linguistic thinking requires language. It has been observed that "the first act of the thinking mind is to make for itself its conceptual atoms or ideas" (Dickoff, James, & Wiedenbach, 1968, p. 420), and these atoms are given names, "whose function is to allow the mind to point out, denote, or attend to conceptually a factor within the mind's consciousness" (p. 420). In the context of linguistic thinking, a thing or a concept does not exist until it is named. For example, the concept of marginalization only became cognizable when it was differentiated from other, similar concepts and given its own label. The word *marginalization* draws attention to and makes connections between a particular set of social phenomena, turning them into a single concept that can be thought about, discussed, and addressed.

Occupational therapists employ both nonlinguistic and linguistic thinking skills in their practice. Some of the specialist thinking skills that make up professional reasoning, such as decision making, theorizing, and ethical reasoning, are explored in this chapter, which is set out in three main sections. The first section reviews issues around occupational therapy terminology and offers a set of definitions of key professional terms. The second section discusses the nature of clinical and professional reasoning in occupational therapy, highlighting the range of thinking skills used in practice. The third section explores the relationship between language and reasoning, finishing with some of the ways in which professional language can support or inhibit the clinical and professional reasoning of occupational therapists.

OCCUPATIONAL THERAPY TERMINOLOGY

Language is a social institution, in that "the individual cannot by himself either create or modify it; it is essentially a collective contract which one must accept in its entirety if one wishes to communicate" (Barthes, 1967, p. 14). Language is made up of words that represent or signify concepts and delineate the relationships between them, and the meanings of words must be agreed on within a linguistic community.

Each group speaking a shared language, such as English or Japanese, accumulates a vocabulary that represents the concepts relevant to everyday thinking and communication; for example, the English language contains many words to describe aspects of our changeable weather. In addition to the everyday language of the community, each discipline, field of practice, or profession has a specialist terminology that represents key concepts. This applies to every type of work, from the production line to particle physics. For example, when a physicist talks about subatomic particles, waves, and photons (Gribbin, 1984), he or she has a clear idea of what these words mean and expects other physicists to share the same understanding. Students of physics must learn the terminology of the field before they can begin to understand or communicate about the subject.

Defining Occupational Therapy Concepts

Occupational therapy has a clearly articulated professional purpose (World Federation of Occupational Therapists [WFOT], 2011), but practitioners often find it difficult to state what we do in ways that differentiate our purpose and practice from the areas of responsibility of other professions or that make clear what is common to occupational therapy practice across multiple fields and cultures (Creek, 1998; Pollard & Sakellariou, 2012). The WFOT (2011) has described occupational therapy as "a client-centred health profession concerned with promoting health and well being through occupation." Understanding this description requires us to know what meaning occupational therapists give to the terms *client centered, health, well being, promoting health,* and *occupation.*

Occupational therapy has its own professional terminology, but many of the key concepts are disputed or ill defined, even within a particular linguistic community. For example, there is no single, accepted definition in English of the word *occupation*, which is central to the field. Different authors and theorists may offer their own definitions or none, assuming that all other occupational therapists share the same understanding, irrespective of their cultural background, work experience, and length of practice (Kantartzis & Molineux, 2012).

Even if occupational therapists within a language group manage to reach agreement on the meaning of key terms, those meanings continue to evolve over time so that new definitions have to be developed continually, because "word meanings are dynamic rather than static formations" (Vygotsky, 1962, p. 124). The word *occupation* would be understood differently in 1915, in 2015, and, we can assume, in 2115. Some words, and the concepts they represent, fall out of fashion or are superseded as new theories are developed or adopted. For example, in some countries the concept of *volunteering* has been replaced by *civic engagement.*

Furthermore, as social needs change and the profession expands into new areas of practice, new words are needed to represent emerging concepts. For example, Galheigo (2005), writing about occupational therapy in the social field, highlighted the need for an occupational therapy vocabulary "to refer to those in need . . . excluded, marginalized, vulnerable, survivors, deviant, under apartheid, disadvantaged, disaffiliated" (p. 87) that would leave no room for misinterpretations of "the phenomenon of inequality" (p. 88).

Another problem we have in trying to understand the intended meaning of a communication, such as the WFOT definition of occupational therapy, is that words often carry personal, cultural, and symbolic meanings that are not found in standard dictionaries. The words that we use can in themselves represent an ideology, a political stance, or a particular worldview. For example, the words occupational therapists use to refer to the people we work with indicate something about how we view our relationship with them; such terms include *patient, client, service user, resident, individual,* or *inmate.* Each of these terms connotes a particular set of expectations about the roles and responsibilities of the therapist and the person.

Professional Knowledge and Language

The words that we use represent particular ways of thinking about the world. At the deepest level, words represent the way we understand the nature of reality. For example, when I talk about *establishing the facts* or *making a firm diagnosis*, I am assuming that illness has an external reality that can be discovered and known. On the other hand, when I talk about *negotiating an understanding of the illness experience*, my words carry the assumption that illness is a social, cultural, and personal construction. These are different epistemological positions, that is, different views about what constitutes knowledge and how its validity can be tested. For example, I can know whether my client's physical function has improved after treatment by using a standardized or individualized outcome measure. I can assume that my client finds occupational therapy intervention helpful if he continues to attend sessions at the day center. The affirmation of this assumption hinges on the co-construction of understanding, knowledge, and meaning between client and therapist through particular forms of communication and language.

The theories that practitioners select give them not only a specialist vocabulary but also a particular way of knowing. For example, the occupational therapist employing a psychoanalytic frame of reference will use words such as *containment, unconscious defenses, denial,* and *transference* (Nicholls, Piergrossi, de Sena-Gibertoni, & Daniel, 2013) and frame what he or she sees in terms of the concepts that these words represent. It is impossible to fully divorce knowledge and understanding from language.

Anna chooses wood carving, a new activity for her, and decides to make a small box. Technically, this is a difficult task; she must gouge with force and precision, and accept the slowness of a long project. Sliver after sliver, she cuts out the inner space of the small container, and towards the end of the session she begins to talk about being hospitalised after the death of her mother for a spinal tap because they thought she had a serious illness. She tells how she became completely blocked, as hard as a piece of wood; that she moved rigidly as if her body were all one piece. She begins to talk about the death of her mother and the shocking scene she remembers having seen. We can hypothesise that the aggressive cutting with the tool in the wood reminded her of the fear of the spinal tap, which for a young child was certainly painful and invasive. It is interesting that she describes herself as "blocked and rigid like a piece of wood." She uses this expression after 30 minutes of concentrated carving in the hard material of wood. We can imagine that, as she transformed the rough material into a small box, gouge after gouge, there was a parallel movement inside herself which transformed an emotional block into a space for being able to remember, to think and to tell. (Piergrossi, 2013, pp. 95-96)

If the occupational therapist thinks that the truth is out there and will be discovered when the appropriate tools have been designed, his or her gaze will be turned toward the patient's signs and symptoms, the patient's functional performance, and the assessment tools by which these can be measured. If he or she thinks that reality is co-constructed in particular situations by particular people, the occupational therapist's attention will turn to the wider context in which he or she and the client are working, including physical, social, and cultural environments and their own relationships to them.

It has been suggested that one reason why occupational therapists have a problematic relationship with our professional terminology is that the profession takes two distinct approaches to conceptualizing and addressing health needs. We take a pragmatic view of the nature of human beings, derived from the profession's founding philosophies, and a structuralist approach to knowledge, influenced by occupational therapy's close relationship with medicine over many years. The development of occupational therapy has been described as a "long conversation" between pragmatist and structuralist discourses (Hooper & Wood, 2002, p. 40). However, it is claimed that these two cultural discourses are discordant and that by attempting to retain both of them, occupational therapy has cultivated "a basic and problematic incompatibility" (p. 46).

The anthropologist Cheryl Mattingly saw occupational therapy's espousal of two very different ways of thinking in a more positive light. She described occupational therapy as a two-body practice because the therapist can "interweave interventions that address both the disease and the illness experience into the same treatment activity" (Mattingly, 1994a, p. 38). One half of the two-body practice works with the body as machine, which involves dealing with functional problems and treating disease with specific techniques. Mattingly (1994a, p. 37) described this as "a practice that occurs in the cultural domain of biomedicine." The other half of the two-body practice works with the lived body, which involves addressing problems that encompass social, cultural, and psychological issues and interrupt people's whole lives, including "their daily practices, life histories, social relationships, and long-term projects, all of which give them a sense of meaning and a sense of personal identity" (Mattingly, 1994b, p. 65).

To work successfully in a two-body practice, occupational therapists need to be aware of which body we are working with at any particular time and to use the appropriate terminology. It may be relevant to talk about *diagnosis, assessment,* and *treatment* when working with the body as machine, but a different vocabulary is needed when the therapist is working with the lived body. This is vividly illustrated in an account by an occupational therapist of going to work in a rural African community. She writes about *alleviating* not *curing*, about *passing on skills* rather than *teaching,* and about *interacting with* instead of *treating.*

So instead of specific remediation I am now involved in alleviating the effects of poverty and deprivation, passing on skills to unskilled but dedicated workers, interacting with crowds of kids instead of one-to-one therapy, accepting third-world solutions rather than expensive first-world ones. (Sherry, 2010, p. 40)

None of the existing occupational therapy terminologies and taxonomies makes explicit the epistemologies implicit in particular terms. Indeed, some authors write as though there is only one professional language for occupational therapy (Davis & Polatajko, 2005), as is evident in discussions about *occupation* and related terms such as *activity, task,* and *skill.* These words represent core occupational therapy concepts, and their meaning has been debated in the professional literature for many years (e.g., Breines, 1984; Katz & Sachs, 1991; Pollard & Sakellariou, 2012). Nonetheless, there have only been limited attempts to locate these concepts and terms within wider social, historical, and political contexts (Kantartzis & Molineux, 2012).

Occupational Therapy Taxonomies

The most commonly seen taxonomy in the occupational therapy literature is the classification of terms related to occupational performance (e.g., Creek, 2003; Hagedorn, 2000; Polatajko et al., 2004). Hagedorn's (2000) Taxonomy of Human Occupation and the Canadian Taxonomic Code for Occupational Performance (Polatajko et al., 2004) organize concepts into hierarchies, based on general systems theory (Boulding, 1968), in which "each higher level [subsumes] all the characteristics of those below it and each higher level [has] one more dimension of complexity than that below it" (Polatajko et al., 2004, p. 263). For example, in the Taxonomic Code for Occupational Performance, an occupation is made up of a set of activities, each of which is made up of a set of tasks, each of which is made up of an action or set of actions, and so on (Polatajko et al., 2004).

An alternative approach to the organization of key occupational therapy concepts, based on complexity theory, was employed in the publication *Occupational Therapy Defined as a Complex Intervention* (Creek, 2003). In this classification, occupations, activities, tasks, and skills do not differ in their degree of complexity. During the course of an intervention, the therapist's attention moves inward from occupations, to activities, to tasks, to skills, and outward again, but the focus of attention is not diluted or simplified; a skill is no more or less complex than a task, an activity, or an occupation. An example of this is given in Box 2-1.

In 2001, the European Network of Occupational Therapy in Higher Education set up a working group to produce a standard terminology of key occupational therapy concepts. This group, representing six European languages, chose complexity theory as the organizing framework for the terminology because it "does not attempt to simplify the complexity of human doing by using words that lock activities and occupations into static categories [but] captures the dynamism and unpredictability of occupation in all its manifestations" (Creek, 2010, p. 12).

The outcome of this project was a conceptual framework made up of 25 terms, each representing an aspect of occupational performance from the perspective of the performer. The 25 terms and their definitions are given in Table 2-1 (ENOTHE Terminology Project 2008, as cited in Creek, 2010). (Note that two of the terms have two definitions each, making a total of 27 definitions.)

Each term in the conceptual framework can be defined only in relation to all the other terms; for example, the definition of *occupation* indicates how it relates to the other 24 concepts—both what it has in common with them and how it differs. The terminology is therefore displayed as a network of relationships between terms, as shown in Figure 2-1. These relationships change depending on the circumstances in which the framework is being used, so the display is not static but has a unique presentation in every situation.

This section discussed some of the issues that occupational therapists are addressing as they continue to refine and extend their professional terminology, including the meaning of key concepts, the evolution of language, multiple epistemologies, and the organization of terminology into taxonomies. The next section defines clinical and professional reasoning and considers the role of language in learning how to reason.

BOX 2-1. OCCUPATIONAL THERAPY AS A COMPLEX INTERVENTION

A young man with long-term mental health problems is preparing to leave the hospital and move into his own place. He and the occupational therapist are considering all the occupations that contribute to independent living and assessing which ones might need intervention at this stage. They take into account not only what the client will need to do, want to do, or be expected to do but also the physical environment in which he will be living; the amount and types of support he can depend on; his cultural background, as it influences what he does and how he does it; his expected income; and a multitude of other factors. Having identified one or more problematic occupational performance areas, the therapist and client carry out an assessment to identify which parts of the occupation he is unable to manage. The problem or deficit might be associated with, for example, the young man's ability to perform a particular activity or activities; his capacity for action, including degree of motivation and volition; the physical environment into which he is moving; or the social context in which he will be living. If the therapist and client identify a problem with the young man's activity performance, the next stage of the assessment will focus on identifying the specific difficulty, which could be inadequate skills to support effective task performance, emotional barriers to performance, lack of knowledge and experience, weak habits and routines, poor social support networks, or many other factors. At each level of assessment, the interactions of a complex range of factors can be seen to shape the young man's occupational, activity, and task performance.

TABLE 2-1
EUROPEAN NETWORK OF OCCUPATIONAL THERAPY IN HIGHER EDUCATION DEFINITIONS

ABILITY	A personal characteristic that supports occupational performance.
ACTIVITY	A structured series of actions or tasks that contributes to occupations.
AUTONOMY	The freedom to make choices based on consideration of internal and external circumstances and to act on those choices.
CONTEXT	The relationships among the environment, personal factors, and events that influence the meaning of a task, activity, or occupation for the performer.
DEPENDENCE	The condition of needing support to be able to perform everyday activities to a satisfactory level.
ENGAGEMENT	A sense of involvement, choice, positive meaning, and commitment while performing an occupation or activity.
ENVIRONMENT	External physical, sociocultural, and temporal factors that demand and shape occupational performance.
FUNCTION	1. The underlying physical and psychological components that support occupational performance. 2. The capacity to use occupational performance components to carry out a task, activity, or occupation.

(continued)

TABLE 2-1 (CONTINUED)

EUROPEAN NETWORK OF OCCUPATIONAL THERAPY IN HIGHER EDUCATION DEFINITIONS

HABIT	A performance pattern in daily life, acquired by frequent repetition, that does not require attention and allows efficient function.
INDEPENDENCE	The condition of being able to perform everyday activities to a satisfactory level.
INTERDEPENDENCE	The condition of mutual dependence and influence between members of a social group.
MOTIVATION	A drive that directs a person's actions toward meeting needs.
OCCUPATION	A group of activities that has personal and sociocultural meaning, is named within a culture, and supports participation in society. Occupations can be categorized as self-care, productivity, and/or leisure.
OCCUPATION/ ACTIVITY/TASK PERFORMANCE	Choosing, organizing, and carrying out occupations/activities/tasks in interaction with the environment.
OCCUPATIONAL PERFORMANCE AREAS	Categories of tasks, activities, and occupations that are typically part of daily life. They are usually called self-care, productivity, and leisure.
OCCUPATION PERFORMANCE COMPONENTS	Abilities and skills that enable and affect engagement in tasks, activities, and occupations. These can be categorized, for example, as physical, cognitive, psychosocial, and affective.
PARTICIPATION	Involvement in life situations through activity within a social context.
ROLE	Social and cultural norms and expectations of occupational performance that are associated with the individual's social and personal identity.
ROUTINE	An established and predictable sequence of tasks.
SETTING	The immediate surroundings that influence task, activity, or occupational performance.
SKILL	An ability developed through practice that enables effective occupational performance.
TASK	A series of structured steps (actions and/or thoughts) intended to accomplish a specific goal. This goal could be either: 1. The performance of an activity, or 2. A piece of work the individual is expected to do.
VOLITION	The ability to choose to do or continue to do something, together with an awareness that the performance of the activity is voluntary.

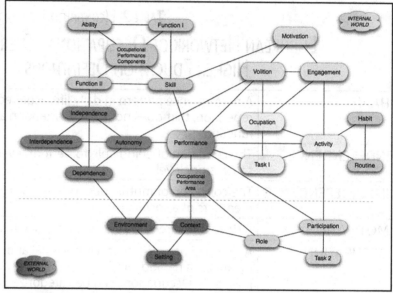

CLINICAL AND PROFESSIONAL REASONING

Clinical reasoning is the term given to the modes of thinking that the therapist uses when trying to understand people's needs and what to do about them, such as defining problems and making judgments (Schell & Schell, 2008; Sinclair, 2007). Two researchers who carried out a 1990s study of occupational therapists' clinical reasoning in the United States observed that

> clinical reasoning involves not one, but several, forms of thinking. Therapists, in other words, think in more than one way. To add to this complexity, clinical reasoning . . . is also a way of perceiving. To talk about how therapists think is necessarily to consider what therapists think about, what they perceive in the way they view their clients, what they focus on as the central problem, what they ignore, how they describe what is physiologically problematic for the client, and even their view of who the client is as a person. (Fleming & Mattingly, 1994, p. 9)

Clinical reasoning is only one aspect of *professional reasoning* and refers to the full range of thinking skills and "cognitive processes used to guide professional actions" (Schell & Schell, 2008, p. 447). Professional reasoning includes the types of thinking used when working with clients, teaching students, establishing new services, developing existing services, negotiating with funders, managing staff, and so on. Occupational therapy practice includes a wide and expanding range of approaches and services, and practitioners need to be able to move among different types of thinking to suit the situation. Thinking consists of both processes and skills, and, like any skill, thinking can be developed and honed with practice so that experienced practitioners are generally more skilled at clinical reasoning than beginners.

Modes of Reasoning

Sinclair (2007, p. 143) carried out research into the development of occupational therapists' clinical reasoning and concluded that thinking skills are "mental processes that become proficient through clinical experience." She identified and named five facets of clinical reasoning used by occupational therapists: evidence discovery, theory application, decision making, judgment, and ethical reasoning.

Evidence discovery is the mode of reasoning the therapist uses when gathering data, carrying out assessments, identifying potential problems, recognizing relevant clinical cues, and defining the problems to be addressed during intervention.

Theory application includes the use of formal theory and the tacit knowledge gained from practical experience. Effective clinical reasoning requires, in addition to thinking skills, a broad range of formal theories and experiential knowledge. A study of the development of expertise in nurses found that one of the key differences between the clinical reasoning of novice and expert practitioners is the latter's ability to know what is possible, based on extensive knowledge embedded in practice (Benner, 1982).

Decision making involves evaluating information, predicting the outcomes of alternative courses of action, planning interventions, setting priorities, and justifying actions taken.

Judgment is the ability to use evidence in drawing inferences and conclusions, weighing arguments, determining the best course of action, recognizing the ramifications of decisions taken, and taking responsibility for them. Good judgments take into account the weight of evidence, the context, the potential utility of solutions, and the pragmatic need for action (Sinclair, 2007).

Ethical reasoning is the process of thinking through the moral dimensions of a situation to reach the best decision. It requires the therapist to recognize that the best clinical course of action may not necessarily be the best moral course of action (Creek, 2008).

The novice practitioner has little or no experience of practice situations and must apply what she has been taught to guide her actions; that is, she depends on context-free rules, protocols, and procedures (Benner & Tanner, 1987). Through practice, she gradually accumulates a store of experience and tacit knowledge based on working with real people and rooted in particular contexts. The expert practitioner does not have to spend time comparing what she is seeing with a set of preexisting rules, and she "no longer relies on an analytical principle (rule, guideline, maxim) to connect her . . . understanding of the situation to an appropriate action" (Benner, 1982, p. 405). "Expertise includes a rich, integrated knowledge base, qualitatively different strategies, automaticity in problem solving, and the ability to reflect on problem solving when necessary" (Carr & Shotwell, 2008, p. 52). The expert practitioner's experiential knowledge gives her an immediate, intuitive grasp of the salient features of the situation, including what further information is needed and what actions should be taken.

Sinclair (2007) pointed out that because occupational therapists employ different modes of reasoning for different tasks, it is possible for them to develop expertise in some forms while remaining a novice in others. For example, a therapist working in an assessment unit might become highly skilled in evidence discovery and decision making but have less experience of judgment or ethical reasoning because of the rapid turnover of patients and lack of opportunities for follow-up.

The same logic applies to professional reasoning as to clinical reasoning: An occupational therapist may be highly skilled in thinking through particular issues, such as those described in many of the chapters in this book, but remain a beginner in other modes of reasoning due to lack of experience. For example, I have taught in many countries and developed reasoning skills that enable me to design and deliver culturally safe and effective teaching sessions. Feeling confident about teaching, I actively seek opportunities to work in different countries and, in turn, the more experience I accumulate the more expert I become in those skills. In contrast, I have little management experience and no confidence in my limited skills for working in such a role. I avoid positions where I would be responsible for managing staff and, consequently, have no opportunities to improve my skills through experience.

Language and Learning

The tacit nature of much expert reasoning, and, hence, the difficulty many practitioners have in finding words to justify their decisions and actions, was mentioned in the introduction to this chapter. Benner's (1982) study of how nurses develop clinical expertise found that it is not possible for expert practitioners to describe in explicit, formal steps all the elements or mental processes that go into their capacity to make rapid and accurate assessments. Expert practitioners are able take actions that they cannot describe and make decisions that they cannot find words to justify (Fleming, 1994).

> For an experienced practitioner what is done is embedded and integrated into a series of reactions, actions and interactions which automatically come into operation when needed. . . . The attempt to unpack practice in order to describe it inevitably carries the risk of diminishing it to oversimplified lists of actions, which, without the context in which they are used, may not carry much relevance or conviction. (Hagedorn, 2000, pp. vii-viii)

The challenge of putting into words the reasoning of experts can mean that their expertise is not as highly valued as formal theory and not taught systematically. This has profound pedagogical implications. Occupational therapy students may not realize that there is more to learn than the abstract, language-based knowledge gained from books and lectures and feel puzzled when their fieldwork educators eschew the use of formal models or procedures for practice. For example, an occupational therapist taught a course in group leadership using a specific, client-centered approach. All the participants became proficient in leading groups of their peers using this approach. Then, after observing therapy groups in fieldwork settings, they became highly critical of the occupational therapy group leaders for not following the format they had been taught, not understanding that the learned techniques of group leadership must be modified to fit the needs of specific client populations and settings.

> Formal models are helpful for teaching the beginner what to consider and how to organize information about patients. Continuing a slavish use of prescribed assessment tools, however, actually can limit the development of more flexible ways to collect and interpret patient information. If a checklist mentality develops instead of active inquiry, the [practitioner] may not advance beyond a competent level of performance. (Benner & Tanner 1987, p. 30)

The novice practitioner gains experience and practical knowledge by participating in communities of practice during periods of fieldwork education. At first, this participation is peripheral, perhaps observing the supervising occupational therapist at work and asking questions. As the novice interacts with colleagues in the context of practice, she begins to share their understandings of what is going on and to participate more fully. Jenkins and Brotherton (1995), in a study of the effectiveness of occupational therapy practice, found that learning happens in context as the fieldwork placement creates a gradually unfolding learning curriculum for the student. These situated learning opportunities are most valuable when students are allowed to participate as fully as possible in all the activities of the community of practice.

> This does not imply access only to the physical activities going on around participants and to the tools of their trade. They must be involved in information gathering and dispersal; they must be in communion with their environment freely and voluntarily; and they must be in a context in which they can make sense of what they see and hear . . . knowledge is neither hidden nor restricted. (Jenkins & Brotherton, 1995, p. 283)

This section has defined and differentiated clinical and professional reasoning. It explained that both involve many different modes of thinking and that a practitioner can have more or less skill in each of these modes, depending on the length and type of her or his experience. The difficulty of putting expert practice into words was highlighted, along with the implications of this for how the theory and practice of occupational therapy are taught. The next section considers some of the ways in which language can influence professional reasoning.

CONNECTION BETWEEN LANGUAGE AND REASONING

*In its public role, [language] is a system of conventions agreed upon by a
speech community for the purpose of effective communication.
But language also has another, private existence, as a system of knowledge
that each speaker has internalised in his or her own mind.*

(Deutscher, 2010, p. 233)

As explained in this chapter, clinical and professional reasoning involve a number of thinking skills and cognitive processes, such as identifying, remembering, problem solving, and decision making. This section looks in more detail at how language and thought interact to shape thinking and reasoning. A summary of current views on the relationship between language and thinking is followed by a discussion about the dynamism of language and some of the various ways in which words come into and out of usage. The influence of context on thought and language is then considered, and the section finishes with a discussion about the use of language as an effective tool to support professional reasoning.

Language and Thinking

In the very young child, thinking begins to develop before language so that cognitive structures are in place to provide the foundation for language acquisition. However, it has been suggested that language starts to influence the continuing development of thinking when the child develops the capacity for symbolic thought (Bloom, 1981). The Russian psychologist Lev Vygotsky argued that it is an error to think of thought and speech as unrelated processes; rather "the meaning of a word represents such a close amalgam of thought and language that it is hard to tell whether it is a phenomenon of speech or a phenomenon of thought" (1962, p. 120).

There has been much discussion and debate about the extent to which language shapes, or even limits, our thinking (Deutscher, 2010), but there is general agreement that none of the languages of different linguistic groups limits their capacity for reasoning. Rather, the words we habitually use, with their repeated connotations and associations, influence our thinking through their effect on our emotions, gut feelings, and intuition.

No evidence has come to light that our mother tongue imposes limits on our intellectual horizons and constrains our ability to understand concepts or distinctions used in other languages. The real effects of the mother tongue are rather the habits that develop through the *frequent use* of certain ways of expression. The concepts we are trained to treat as distinct, the information our mother tongue consciously forces us to specify, the details it requires us to be attentive to, and the repeated associations it imposes on us—all these habits of speech can create habits of mind that affect more than merely the knowledge of language itself. (Deutscher, 2010, p. 234)

The ways that people see the world are subject and culture bound and are influenced, at least in part, by the language they habitually use. For example, within English culture, people habitually complain about the weather: when it is warm, they say it is too hot for comfort; when it is cold, they feel too cold; when it is dry, they worry about water shortages; when it is wet, they say the rain interferes with what they want to do. This discourse expresses and shapes the tendency of English people to think of their mild, temperate climate as hostile and unpredictable.

In occupational therapy, it is possible to trace through the professional literature how the word *occupation* went into and out of fashion during the 20th century (see, for example, Blom-Cooper, 1989; Creek, 1998; Nelson, 1997) and how its increased usage in the 21st century is shaping occupational therapy discourse, practice, and professional identity (see, for example, Watson & Swartz, 2004; Whiteford & Wright-St Clair, 2005; Wilcock, 1998).

Where Words Come From

Language, by which is meant words, their meanings, and how they are expressed, derives from many sources. The everyday language of communities comes from their shared history, culture, and environment and evolves over time. As the pace of social change accelerates, in part due to urbanization and technological developments, so language has to keep up. New words are coined to refer to new developments, and some words fall out of use because the concepts they represent are no longer relevant. For example, when I was a student, occupational therapists in physical rehabilitation used a piece of equipment that determined what type of wrist movements a person could employ in performing a manual task. It was called a FEPS, an acronym for flexion, extension, pronation, and supination. Because this piece of equipment is no longer in use, its name has been dropped from the occupational therapist's vocabulary.

New words may come into a community from outside, for example, via the global media or the Internet. Indeed, the wide use of social media may be accelerating the rate of evolution of language. Some words come into use as circumstances change. For instance, few people in Europe knew the meaning of the word *tsunami* before the disastrous earthquake and tidal waves of 2004 killed tens of thousands of people across Asia. New words may be coined to refer to new technology, newly discovered species, or new illnesses, such as acquired immune deficiency syndrome (AIDS). Some words first come into use in a single locality or a particular group of people and may or may not be taken up more widely. When a community of people uses its own vocabulary that is not understood outside the group, a newcomer has to become familiar with the words and their meanings to fit in; language is part of the group identity. For example, street gangs in New York have their own language that represents who they are and shows their camaraderie (Savelli, 2006).

Some words change their meaning over time; for example, the word *gay* is now commonly used to mean homosexual and rarely used in any of its other senses. Words sometimes become unacceptable, either because the meaning has changed or because society's values have changed. An example of this is the word *lunatic*, which was once used to refer to a person with mental illness and is now thought of as a term of abuse. The words that people use to refer to themselves form part of their individual or group identity; for example, I call myself eccentric and am comfortable if other people describe me as such. However, a person or group of people may use words for themselves that outsiders are not allowed to use, such as *nutter* or *witch*. The subtle dynamics of language can become a minefield for someone attempting to communicate with people from a different social or cultural background.

Labeling means describing someone in such a way that the descriptor comes to dominate over other aspects of the person. For example, when a person is diagnosed as mentally ill she may find that everything she does is seen through the lens of that label, and even actions that were previously considered normal are now seen as signs of illness; the illness is seen before the person (History Learning Site, 2014). An example of labeling is provided in Box 2-2. Using words as labels acts as a barrier to thinking more broadly about what is going on. For example, calling a person noncompliant because she does not want to join in occupational therapy can prevent the therapist from exploring with the client why she is refusing to engage when such an exploration could open the door to an effective, collaborative intervention.

The term *politically correct* is sometimes used to refer to language that is carefully selected with the purpose of not offending or upsetting a particular group of people. For example, the different words used to refer to people with disabilities may be described as politically correct or incorrect, depending on the time and place. Language that is thought to be inoffensive in one era may be considered politically incorrect at another time or in a different cultural context. In the modern world, a celebrity or politician who is heard using a politically incorrect term is likely to be vilified in the media. An example of this is the UK politician who was alleged to have called a policeman a *pleb* (from the Latin *plebeian*, meaning a commoner and used here as an insult) when the man

---

Box 2-2. The Effects of Labeling

A young man experiencing an acute psychotic episode was admitted to the hospital for assessment. One night, he left the ward without telling the staff and went out for a drink with some friends. When he returned, the male night nurse told him off, and the young man lost his temper. This was interpreted by the team as a sign of mental illness. Alternative interpretations might have been that anger was the natural reaction of a young man who had been drinking or that it was a response to the perceived aggression of the night nurse.

---

prevented him from going through a gate on his bicycle; the politician was subsequently forced to resign his position after a media outcry.

The Influence of Context

The language we use to refer to others is important because it reveals both how we perceive them and the nature of our relationship to them. As mentioned earlier, the word *patient* carries connotations about the roles and relationship of person and health care professional that are very different from those of the term *service user*. When we take words out of the business sector and use them in the health care context, or when we bring medical terminology into the occupational therapy context, we are at the same time carrying with us the perspectives and expectations that those words connote. This was pointed out by a professor of nursing, as the marketization of health services gathered pace in the United Kingdom at the end of the last century.

> Why have we failed to notice that we are adopting more than just the language [of the marketplace]? It seems we have been anaesthetised in order to have our philosophy surgically removed and a donor philosophy implanted. And this donor philosophy is not about care, patients or people but about . . . money. (Webb, 1990, p. 414)

It is important to think about the language we use when talking of other people because it both indicates and affects how we feel about them. But we must also be aware of the words we apply to ourselves because they inform others how we think about ourselves and this, in turn, influences how others see us (Creek, 1998). In the work setting, for example, the language occupational therapists use about themselves and what they do can affect their credibility and status. It can even be a contributing factor in whether their services attract funding; for example, in the United States, occupational therapy services in public schools always need to be described as relating to academic performance or observable social behavior. Occupational therapists have to think politically and strategically about what words to use if their professional communications are to be understood in the way intended.

Because language is a tool for communicating and connecting with others, the way that we speak it changes depending on who we are talking to—not only the words we select but also our style of speech. When we know a person or a group of people well, it is usually possible to engage them immediately in discussion because we are familiar with their vocabulary, interests, favorite style of communication, and so on. When meeting someone for the first time, most people are adept at picking up verbal and nonverbal cues and progressively shaping their responses until the interaction flows in the way they want.

The way we speak also changes with the purpose of the communication. Seeking to engage someone's interest or cooperation requires a different use of language from "attempting to ram home your case as though its content is all that counts" (Sennett, 2012, p. 18). Language can be used in ways that create connections with other people by demonstrating respect and responsiveness. It can also be used in ways that are deliberately exclusionary—for example, using highly specialized words that most people cannot be expected to understand or making allusions to events or litera-ture with which they are unlikely to be familiar.

Language as a Reasoning Tool

The subtlety and complexity of language, which can make communication seem challenging, also make it an effective tool to support different modes of reasoning. The occupational therapist has a vast array of words from which to choose but, to reason effectively, it is important to select the most appropriate language to suit the situation. The words we use are not merely descriptive but shape how we frame situations and how we respond to them

The problems addressed by occupational therapists are often messy and ill defined, so they need to be framed in terms that suggest possibilities for appropriate action. In other words, the way that we define a problem influences the solutions open to us. For example, if we say that a man is unable to work because he has an illness, this suggests that medical treatment would be appropriate. If we say the man cannot work because there are no jobs available in his locality, a social or political approach is indicated. Saying that the man cannot find a job because he does not know how to go about it points to a need for occupational therapy intervention. Sometimes, changing the words we use to describe a situation can change how we see it and indicate alternative strategies.

Occupational therapy is most effective when it is a collaborative process that includes a number of stakeholders, such as "people with disabilities, their families, their communities, governments (local, regional, national), NGOs [nongovernmental organizations], and organizations of people with disabilities, professionals (medical and allied health professionals, educators, social scientists, and others), and the private sector" (Fransen, 2005, pp. 167-168). A research study carried out in the United Kingdom looked at the multifaceted and sometimes conflicting factors that confronted the occupational therapist in making clinical decisions in the context of a wheelchair seating clinic (White, 2007). Stakeholders included service users, carers, health care staff, teaching staff, and ser-vice funders. The investigator concluded:

> The findings of the research provided a fascinating insight into a range of individual values and motivations. Perhaps the most significant finding was that the provision of a single wheelchair and seating system to an individual provoked an enormous range of perspectives as to its purpose and function. (White, 2007, p. 121)

To achieve cooperation between people with different goals and interests requires sophisti-cated communication skills, including the ability to find appropriate, inclusive language. Such language makes it possible to create meaning and understanding through dialogue, negotiate and define goals, reach agreement about the best course of action, and engage everyone in the process. Collaborative reasoning through dialogue is a necessary part of collaborative practice.

In this chapter, it has been argued that occupational therapists need a wide vocabulary and a deep understanding of the different ways in which words can be understood in particular contexts. Words represent concepts; therefore, having more words in their professional vocabulary enables therapists to differentiate more precisely between related concepts, which, in turn, allows for more precise communication and greater flexibility in reasoning. For example, a sound comprehension of the nature of motivation and volition enables the occupational therapist to assess which of these areas is the primary problem and plan the most appropriate intervention (Creek, 2007a).

Conversely, the therapist who has access to a limited vocabulary or does not fully understand the concepts it represents may oversimplify the client's situation by using structuralist language that does not capture the complexity and dynamism of occupational needs and strategies. This was illustrated in the story at the beginning of this chapter. Using a small vocabulary or using words without fully understanding their meaning reduces the occupational therapist's capacity for clini-cal and professional reasoning.

The first section of this chapter discussed occupational therapy terminology; the second explored the nature of clinical and professional reasoning in occupational therapy. This third section brought together some of the themes covered in the first two, looking at the nature of the relationship between language and professional reasoning as it affects therapeutic practice.

CONCLUSION

This chapter has emphasized the importance to the occupational therapist of having a wide professional vocabulary and an explicit understanding of the systems of knowledge represented by different terminologies. Language allows occupational therapists to explain their role and to differentiate it from those of other professions. Language is also an essential tool for effective clinical and professional reasoning, but more work is needed to reach agreement on the meaning of key terms and to clarify the epistemological implications of the words we use.

Language is inseparable from thought; it directs our attention to what is significant in any situation and suggests possible ways of responding. The words that we use can illuminate or disguise possibilities for action. Clear and logical professional reasoning is based on a deep understanding of what words represent—not just their intended professional meanings, but also their social, cultural, and symbolic meanings. Language is a social institution, and the meanings of words have to be negotiated and agreed on within particular communities.

Occupational therapists work across different communities: their own professional community, health and social care communities, and the communities where their clients live and work. They often need to adapt their language to suit the settings in which they are working to communicate effectively. Meaning and understanding can be negotiated through dialogue, using appropriate and inclusive language in a process of collaborative reasoning.

Professional reasoning is both a skill and a process. It includes many ways of reasoning, some of which are described in the following chapters.

REFERENCES

Barthes, R. (1967). *Elements of semiology.* London, England: Jonathan Cape.

Benner, P. (1982, March). From novice to expert. *American Journal of Nursing,* 402-407.

Benner, P., & Tanner, C. (1987, January). How expert nurses use intuition. *American Journal of Nursing,* 23-31.

Blom-Cooper, L. (1989). *Occupational therapy: An emerging profession in health care.* London, England: Duckworth.

Bloom, A. H. (1981). *The linguistic shaping of thought: A study in the impact of language on thinking in China and the West.* Hillsdale, NJ: Lawrence Erlbaum.

Boulding, K. E. (1968). General systems theory—the skeleton of science. In W. Buckley (Ed.), *Modern systems research for the behavioural scientist* (pp. 3-10). Chicago, IL: Aldine.

Breines, E. B. (1984). An attempt to define purposeful activity. *American Journal of Occupational Therapy, 38,* 543-544.

Carr, M., & Shotwell, M. (2008). Information processing theory and professional reasoning. In B. A. B. Schell & K. W. Schell (Eds.), *Clinical and professional reasoning in occupational therapy* (pp. 36-68). Philadelphia, PA: Lippincott Williams & Wilkins.

Creek, J. (1998). Communicating the nature and purpose of occupational therapy. In J. Creek (Ed.), *Occupational therapy: New perspectives* (pp. 114-141). London, England: Whurr.

Creek, J. (2003). *Occupational therapy defined as a complex intervention.* London, England: College of Occupational Therapists.

Creek, J. (2007a). Engaging the reluctant client. In J. Creek & A. Lawson-Porter (Eds.), *Contemporary issues in occupational therapy: Reasoning and reflection* (pp. 127-142). Chichester, England: Wiley.

Creek, J. (2007b). The thinking therapist. In J. Creek & A. Lawson-Porter (Eds.), *Contemporary issues in occupational therapy: Reasoning and reflection* (pp. 1-21). Chichester, England: Wiley.

Creek, J. (2008). Approaches to practice. In J. Creek & L. Lougher (Eds.), *Occupational therapy and mental health* (4th ed., pp. 59-79). Edinburgh, Scotland: Churchill Livingstone Elsevier.

Creek, J. (2010). *The core concepts of occupational therapy: A dynamic framework for practice.* London, England: Jessica Kingsley.

Davis, J. A., & Polatajko, H. J. (2005). Letter to the editor. *Canadian Journal of Occupational Therapy*, 72, 125-127.

Deutscher, G. (2010). *Through the language glass: Why the world looks different in other languages.* London, England: Random House.

Dickoff, J., James, P., & Wiedenbach, E. (1968). Theory in a practice discipline: Part 1. Practice oriented theory. *Nursing Research*, 17, 415-435.

Fleming, M. H. (1994). The search for tacit knowledge. In C. Mattingly & M. H. Fleming (Eds.), *Clinical reasoning: Forms of inquiry in a therapeutic practice* (pp. 22-34). Philadelphia, PA: F. A. Davis.

Fleming, M. H., & Mattingly, C. (1994). Giving language to practice. In C. Mattingly & M. H. Fleming (Eds.), *Clinical reasoning: Forms of inquiry in a therapeutic practice* (pp. 3-21). Philadelphia, PA: F. A. Davis.

Fransen, H. (2005). Challenges for occupational therapy in community-based rehabilitation. In F. Kronenberg, S. S. Algado, & N. Pollard (Eds.), *Occupational therapy without borders: Learning from the spirit of survivors* (pp. 166-182). Edinburgh, Scotland: Elsevier Churchill Livingstone.

Galheigo, S. M. (2005). Occupational therapy and the social field: Clarifying concepts and ideas. In F. Kronenberg, S. S. Algado, & N. Pollard (Eds.), *Occupational therapy without borders: Learning from the spirit of survivors* (pp. 87-98). Edinburgh, Scotland: Elsevier Churchill Livingstone.

Gribbin, J. (1984). *In search of Schrödinger's cat: Quantum physics and reality.* London, England: Black Swan.

Hagedorn, R. (2000). *Tools for practice in occupational therapy: A structured approach to core skills and processes.* Edinburgh, Scotland: Churchill Livingstone.

History Learning Site. (2014). *The labelling theory.* Retrieved from http://www.historylearningsite.co.uk/sociology /crime-and-deviance/the-labelling-theory

Hooper, B., & Wood, W. (2002). Pragmatism and structuralism in occupational therapy: The long conversation. *American Journal of Occupational Therapy*, 56, 40-50.

Jenkins, M., & Brotherton, C. (1995). In search of a theoretical framework for practice, part 1. *British Journal of Occupational Therapy*, 58, 280-285.

Kantartzis, S., & Molineux, M. (2012). Understanding the discursive development of occupation: Historico-political perspectives. In G. E. Whiteford & C. Hocking (Eds.), *Occupational science: Society, inclusion, participation* (pp. 38-53). Chichester, England: Wiley-Blackwell.

Katz, N., & Sachs, D. (1991). Meaning ascribed to major professional concepts: A comparison of occupational therapy students and practitioners in the United States and Israel. *American Journal of Occupational Therapy*, 45, 137-145.

Mattingly, C. (1994a). Occupational therapy as a two-body practice: The body as machine. In C. Mattingly & M. H. Fleming (Eds.), *Clinical reasoning: Forms of inquiry in a therapeutic practice* (pp. 37-63). Philadelphia, PA: F. A. Davis.

Mattingly, C. (1994b). Occupational therapy as a two-body practice: The lived body. In C. Mattingly & M. H. Fleming (Eds.), *Clinical reasoning: Forms of inquiry in a therapeutic practice* (pp. 64-93). Philadelphia, PA: F. A. Davis.

Nelson, D. L. (1997). Why the profession of occupational therapy will flourish in the 21st century. *American Journal of Occupational Therapy*, 51, 11-24.

Nicholls, L., Piergrossi, J. C., de Sena-Gibertoni, C., & Daniel, M. (2013). *Psychoanalytic thinking in occupational therapy.* Chichester, England: Wiley-Blackwell.

Piergrossi, J. C. (2013). Re-awakening psychoanalytic thinking in occupational therapy: From Gail Fidler to here. In L. Nicholls, J. C. Piergrossi, C. de Sena-Gibertoni, & M. Daniel (Eds.), *Psychoanalytic thinking in occupational therapy* (pp. 87-101). Chichester, England: Wiley-Blackwell.

Polatajko, H. J., Davis, J. A., Hobson, S. J. G., Landry, J. E., Mandich, A., Street, S. L., et al. (2004). Meeting the responsibility that comes with the privilege: Introducing a taxonomic code for understanding occupation. *Canadian Journal of Occupational Therapy*, 71, 261-264.

Pollard, N., & Sakellariou, D. (2012). Introduction. In N. Pollard & D. Sakellariou (Eds.), *Politics of occupation-centred practice: Reflections on occupational engagement across cultures* (pp. 1-24). Chichester, England: Wiley-Blackwell.

Savelli, L. (2006). *Gangs across America and their symbols.* Flushing, NY: Looseleaf Law.

Schell, B. A. B., & Schell, K. W. (2008). *Clinical and professional reasoning in occupational therapy.* Philadelphia, PA: Lippincott Williams & Wilkins.

Sennett, R. (2012). *Together: The rituals, pleasures and politics of communication.* London, England: Penguin.

Sherry, K. (2010). Voices of occupational therapists in Africa. In V. Alers & R. Crouch (Eds.), *Occupational therapy: An African perspective* (pp. 26-47). Johannesburg, South Africa: Sarah Shorten.

Shorter Oxford English Dictionary. (2002). Oxford, England: Oxford University Press.

Sinclair, K. (2007). Exploring the facets of clinical reasoning. In J. Creek & A. Lawson-Porter (Eds.), *Contemporary issues in occupational therapy: Reasoning and reflection* (pp. 143-160). Chichester, England: Wiley.

Vygotsky, L. S. (1962). *Thought and language.* Cambridge, MA: MIT Press.

Watson, R., & Swartz, L. (Eds.). (2004). *Transformation through occupation.* London, England: Whurr.

Webb, C. (1990). *Nursing as a profession—Towards a new model.* University of Manchester, inaugural lecture.

White, E. (2007). When service users' views vary from those of their carers. In J. Creek & A. Lawson-Porter (Eds.), *Contemporary issues in occupational therapy: Reasoning and reflection* (pp. 115-126). Chichester, England: Wiley.

Whiteford, G., & Wright-St Clair, V. (Eds.) (2005). *Occupation in practice and context.* Sydney, Australia: Elsevier Churchill Livingstone.

Wilcock, A. A. (1998). *An occupational perspective of health.* Thorofare, NJ: SLACK Incorporated.

World Federation of Occupational Therapists. (2011). *Statement on occupational therapy.* Retrieved from http://www.wfot.org/Portals/0/PDF/STATEMENT%20ON%20OCCUPATIONAL%20THERAPY%20300811.pdf

3

Strategic Thinking and Reasoning in Occupational Therapy

Hanneke van Bruggen, Bsc OT, Hon.Dscie, FWFOT

This chapter provides an intellectual challenge for those who are engaged in strategic development and innovation and who expect to operationalize these ideas in their respective organizations or new practice area. It enables occupational therapists to deepen their understanding of national and international social, health, and educational policies in relation to the development of occupational therapy education and practice.

The chapter begins with an introduction to strategic thinking and an explanation of different perspectives, such as systems thinking, envisioning, and creative thinking. This is followed by case examples and discussion of a synthesis, strategic choices, and alliances for development. The importance of thinking strategically in wider policy contexts is illustrated through an account of the foundation and development of the European Network of Occupational Therapy in Higher Education (ENOTHE) and two related projects: establishing occupational therapy in Georgia and Armenia and creating occupational justice and social inclusion in community projects.

Within the chapter, the terms *thinking* and *reasoning* are conceptualized as being on a continuum toward planning. Strategic thinking leads to strategic reasoning, which, in turn, leads to planning; in this chapter, however, attention is paid only to the first two terms.

DEFINING STRATEGIC THINKING AND REASONING

Strategy is an abstract concept that we cannot just reach out and touch, and this makes the process of thinking about it much more difficult. Too often in the "action is everything" world we live in, we are hamsters running on a wheel. Day in and day out, we run faster and faster, doing the same things in the same ways we have always done them. The trouble is, we are often doing the wrong things.

Cole, M. B., & Creek, J. (Eds.).
Global Perspectives in Professional Reasoning (pp. 25-43).
© 2016 Taylor & Francis Group.

As an example, for the past decade, the World Health Organization (WHO) has been asking health care professionals and policy makers the question: "Why are we treating people's illnesses and then sending them back to the living and social conditions that made them sick in the first place?" (WHO, 2008). Nowadays, much more is understood about the extent and social causes of health inequities. Action is needed on the social determinants of health, across the life course and in wider social and economic spheres, to achieve greater health equity and protect future generations. "Do something, do more, do better" is the concluding recommendation in the European WHO Review of the social determinants of health and the health divide (WHO, 2013).

If occupational therapists are concerned about health inequities and the social determinants of health, then why are they mostly still working in the health sector on individual treatment? There is a reciprocal relationship between poverty and disability. In 2009, an ENOTHE survey was undertaken among occupational therapists for a grant on poverty reduction competences (unpublished). The majority of respondents expressed the opinion that occupational therapy had nothing to do with poverty reduction strategies.

Health inequities or poverty cannot be reduced by individual treatment plans or by traditional clinical reasoning. Those occupational therapists who are concerned with these issues, occupational justice (Wilcock & Townsend, 2000), or community development through occupation have to use a different kind of thinking and reasoning. Where do occupational therapists want to be in 10 or 15 years, and how can they contribute to reducing health inequities and poverty to prevent disability? How can they position themselves in a constantly changing world?

These are complex questions that ask for creative and strategic thinking and not only for strategic planning or a rational, straightforward project plan. Mintzberg (1994) postulated that the concept of strategic planning is built on a contradiction: on the one hand, planning is analytic and rational, involving a conscious breakdown of tasks and activities; on the other hand, strategy development is a complex, holistic, and creative process. However, creativity alone cannot ensure that an organization, a professional body, or a network is managing well in the strategic sense. Complementary analysis and rational thinking are just as important. In the view of Graetz (2002), the role of strategic thinking is to seek innovation and imagine new and different futures that may lead to redefining the core strategies of an association or institution and even its products. The role of strategic planning is to realize and support strategies developed through strategic thinking and to integrate these back into the association, network, or other entity.

There is agreement among researchers (Bonn, 2005; Liedtka, 1998; Pisapia, 2009; Senge, 1990) that systems thinking, creativity, and vision are key elements of strategic thinking. Systems thinking enables the identification and clarification of patterns and supports effective change, thereby increasing creativity. Vision helps provide meaning and gives a sense of direction in the decision-making process. Strategic thinking is at the intersection of these three elements (Bonn, 2005); it is not just an individual activity but is influenced by the individual's environment and social interactions (Figure 3-1).

Bonn's theoretical framework of strategic thinking incorporates a multilevel approach in which strategic thinking is defined as an integrative process that crosses interorganizational boundaries and spans multiple levels of analysis. A systems perspective also demands that the strategic thinker has knowledge of the external environment as well as the internal environment of the organization, community, or professional association. "The strategic thinker sees vertical linkages within the system from multiple perspectives" (Liedtka, 1998, p. 122; Figure 3-2).

This thinker sees relationships among the following:

- The organization and functional strategies
- The external context
- The personal choices the thinker makes on a daily basis
- Departments, units, or parts of the network and functions
- Communities of stakeholders

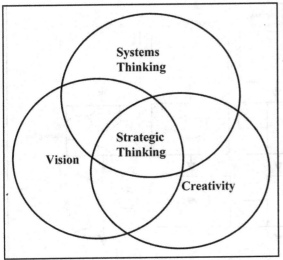

Figure 3-1. Strategic thinking. (Republished with permission of Emerald Group Publishing Ltd., from Improving strategic thinking: A multilevel approach, Bonn, I., *Leadership and Organization Development Journal*, 26, 336-354, 2005; permission conveyed through Copyright Clearance Center.)

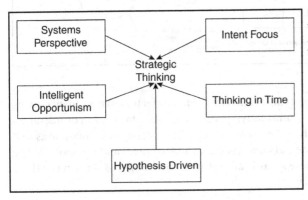

Figure 3-2. Liedtka's elements of strategic thinking. (Reprinted from *Long Range Planning*, *31*, Liedtka, J., Strategic thinking: Can it be taught?, 120-129, 1998, with permission from Elsevier.)

For those who now think, on the basis of the two models, that strategic thinking is linear, the complexity of strategic thinking is presented in Figure 3-3. Strategic thinking is action oriented and concerned with identifying how to resolve ambiguity and make sense of a complex world. Or, as John Pisapia (2006) said, "learning the labyrinth" means studying and understanding the internal and external environments in which strategic thinking is practiced.

The rest of this section takes a more detailed look at three key elements of strategic thinking: systems thinking, formulating a vision, and using creativity. A fourth element, thinking in time, seeks to connect past, present, and future.

Systems Thinking

Strategic thinking is built on the foundation of a systems perspective from which a problem or opportunity is seen as a part of the whole situation or system (Bonn, 2005; Liedtka, 1998). This way of thinking requires that people deviate from paying attention to daily affairs and instead look at how different issues are interconnected, how they influence each other, and how a solution in one part of the system affects the other parts (Bonn, 2005; Liedtka, 1998). Strategic thinking does not just involve pattern recognition but being able to look at things from many angles. It requires one's mind to be open to alternative perspectives, perhaps even ones that diverge from what one believes or run counter to what one has seen before.

Figure 3-3. Complex strategic thinking. (Reprinted with permission from Ohmae, K. [1982]. *The mind of the strategist the art of Japanese business.* New York, NY: McGraw-Hill. Reproduced with permission from McGraw-Hill Education.)

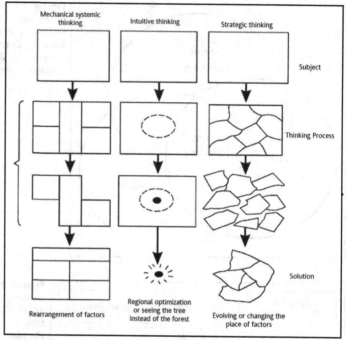

Strategic thinkers also have to understand the internal and external factors that influence cooperation among parts of the organization, community, or network. They take into consideration many contexts (representing systems), such as the scientific, technical, social, and economic as well as the local, regional, national, and continental contexts (e.g., the European and the global). The motivation for strategic thinking in all these areas is always an intrinsic one, as seen in the three examples that make up the bulk of this chapter.

Formulating a Vision

Strategic thinking should be accompanied by a powerful understanding of the future goal. In other words, it should be vision driven or, as Liedtka (1998) called it, intent-driven.

Strategic thinking requires the ability to look forward, look ahead, and look around to anticipate possibility. Change is a constant in the world so how, as an occupational therapist, are you looking for potential disruptions, opportunities, signals, or change? This is not just about recognizing trends; it is about dealing with uncertainty, taking in the most important shifts, and thinking about what they might mean for your organization, the community, or your profession.

Professional leaders can develop forward thinking by reading national, European, and world policies on human and social rights, health, education, labor, and so on and by anticipating the future implications of these policies for occupational therapy. Having vision, or an intent-focus, implies a particular point of view about the future; hence, it conveys a sense of direction and discovery. Values and vision are closely connected concepts in strategic thinking.

Using Creativity

Creativity is considered to be an essential principle of strategic thinking (Mintzberg, 1994). Teaching creativity often emphasizes the importance of production and of paying attention to different solutions that can increase the quality of the final solution (Raimond, 1996). For each individual, creativity is a combination of three components: area of expertise, creative thinking skills, and motivation.

Rather than accept conventional wisdom in their area of expertise, creative thinkers challenge long-standing assumptions and examine sources of uncertainty to understand how these may impact on expected results. They apply creativity to reframe a problem from several angles, to understand its root causes, to seek out diverse views, and to see multiple sides of an issue.

In a rapidly changing world, strategy and creativity are necessities for occupational therapy to survive as a discipline. *Strategic thinking* hinges on creativity—connecting disparate issues and events and ultimately rewriting the rules. *Critical thinking* hinges on improving reasoning by questioning and highlighting innate biases, beliefs, assumptions, and perceptions. Unless both these hinges are on the door to your strategy, it will not open very wide or allow your organization to move into a new, success-oriented environment. Both hinges rely on people with different perspectives and experiences conversing, considering, and creating.

Strategic thinking is much more than simply having a new idea; that idea must have a context, one in which the idea has a meaning defined by the specific aims of the activity.

Thinking in Time

The model of strategic thinking presented by Liedtka (see Figure 3-2) includes an element that is particularly important in developing and managing projects and organizations or associations: thinking in time. Strategic thinking links past, present, and future because it is the gap between today's reality and our intent for the future that is critical. Strategy focuses on the degree of fit between existing resources and current opportunities, but strategic thinking always involves thinking in time. The thinker needs both a sense of continuity with the past and a sense of direction for the future in order to maintain a feeling of control in the midst of change.

CASE EXAMPLE 1: THE FOUNDING OF THE EUROPEAN NETWORK OF OCCUPATIONAL THERAPY IN HIGHER EDUCATION

This section demonstrates the application of strategic thinking in the founding of ENOTHE, which incorporated multiple contexts. These included the importance of internationalization and harmonization in the European higher education area, the European labor market, the enlargement of the European Union (EU) with the accession of new member states, and the growing inequities in health, social injustice, and poverty. The process begins with developing an understanding of all these external contexts and systems as well as the internal European occupational therapy context. Formulating a vision and using creativity in positioning the European occupational therapy profession leads to the outcome of strategic thinking: the establishment of a disciplinary network with the general aim of developing opportunities for occupational therapists to improve standards of practice and education and advance the theory and practice of occupational therapy.

Systems Thinking

To attract the main European occupational therapy schools to become members of this new network and to collaborate on a common strategy, it was first necessary to better understand the European occupational therapy internal world and the external contexts (systems). From this foundation, leaders together with the members could then formulate a common vision and use creativity in positioning the network within the systems and combine all these factors.

Internal Situation of Occupational Therapy in Europe

How was occupational therapy positioned in Europe and under which systems were most occupational therapists functioning in 1995? The number of working occupational therapists per capita in European countries differed enormously, between 1 (Italy) to 75 (Denmark) therapists per 100,000 inhabitants. Most occupational therapists were employed by national or local health authorities. The profile of the occupational therapist was changing rapidly due to changes in health and social care and scientific and technical developments. Therefore, decisions had to be made about the core skills to be taught in regular education and the development of continuing professional education.

In which system was occupational therapy education embedded in the different countries? The facts and figures showed enormous differences from small private vocational schools with an annual intake of 20 students to university-level programs with an annual intake of more than 100 to 150 students. Only two countries offered occupational therapy education at doctorate level and in three countries at master's level. The majority of occupational therapy education in Europe was not embedded in the higher education system.

A great number of new occupational therapy educational institutes had started in Spain, Italy, and Eastern/Central Europe, and their leaders had asked for assistance in curriculum development. In occupational therapy education, new technologies in teaching were hardly introduced on a large scale. One of the conclusions of the European HEART (Horizontal European Activities Rehabilitation Technology) project (E.Com, 1994) was that occupational therapists needed to be trained in the latest assistive technology so that they could advise persons with disabilities in the use of computers.

The mobility of occupational therapists from one European nation to another was limited, partly because of recognition problems of curricula and partly due to different autonomy levels on which professionals were able to perform in practice. Student exchange within the discipline was minuscule. Most occupational therapy programs did not offer much flexibility and were subject based.

In light of the unified European labor market and developing standardization of the European higher education and research areas, these differences posed an enormous risk for the profession. With more than three quarters of the occupational therapy education still not functioning at a higher education level, ministers could easily decide that the profession in the whole of Europe could be at vocational level and that it should be much cheaper. Before strategic reasoning or action, organizers needed to have a more detailed idea of the systems surrounding occupational therapy.

External Global/European Context

Current initiatives such as the *Universal Declaration of Human Rights* (UN Commission on Human Rights, 1948) and the European Charter (and drafts) of Fundamental Rights (E.Com, 2000) promoted the same ideals as those central to our profession. These include the recognition of dignity, equality, and citizen's rights, which form the foundation of freedom, peace, solidarity, and justice. Although most occupational therapists recognize these ideals, few are currently working on improving health inequalities or occupational justice. Also the European social agenda focused on strengthening citizenship by employment and equal opportunities in all life areas.

The WHO and European health policy specifically focused on health promotion and prevention within community or primary health care settings. The United Nations Educational, Scientific and Cultural Organisation and later the European Bologna Process[1] recommended implementing a three-cycle degree system, quality assurance and recognition of degrees, and study periods of all academic disciplines across Europe. Furthermore, higher education should be relevant, address social needs, and collaborate internationally. During the 1990s, the European Commission launched several stimulation programs for student and teacher exchange, for the development of joint intensive courses and master's programs.

---

[1] The Bologna Process is a series of ministerial meetings and agreements among European countries designed to ensure comparability in the standards and quality of higher education qualifications.

The European freedom of mobility within one unified labor market had existed for about 10 years. Europe was about to enlarge, adding several countries that had been part of the former Soviet Union. Everywhere, the technical possibilities were growing and communication systems were changing considerably. Vulnerable groups such as persons with disabilities, elderly, people with a mental illness, migrants, homeless, and street children were on the rise.

Summary of Systems Perspective

Looking at these many systems and influences, we can conclude that the European context during the 1990s was complex and uncertain and not easily navigated for a rather small profession. So what could be done to improve on an internally diverse professional practice and educational discipline with a lot of external challenges? Where should the occupational therapy professional education and practice go next?

Formulating a Vision

The long-term vision of ENOTHE was to develop and maintain an evidence-based academic discipline rooted in occupational science, which could contribute to the six values of dignity, freedom, equality, solidarity, citizens' rights, and justice promoted by the United Nations and contained in the European Charter of Fundamental Rights. Occupational therapy practice and education could address these key values through the following:

- Strategies/interventions to limit the impact of occupational injustices experienced by individuals or groups
- Promotion of equal occupational opportunities for all and full participation in all life areas
- Advocacy with groups who are occupational deprived (elderly, migrants, street children, persons with disabilities, etc.) for their occupational rights
- Designing and developing full accessibility (combating physical and attitudinal barriers)
- Influencing policy making toward inclusive development (van Bruggen, 2012)

However, the fundamental underlying conditions for free movement of occupational therapists from country to country with academic and professional recognition were yet to be fulfilled.

Equalizing the Status of the Occupational Therapy Profession

Because in most countries at that time occupational therapy was not an academic discipline, it was important to choose a European approach that could put pressure on governments, universities, professional bodies, and other decision makers to equalize the status of occupational therapy. To do so, the profession needed to develop a strong body of knowledge that could earn its place in the European Higher Education area and in the different health and social systems.

Choosing a European approach to strengthen the profession came partly from questions and issues that came up within the Committee of Occupational Therapists for the European Communities (COTEC), now the Council of Occupational Therapists for the European Countries, around diploma recognition, which could not easily be accomplished without involving educational institutions.

Taking Advantage of Personal Opportunities

A personal motivation to develop the network came from my position as the chair of COTEC and a leader in an occupational therapy educational department in Amsterdam. In that role, I had just started to work with the Socrates-Erasmus programs (parts of the European lifelong learning program, stimulating mobility and internationalization in higher education) and discovered a chance to obtain a grant for establishing a European network.

In 1994, a new funding program was about to start, and there were some signals that it should contain a program to establish networks. I communicated with a representative of the European Commission, discussed the problems in our discipline, and asked him whether we could be financed to start a network. He told me that the conditions to become an international network were complicated and advised me to apply first for a smaller action (Action 4) under the Erasmus program, which had less strict conditions. I asked him if I could mention his name when I applied, and he agreed (a strategic action—referring to influential people).

The Vision Takes Shape

ENOTHE was established in 1995 with support of Erasmus, and 2 years later, we became an official Thematic Network, one of the main innovations of the Socrates-Erasmus programs at that time. Networks were created to deal with forward-looking, strategic reflection on the scientific, educational, and institutional issues in the main fields of higher education. Normally, all countries participating in the Socrates-Erasmus programs (EU, European Free Trade Association, and Candidate Countries) should be represented in a Thematic Network. The main aim of a Thematic Network was to enhance quality and to define and develop a European dimension within a given academic discipline or study area.

We consciously and strategically chose to be a network rather than a formal association because a network is dynamic, flexible, adaptable, and easily extended or connected with communities of practice and other networks and also allows for diversity. ENOTHE aimed to be an open knowledge network. Furthermore, an important reason was the availability of grants, although limited, for some networks in higher education in Europe.

Using Creativity and Innovation

Jeanne Liedtka (1998) highlighted that strategic thinking is not "thinking about strategy" but about building a capability for real strategic thinking, which produces an innovative response and an efficient organization to capitalize on that innovation. She explained that strategic thinking breeds inventiveness and innovation. It engenders speed and flexibility. It invites members at all levels into the strategic conversation and engages them as a result. Establishing a network seems quite in line with these characteristics of strategic thinking. However, creating a future vision and being aware of the internal and external systems is not enough to achieve change. For strategic thinking, a third aspect, creativity, is also necessary and a combination of the three aspects.

Using Creativity to Position the European Network of Occupational Therapy in Higher Education Within the Different Systems

Defining how we position occupational therapy within these converging internal and external systems in the long-term vision requires creativity—moreso if ENOTHE wanted to become an official subsidized European Thematic Network. The following questions around the conditions for official Educational Networks emerged:

- How could we say occupational therapy is academic, if more than half of the education was not?
- How could we say that we were one of the main fields in higher education? Could we compete with medicine, engineering, business, or humanities studies such as history and law?
- Should we pretend to be one of them, or could we present ourselves from a different angle?
- How could we have representation of occupational therapists/educators from all European countries when the new accession countries did not have any occupational therapists?

Deciding how to position oneself or one's organization in context is crucial to be successful and to receive a grant.

Considerations Contributing to a Creative Solution

We decided to position ENOTHE as a disadvantaged network and appeal to the European principle of equality or equal opportunity in different aspects as follows:

- Occupational therapy is a rather new academic discipline and yet a fast-growing profession (increase of 50% over the past 5 years).
- Theories underpinning occupational therapy are changing from purely medical and impairment directed toward more psychosocial and occupation based, directed toward the participation of persons with disabilities and/or older people in society, but there is need for further development (gap 1).
- All curricula in occupational therapy in Europe need to change to more occupation and research based and require a strong relation to the generic academic competences and with the new policies/trends in approaching people with disabilities (participation) (gap 2).
- The position and status of occupational therapy education throughout Europe is not yet harmonized. This is a barrier in the mutual professional recognition and mobility of occupational therapists (free movement). Particularly in Germany, most occupational therapy educational institutes (more than 160) are not yet included in higher education (gap 3).
- In several southern European countries, the numbers of occupational therapy educational institutes is low compared with the demand, and in several of the associate countries, occupational therapy education is not yet provided or is offered only as one module within a curriculum of another discipline (gap 4).
- In most countries (except Sweden, Finland, and the United Kingdom), occupational therapists have little opportunity to enter formal continuing education at a master's or doctoral level (gap 5).
- Currently the entry level into the profession for occupational therapy in United States and Canada is at a master's level. To be competitive, Europe must prove that their bachelor competencies as entry level in the profession are equal to the US and Canadian master's level. Global discussions on the competences of occupational therapists are necessary to raise their competitive position of Europe.
- In southern, eastern, and central Europe, the focus on inclusion and rehabilitation toward empowerment of disabled and/or older people is new or less developed than in the rest of Europe. In several countries, occupational therapy service is scarce or simply not provided, even as client groups are asking for it (e.g., Italian patients with multiple sclerosis, war victims in the Balkans, parent groups of children with disabilities in Bulgaria, Turkey, Georgia, and Armenia) (gap 6).
- ENOTHE has been approached for support in setting up occupational therapy education by several institutes in Romania, Hungary, Bulgaria, Poland, Lithuania, and Turkey—the demand is there.
- Most of the professional literature comes from the United States and the United Kingdom, and little of it has been translated into other languages. Because occupational therapy is not always taught in an academic environment, the use of English is not yet common in all countries. Thus, the knowledge about occupational therapy is not equally spread over Europe. More possibilities for translation of ENOTHE publications should be created (in particular, curriculum guidelines, competencies, and teaching materials), and further discussions on unifying terminology in diversity should be developed (related to the strong European value of diversity).
- Students in occupational therapy are rather isolated in an international context because their institutions are too small to provide international services; they have requested the support of ENOTHE. Annually, more than 150 students are actively involved at the ENOTHE meeting, and before and after in projects related to the meeting (gap 7).

Positioning your profession or discipline as disadvantaged is not strategic unless you can give evidence of an internal system that is strong enough to fight these inequalities. Strategic thinkers must appreciate the interrelationship among the internal pieces that, taken together, comprise the whole (Liedtka, 1998).

Using Creativity to Structure the Network Toward the Outside World and to Unite Internally

Much creativity was needed to unite the greatly divided European occupational therapy world into a single strong organization with diverse directions connected to the external systems. Such a network defines roles for individual members within the larger system and clarifies for them the effects of their behavior on various parts of the system, as well on its final outcome. ENOTHE can be seen as a complex system in which patterns of interaction and hence roles change over time so that the system evolves in a nonlinear way (Creek, 2010). ENOTHE has been organizing itself in various ways in line with the dynamics of a learning network in relation to a rapidly changing outside world.

An example of one of these structures of ENOTHE in line with the Bologna and TUNING Educational Structures[2] and several social policy documents (e.g., the Social Agenda, "Towards a Europe for All Ages," E.Com, 1999) and the enlargement of Europe was as follows:

- TUNING and quality assurance in occupational therapy education:
  - Develop first-, second-, and third-cycle subject-specific competencies (following the TUNING methodology, 2008)
  - Create uniformity in professional and educational terminology and context relevant translations, with a book presenting a conceptual framework for occupational therapy in six languages as the final outcome
  - Develop an international peer review system
  - Support the implementation of occupational therapy education in an enlarged Europe
- Development of the European Dimension in Occupational Therapy Education
  - Identify and encourage implementation of learning outcomes concerning the European Dimension of Occupational Therapy and develop an Internet course concerning occupational therapy in Europe
  - Encourage student and teacher mobility
- Development of Continuing Education and Training in Occupational Therapy Research
  - Encourage joint master's education in occupational therapy and formulate guidelines
  - Establish synergy between the occupational therapy education and research areas
  - Develop an Internet self-study package on occupational science
  - Support the development of an application for Early-Stage Training for young researchers, 6th/7th Framework,[3] and make links to research networks
- Development of Innovative Teaching Methods
  - Concerning problem-based learning, produce "signposts" and stories about problem-based learning
  - Develop guidelines for innovative teaching of practical skills in an academic environment

Under each of these above categories, many projects, which were suggested by the members themselves, could be scheduled and together they formed a process of capacity development and reform in occupational therapy education, practice, and research. Most lecturers and students of the member institutions of the network could find their role and place or were engaged in the network. In the foregoing structure, we see that strategic thinking is closely connected with strategic planning that is outcome related.

---

[2] TUNING Educational Structures in Europe is a university-driven project that aims to offer a universal approach to implementing the Bologna Process at the level of higher education institutions and subject areas. The TUNING approach consists of a methodology to (re)design, develop, implement, and evaluate study programs for each of the three Bologna cycles.

[3] The 6th and 7th Framework Programmes were European funded for research and technological development from 2002 until 2013.

The Innovative Aspects of This Structure

Some of the identified problems and their proposed solutions or objectives were as follows:

- Occupational therapy curricula and teaching materials were/are predominately in the English language. It was important to develop terminology in the professional language that is understood throughout Europe in a similar way but expressed in students' and researchers' own languages (uniformity in diversity).

- The network was aiming for research- and policy-driven curricula focusing at social inclusion in an enlarged Europe. Enablement and participation of persons with disabilities and older people in society is still not common throughout Europe. Introduction of occupational therapy education in several east, central, and southern European countries is (totally) new and will support the empowerment of persons with disabilities. The occupational therapy education is in line with the idea of participation described in the WHO's *International Classification of Functioning, Disability and Health*, the EU Disability Action Plan, and policies such as Towards a Europe for All Ages (E.Com, 1999).

- The profession of occupational therapy is still relatively new in Europe. Comparative studies, research, and introduction of the European dimension in the occupational therapy curricula are necessary to improve the standards of occupational therapy education and practice throughout Europe in a more equal way.

- The academic discipline of occupational science must be introduced and developed in a European way and must underpin the undergraduate and graduate curricula.

- There is a great need to change occupational therapy education from subject to problem based, to provide more project-oriented and student-centered education, and to ensure the implementation of new technologies.

- Teaching methods must be carefully chosen and clearly connected with competencies and the learning outcomes. Development of examples of good practice of teaching activities in an academic environment will be welcomed by occupational therapy educators.

Summary of Application of Strategic Thinking With the European Network of Occupational Therapy in Higher Education

ENOTHE demonstrates the vision of occupational therapy as an academic discipline advocating for equal services for people with disabilities in all European countries. It gives occupational therapy students and lecturers the chance to develop internationalization and scientific skills based on a strong network structure. These strategic arguments were highly valued by an independent expert assessment of the European Commission, which commented as follows on the grant application: "It is obvious that the societal demand is great for developing an academic based discipline as Occupational Therapy with impact on a European scale" (van Bruggen, personal communication, grant 223102-CP-1-2005-1-NL-ERASMUS-TN).

Should we always position occupational therapy as a disadvantaged discipline? Of course not. The next example takes a completely opposite approach.

CASE EXAMPLE 2: POSITIONING OCCUPATIONAL THERAPY AS A STRONG ACADEMIC PROFESSION IN GEORGIA AND ARMENIA

Next we look at introducing occupational therapy for the first time in Georgia and Armenia. These are two relatively new member countries in the European Higher Education Area, the law of which stipulates that the governments of member countries should ensure, in accordance with the *United Nations' World Programme of Action Concerning Disabled Persons* (1983), the accessibility of the outside world to persons with disabilities. New criteria for the (re)construction of buildings and transportation includes making these accessible for persons with disabilities. Standards also must guarantee a social safety net and provide social services and employment for persons with disabilities.[4] The amendment to the legislation will contribute to the integration into the society of people with disabilities. The long-term goal is to create conditions that enable participation in society of children and adults with physical and mental disabilities. The development of health promotion and education and the new context of education, habitation, and rehabilitation have become a priority.

Systems Thinking

The governments of Armenia and Georgia are committed to reform higher education as well as the health and social sector toward systems and standards that are more comparable to those of Europe. The introduction of the education and profession of occupational therapy could play an important role in these reform processes. Occupational therapy is taught all over Europe in higher education, mainly at bachelor's and master's levels and in the United Kingdom and in Sweden at the PhD level as well. The discipline is following the Bologna Process supported by the European Commission and focuses on participation of all people in society. Over the past 5 years, there has been a 50% increase in occupational therapists in Europe. This shows that the profession has a valuable and distinctive contribution to make to society.

However, being a strong and useful profession that can contribute to social and educational reform does not immediately predict that countries such as Georgia or Armenia will introduce such a profession in its rightful place within their social, health, and educational systems. Often occupational therapy is introduced in a country when a rehabilitation center or an orphanage or a single doctor is asking for an occupational therapist to help. In Georgia, it was an enthusiastic neurologist who had seen occupational therapy in North America and was asking for an organization who was willing to educate 10 occupational therapists within 2 years (that was the funding condition) for his children's rehabilitation center.

What, then, is the wise answer if you know that there is no occupational therapy and rehabilitation in that country? Rehabilitation of persons with disabilities has been strongly based on "defectology," meaning that only corrective measures were applied. People with disabilities were more than likely excluded from full participation in society, denying them human rights. In addition to the approximately 10% of the population that was disabled, another 10% was internally displaced and perhaps occupationally deprived because of several wars. Between 13% and 15% of the labor force was unemployed (Eurostat, 2013), and 41% of the population lived below the poverty line (World Bank, 2010). The country continues to move toward a market economy and greater integration with Western institutions. The social institutional arrangements and policies, which provided "cradle to grave" protection to the total population, had been designed for a very different economic system and was severely affected by the transition process.

---

[4] This is before the *Convention on the Rights of Persons with Disabilities* (signed in 2009).

Formulating a Vision

Some occupational therapists will argue that doing something is better than nothing. But the present position of occupational therapy in several countries is still problematic because the profession once was started as a private or voluntary undertaking and not a structural one. This results in a long and difficult road to achieve a recognized academic status. In this case, however, we thought strategically about the long-term vision: developing the academic discipline and profession of occupational therapy in close collaboration with all stakeholders to facilitate participation of persons with disabilities and other disadvantaged groups in the society. This could not be a single disciplinary action from outside; it needed a core organization in Georgia, which was embedded in different systems, such as health, education, social affairs, and labor.

The Vision Takes Shape

Now we consider a more specific aspect of system thinking: partnerships. The creative aspect in this case is identifying and building effective partnerships for sustainable development. "Partnering is easy to talk about but invariably somewhat harder to undertake. It requires courage, patience, and determination over time. It is rarely a 'quick fix' solution to a problem and can sometimes be a frustrating and disappointing experience" (Tennyson, 2011, p. 1). There is mounting evidence from many partnership initiatives under development in different parts of the world that such cross-sector collaboration can be highly effective and sustainable when it is designed, developed, and managed in a systematic way. A partnership is a cross-sector collaboration in which organizations work together in a transparent, equitable, and mutually beneficial way toward a sustainable development goal and those defined as partners agree to commit resources and share the risks as well as the benefits associated with the partnership (Tennyson, 2011). Cross-sector (business, not-for-profit organizations, government, academia, media) partnering is an important mechanism for addressing critical and sustainable development issues such as health, employment, social inclusion, and development.

The full partnering process consists of 12 steps following the partnering method of Tennyson (2011). In the framework of strategic thinking, particularly the first three steps—scoping, identifying, and building the right partnerships within different sectors/systems, including all stakeholders—is essential. The other nine steps (planning, structuring, mobilizing, delivering, measuring, reviewing, revising, scaling, and moving on) are parts of strategic planning and managing.

Developing Partnerships in Georgia

Now I return to the neurologist in Georgia, who was still waiting for our answer. After having investigated the context and having learned that this doctor and his staff had some experience doing projects with Western organizations, I decided to involve him directly in our strategic thinking process. So I answered, "I can see the need in your center for 10 occupational therapists, but what about the recognition of their education and the legal status of the profession? And how do we provide occupational therapists for the whole town, region, and country in the future?" He concluded that occupational therapy should become an integral part of the curricula in academic institutions to ensure an adequate number of trained professionals as well as unification of education in occupational therapy, encompassing a uniform knowledge base, philosophy, theory, and practical training.

Using Creativity

We anticipated some difficulties persuading the Georgian government that occupational therapy is much needed for persons with disabilities and finding a university that wanted to be involved in curriculum development. This process would likely take more than 2 years. So what to do in the short term? We decided to create a pilot project with the following aims:

- Educating and supervising the first group of 8 to 10 Georgians (who had a degree in psychology or medicine and were unemployed) to become lecturers and/or clinical supervisors in occupational therapy
- Searching for a university that was willing to develop a bachelor's program following European standards (as a condition for funding) in collaboration with stakeholders and the first occupational therapists and issue their diplomas with a degree
- Promoting public awareness of persons with disabilities as equal citizens and developing inclusion programs
- Establishing and legalizing an association for occupational therapists
- Looking for the "right" partners to establish the profession in a sustainable way
- Looking for funding for further development of occupational therapy in the country, contributing to social reform and human rights

While we performed a pilot project, we constantly searched for new partners and worked to build a sustainable network. At the end of the pilot, we had identified more than 20 partners who were willing to sign an application for funding and to commit themselves to developing occupational therapy to contribute to an inclusive society. In searching for partners, it was important to consider the various sectors and the external systems where occupational therapy should be embedded and the scale of partnership connected with the future vision that the profession should contribute to inclusion and human rights.

During the period of the pilot project, we found the following partners ready to collaborate in a project with the following aim: facilitate participation of disadvantaged groups in society through the development of occupational therapy practice and education:

- The Ministries of Education, Health, Social Affairs, and Labour (agencies) from Georgia as well as Armenia. We wanted to apply for European funding that supports countries that wish to join the European Higher Education Area, and it turned out that working with two Caucasus countries together was a condition of such funding. Thus, we began involving several Armenian partners in the project. However, this made it complicated because the two countries have different political orientations, different languages, and even different alphabets. And why did we have to involve so many ministries? We were not sure whether the profession should be a pure health or social profession or a mixture of these contexts, and thus we needed jobs in both sectors. The Ministry of Labor in both countries was involved to make sure that once the Ministry of Education agreed to accredit the discipline, the profession would be accepted in the list of officially recognized professions of both states.
- Faculties of two universities in each country (total of 4), again a mixture of medical-oriented and sociopedagogical faculties; different universities and faculties could contribute to the development of a curriculum.
- Three European Universities, which had experience with such a project (the grant condition was not to develop a total new curriculum but to use the experience of a more or less identical project, which in our case had taken place in Prague, Czech Republic). In addition, a Japanese university was ready to contribute to the project because it had a lecturer who had experience working in Armenia.
- Stakeholders, such as disability organizations, parent organizations, and rehabilitation centers.
- Centre for Training and Consulting Foundation, Norwegian Refugee Council, and the Global Initiative on Psychiatry: All three organizations were well acquainted with project development, the situation of migrants, conflict zones, and mental health, which should all be part of a occupational therapy curriculum.

The strategy chosen in the pilot project turned out to be the right one. It quickly became clear that the project could have great influence beyond its original intention of training occupational therapists to assist children: The project also created a growing demand for occupational therapy.

Many nongovernmental organizations became interested in learning more about occupational therapy and using trained staff.

The minister of health put occupational therapy in the standards list of activities covered by state programs and allocated money for occupational therapy activities as well. Representatives of different ministries attended conferences organized by the children's rehabilitation center as well. "The pilot project seems to be well designed and implemented both concerning content and approach," concluded the official evaluator from the funding organization after a year and a half.

Thinking in Time

Together with the various partners, we were fortunate to apply for European funding at the right time, because it was the European Year of Disability, and we were one of three projects approved for Georgia and Armenia. Now full bachelor's courses following the Bologna/TUNING Process in occupational therapy have been developed in both countries. Three occupational therapists from the first cohort became policy makers within the government, advocating for inclusive education, human rights for people with disabilities, and inclusion of internally displaced people after war.

The Georgian neurologist, Dr. Z. Kakushadze, stated: "One of the major impacts is that occupational therapy is contributing to social reform in the sense that the occupational therapists have created awareness for equal opportunities for persons with disabilities at different levels" (van Bruggen, 2011). One of the ministers asked: "Can you please give us 50 more of these occupational therapists?" From this example, we can learn how vision was connected to an analysis of reality in time and contexts, demonstrating the principle of thinking in time. The gap between vision and reality creates an emotional and energetic tension that seeks to be resolved. This is what Peter Senge (1990) called the "principle of creative tension."

CASE EXAMPLE 3: SEEING THE BIGGER PICTURE IN OCCUPATIONAL THERAPY PRACTICE: HOW BIG SHOULD THE PICTURE BE?

The two previous examples of strategic thinking and crossing borders may not be relevant to the daily practice of many occupational therapists. Therefore, an example from occupational therapy practice follows.

Systems Thinking

The context is Georgia, where, as mentioned earlier, more than 60% of the population is living below the poverty line. Occupational therapy is subsidized in part by the government, but it also requires a contribution from the individual client for each session. This case discusses a single mother and her 7-year-old child with learning disabilities who came to the children's rehabilitation center in Tbilisi, Georgia, the only one where occupational therapy services are provided. After three sessions, she told the occupational therapists that she could not return with her child—not because she does not value the therapy. The mother began to cry and said she could not disclose the reason why they would not be returning.

What could be the cause for this? What is the bigger picture here? What different perspectives can we look at? How can the mother and her child be understood in their situation? Is looking at the family situation a big enough picture? Or should we look at the neighborhood? Or other, broader systems? If our vision is social inclusion through occupational participation for all, how can we improve this situation?

Figure 3-4. Levels involved in a social inclusion process. (From *Creating an inclusive society: Practical strategies to promote social integration*, by United Nations Department of Social and Economic Affairs, © 2009 United Nations. Reprinted with the permission of the United Nations.)

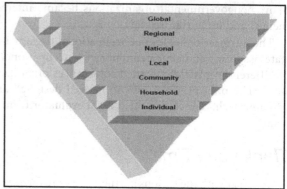

Figure 3-5. Layers of factors affecting health. (Reprinted with permission from Dahlgren, G., & Whitehead, M. [1993]. *Tackling inequalities in health: What can we learn from what has been tried?* Working paper prepared for the King's Fund International Seminar on Tackling Inequalities in Health, September 1993, Ditchley Park, Oxfordshire. London, England: King's Fund. Accessible in Dahlgren, G., & Whitehead, M. [2007]. *European strategies for tackling social inequities in health: Levelling up. Part 2.* Copenhagen, Denmark: WHO Regional office for Europe. Retrieved from http://www.euro.who.int/__data/assets/pdf_file/0018/103824/E89384.pdf)

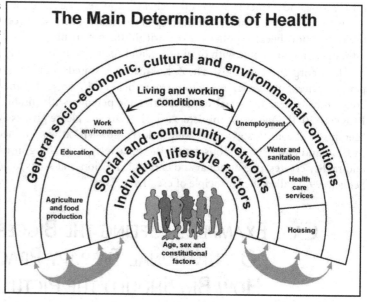

Social inclusion is understood as a process by which efforts are made to ensure equal opportunities for all, regardless of their background, so that they can achieve full potential in life. It is a multi-dimensional process aimed at creating conditions which enable full and active participation of every member of the society in all aspects of life, including civic, social, economic, and potential activities, as well as participation in decision making processes. (United Nations Department of Social and Economic Affairs [UN DESA], 2009, p. 3)

Social inclusion needs to occur at various dimensions and multiple levels, as defined in Figure 3-4 (UN DESA, 2009).

Should the occupational therapist look at all these levels? If so, how, and what can he or she do? What factors are barriers in occupational participation at the different levels?

The occupational therapist looks at the social determinants of health depicted in Figure 3-5 and finds the following individual-, household-, and community-level barriers to occupation for both the mother and the child: lack of money, lack of a social network, lack of employment, and lack of accessibility to education and adequate rehabilitation.

The mother did not have enough money for further occupational therapy; she had been working but was now unemployed because she had to look after the child. The child could not go to school because the law did not provide any opportunities for children with disabilities. The mother tried through occupational therapy service to rehabilitate her daughter so that she could go to school and the mother could return to work. However, she quickly realized that her child could not easily achieve primary school–level functioning. Furthermore, at the local and national levels, it seemed that children with disabilities had by law no opportunity to enter school, and what little day care was provided was not free. Nor were there social services provided for unemployed people.

At European and global levels, the disability rights and millennium goals supported by the Georgian government (United Nations Development Programme, 2004), in particular the goals of eradicating extreme poverty and improving the quality of Georgian educational systems to ensure equivalence with the educational systems of developed countries, should work as facilitators in the process.

Formulating a Vision

Here we return to the question at the beginning of the chapter: Why treat the child individually and then send the mother and child back to their more or less impossible situation? How can an occupational therapist reason strategically in this situation? What are the various perspectives and contexts? Looking at the social determinants of health, one of the biggest issues is poverty and unemployment, which for this family needed to be solved first to prevent illness.

Initially, we looked at their social networks. Were there other persons in the family or neighborhood who could look after the child with disability? In this case, we found four mothers in the same situation who decided to share caregiving. Each took 1 day to care for all four children, allowing the mothers several days each week to do paid work.

Is this enough? What is the future vision for this situation? At the same time, the mothers could be empowered to start, together with other parents, an advocacy group. The mothers involved the media and began to create awareness about the situation of their children and lobbied for inclusive education. The group, together with the occupational therapists, partnered with a primary school that was willing to be a pilot school in a process toward inclusion.

Using Creativity

Furthermore, in line with the convention of rights of persons with disabilities and the millennium goals, discussions with the Ministry of Education took place about universal primary education for all. As a result, all stakeholders participated in developing an inclusive school as a pilot project, along with guidelines for further inclusive education.

The final result of the entire strategic thinking, planning, and implementation was as follows:

- A member of the first cohort of occupational therapists became a policy maker at the Ministry of Education.
- In collaboration with the disciplines of occupational therapy and psychology, the pedagogical faculty introduced into the curriculum for primary school teachers a full year of instruction in inclusive education.
- After 3 years, there were 10 inclusive primary schools in Tbilisi, the law for primary education was changed toward inclusive education, and a multidisciplinary team for inclusion was established to advise and support schools and parents in the process of inclusiveness.

These results followed directly from occupational therapists looking beyond the immediate problem, considering the broader picture, and thinking strategically.

CONCLUSION

From the examples described in this chapter, we can conclude that strategic thinking consists of various attributes that overlap with cognitive dimensions of leadership. Exploratory studies on strategic thinking (Amitabh & Sahay, 2008) confirm this overlap with leadership skills.

Townsend and Polatajko (2007) have also encouraged occupational therapists "to immerse themselves in leadership strategies and consider potential allies in occupational enablement to benefit society through clinical services, consulting, management, education, research and policy development in public and private sectors" (p. 275).

The strategic skills demonstrated in this chapter are the ability to:

- See the big picture
- Visualize long-term future scenarios
- Initiate innovative ideas
- Conceptualize complexity
- Know the right questions to ask
- Think horizontally and simultaneously
- Form a broad strategy and allow specifics to emerge with time
- Look for environmental cues to develop "what ought to be"
- Identify partners for sustainable networks
- Embrace alternatives and uncertainties
- Challenge current processes, practice, and strategy

Good strategic thinking flows from understanding the nature of the environment and creating a symmetry and synergy of vision, intents, concepts, and resources that offers the best probability of achieving policy aims. Good strategy development provides for flexibility and adaptability so that planning and execution can be tailored to more immediate circumstances and respond to unanticipated opportunities and constraints. Good strategy remains valid in its focus and direction and achieves its intent even when these opportunities and constraints are taken into account, however.

This chapter does not intend to give a full international policy context, nor does it include strategic planning, which is a process in which long-term goals are transformed into short-term tasks and objectives; this relies on linearity and rationality and would require a separate chapter.

In essence, occupational therapists work in a multifaceted reality and need to learn strategic thinking and to apply a multifaceted set of leadership skills. Are occupational therapists prepared for the future and able to work on inequalities in complex communities?

REFERENCES

Amitabh, M., & Sahay, A. (2008). *Strategic thinking: Is leadership the missing link? An exploratory study.* Retrieved from http://www.iitk.ac.in/infocell/announce/convention/papers/Strategy-01-Manu%20Amitabh%20final.pdf

Bonn, I. (2005). Improving strategic thinking: A multilevel approach. *Leadership and Organization Development Journal, 26,* 336-354.

Creek, J. (2010). *The core concepts of occupational therapy, a dynamic framework for practice.* London, England: Jessica Kingsley.

Dahlgren, G., & Whitehead, M. (1993). *Tackling inequalities in health: What can we learn from what has been tried?* Working paper prepared for the King's Fund International Seminar on Tackling Inequalities in Health, September 1993, Ditchley Park, Oxfordshire. London, England: King's Fund. Accessible in Dahlgren, G., & Whitehead, M. (2007). *European strategies for tackling social inequities in health: Levelling up. Part 2.* Copenhagen, Denmark: WHO Regional office for Europe. Retrieved from http://www.euro.who.int/__data/assets/pdf_file/0018/103824/E89384.pdf

E.Com. (1994). HEART (Horizontal European Activities Rehabilitation Technology) Study. *European Service Delivery Systems in Rehabilitation Technology*, IRV, the Netherlands.

E.Com. (1999). *Towards a Europe for all ages*. Retrieved from http://ec.europa.eu/employment_social/social_situation/docs/com221_en.pdf

E.Com. (2000). Charter of fundamental rights of the European Union. *Official Journal of the European Communities*. 2000/C 364/01. Retrieved from http://www.europarl.europa.eu/charter/pdf/text_en.pdf

Eurostat. (2013). *European Neighbourhood Policy—East—labour market statistics*. Retrieved from http://ec.europa.eu/eurostat/statistics-explained/index.php/European_Neighbourhood_Policy_-_East_-_labour_market_statistics

Graetz, F. (2002). Strategic thinking versus strategic planning: Towards understanding the complementarities. *Management Decision, 40*, 456-462.

Liedtka, J. (1998). Strategic thinking: Can it be taught? *Long Range Planning, 31*, 120-129.

Mintzberg, H. (1994). *The rise and fall of strategic planning*. Englewood Cliffs, NJ: Prentice-Hall.

Ohmae, K. (1982). *The mind of the strategist the art of Japanese business*. New York, NY: McGraw-Hill.

Pisapia, J. (2006). *Mastering change in a globalizing world: New directions in leadership*. Education Policy Studies Series No. 61. The Hong Kong Institute of Educational Research, the Chinese University of Hong Kong. Retrieved from http://www.academia.edu/186994/Mastering_Change

Pisapia, J. (2009). *The strategic leader*. Charlotte, NC: Information Age.

Raimond, P. (1996). Two styles of foresight: Are we predicting the future or inventing it? *Long Range Planning, 29*, 208-214.

Senge, P. (1990). *The fifth discipline*. New York, NY: Doubleday.

Tennyson, R. (2011). *Partnering toolbook*. London, England: International Business Leaders Forum.

Townsend, E. A., & Polatajko, H. J. (2007). *Enabling Occupation II: Advancing an occupational therapy vision for health, well-being, & justice through occupation*. Ottawa, Canada: Canadian Association of Occupational Therapists.

TUNING Occupational Therapy Project Group. (2008). *Reference points for the design and delivery of degree programmes in occupational therapy*. Universidad de Deusto, Spain.

United Nations Commission on Human Rights. (1948). *Universal declaration of human rights*. General Assembly adopted on 10 December 1948.

United Nations. (1983). *World programme of action concerning disabled persons*. Retrieved from http://www.independentliving.org/files/WPACDP.pdf

United Nations Department of Social and Economic Affairs. (2009). *Creating an inclusive society: Practical strategies to promote social integration*. Retrieved from http://www.un.org/esa/socdev/egms/docs/2009/Ghana/inclusive-society.pdf

United Nations Development Programme. (2004). *Millennium development goals in Georgia*. Retrieved from http://www.undp.org/content/dam/georgia/docs/mdgrep/GE_mdg_2004.pdf

van Bruggen, H. (2011). Eastern European transition countries: Capacity development for social Reform. In F. Kronenberg, N. Pollard, & D. Sakellariou (Eds.), *Occupational therapy without borders: Volume 2. Towards an ecology of occupation-based practices* (pp. 295-304). London, England: Churchill Livingstone/Elsevier.

van Bruggen, H. (2012). The European employment strategy and opportunities for occupational therapy. *Work, 41*, 1-7.

Wilcock, A., & Townsend, E. (2000). Occupational terminology interactive dialogue: Occupational justice. *Journal of Occupational Science, 7*(2), 84-86.

World Bank. (2010). *Georgia—poverty headcount ratio*. Retrieved from http://www.indexmundi.com/facts/georgia/poverty-headcount-ratio

World Health Organization. (2008). *Closing the gap in a generation: Health equity through action on the social determinants of health*. Retrieved from http://www.who.int/social_determinants/thecommission/finalreport/en/index.html

World Health Organization. (2013). *Review of social determinants and the health divide in the WHO European Region*. Copenhagen, Denmark: WHO Regional Office for Europe.

Collaborative Reasoning
Working in Partnership With Third Sector Organizations

Angela Birleson, Dip COT, MSc, PhD

Occupational therapists, whatever their grade or whoever their employer, are often in the position of making daily decisions regarding how they manage their time in the workplace. These decisions can be around how they utilize their clinical time, frequently having to decide how they divide this limited resource among the people who use their services. The decisions can also involve how nonclinical time should be spent, what tasks to achieve, or which networks to establish. Reasoning with yourself about how to invest your time, or justifying to others why you have invested your time as you have, can be difficult and may result in occupational therapists being overcautious with their time rather than being innovative. Understanding how to reason time investment can enable occupational therapists to be more confident in exploring new ventures for service development.

The National Health Service (NHS) is the publicly funded health care organization that operates in the United Kingdom. It is funded mainly through general taxation and allows people who are legally resident in the United Kingdom to receive health care free at the point of use in primary, secondary, and tertiary care. Acute specialist services and general health care services for people in the United Kingdom are commissioned by separate agencies within the NHS and are often provided by organizations such as Foundation Trusts. A Foundation Trust is a corporation responsible to a board of governors that typically provides hospital, mental health, or ambulance services within a local area.

Social care services in the United Kingdom are provided by local authorities, which are local government organizations, often called county councils, that are also responsible for providing a range of services such as housing and refuse collection. Local authorities receive funding through general taxation but they can means test people for the provision of care; the rules for this differ across areas of the United Kingdom.

Third sector organizations differ from public organizations, such as the NHS and local authorities, as they are nongovernmental and, therefore, not funded through taxation. Third sector

Cole, M. B., & Creek, J. (Eds.).
Global Perspectives in Professional Reasoning (pp. 45-55).
© 2016 Taylor & Francis Group.

organizations, in contrast to government-funded or private sectors, are not for profit and are typically charities or community organizations, each one established to help tackle a particular issue, such as supporting people with a health condition, addressing a local community problem, or raising funds for research. The public can become members of these organizations, sometimes for a donation or joining fee. Typically, members may either be people with the condition that the organization supports, such as a head injury, or their families or professionals with an interest in that issue or condition. Often, organizations that cover the whole of the United Kingdom are divided into local branches to better address the needs of the local population. Third sector organizations that deliver support and research for health care issues have become a force in influencing and directing statutory services for their members. They are often called on to inform government organizations of their members' health and therapy needs, both within local areas and nationwide.

Most occupational therapists working in the United Kingdom are employed by either the NHS or local authorities. However, the NHS is struggling to fund the cost of required health care for the population (NHS Confederation, 2013) and a similar situation can be found in local authorities. Government austerity measures are affecting health and social services in ways never before experienced. Staff development has become increasingly difficult to fund, so occupational therapy managers must look toward new and alternative methods of developing staff to maintain and improve their service delivery.

I work as an occupational therapy manager for an NHS Foundation Trust, leading a team of neurosciences occupational therapists who work with patients in acute neurology and neurosurgery, inpatient neurorehabilitation, and community neurorehabilitation. The specialist inpatient neurosciences unit admits patients from across a wide geographic region made up of several localities, while the community neurorehabilitation team covers a single locality within this region. I am accountable to both the Director of Occupational Therapy and the Neurosciences Service Manager within the Trust for the performance of my team but have autonomy regarding operational decisions, development of my team, and service development. For many years, I have fostered relationships with third sector organizations concerned with neurological conditions in the United Kingdom, such as Parkinson's UK, Headway, and the MS Society, because I have found these connections to be immensely beneficial for service and staff development.

This chapter describes the professional reasoning that was involved in developing a particularly strong relationship with Headway. Headway is a registered charity that works to improve the lives of those affected by head injury. The organization has branches across the United Kingdom that offer a range of services. This chapter explores the influence that this relationship has had on service and staff development within the occupational therapy service I lead. However, my challenge is to describe an essentially implicit process that has become progressively established over time. So implicit is this process in my working practices that it now seems like an obvious choice for occupational therapists in positions similar to mine. When I reflect on what brought me to this conclusion, I recognize that I have had to make a series of calculated choices about how to invest time in developing this relationship.

Time is a valuable resource, and all occupational therapists have to be mindful of how they spend this resource, whether in practice, education, or management activities. To invest time in developing a relationship with Headway, I had to allocate time for this activity rather than investing it in other activities. Working with third sector organizations is not a mandatory part of my job description and, with the pressures on time management that most occupational therapists will recognize, any allocation of time outside of normal day-to-day practice needs to be justified and defended. I have justified my time investment in developing a relationship with Headway through the benefits that it brings to my service.

This chapter describes four events that occurred over a 4-year period that, together, firmly established a partnership between Headway and the neurorehabilitation service within the NHS Foundation Trust in which I work. Each event is described in chronological order and presented with my reflections on the effect that the event has had on staff and service development. The chapter ends with a summary of the impact this partnership has had on service quality and delivery.

A MENTORING OPPORTUNITY

Five years ago, I was offered the chance to be seconded from my permanent post for 2 days a week for a 2-year period to become a mentor on a newly developed program funded by the NHS in the North East of England. This program was created to promote the development of skills and knowledge in practitioners working in health and social care settings with people affected by long-term neurological conditions. The program used an innovative approach to improve practice in neurorehabilitation, both through the use of a mentoring process and by developing partnerships or communities of practice with peers. Experienced practitioners from the NHS, social care settings, and third sector organizations were sought to be mentors, and the organizers of the program matched these experienced clinicians with mentees who were new to, or less experienced in, neurological practice in order to help them develop specialist skills and knowledge. Mentorship posts were offered as secondments from practitioners' substantive posts and backfill funds were offered.

I had to weigh the pros and cons of this secondment as, although it would be an exciting opportunity, it involved me taking time out of my already demanding post. However, since it was a funded secondment, my employer would be reimbursed for my time and I realized that I could negotiate to use this backfill funding to employ a junior occupational therapist on a temporary contract in the neurosciences occupational therapy team. Junior posts are rarely available in neurosciences, so this would be a sought-after opportunity, enabling succession planning in the team.

Another factor in favor of the program was that it offered me the experience of working with a range of neurosciences professionals from across the North East of England, an opportunity that I acknowledged would enable me to compare my practice with that in other hospitals and community services. This benchmarking could facilitate practice improvement through the implementation of successful developments and ideas taken from these other services. The program would also give me the opportunity to develop mentoring skills, which I could then utilize in my permanent NHS post.

My application was successful and I was recruited as a mentor, together with nine other experienced neurological practitioners who came from a range of professional backgrounds and were working in a variety of organizations, including NHS and third sector.

I was matched as a mentor to a Headway area organizer for a Headway branch in the North East of England who was new in post and, although having had extensive experience of working within charities, had little experience of the impact of head injury on individuals and their families. The funding for the area organizer's post had been achieved through a successful bid by a branch of Headway to their local Primary Care Trust. Primary Care Trusts in England were abolished in 2013 but, at that time, were an administrative body, part of the NHS, that provided and commissioned community health services.

As I developed an understanding of what my mentee needed to learn about head injuries and why, an appreciation of the context in which my mentee worked began to emerge, including Headway's priorities for this post. These priorities included securing continued funding for the post and for the post to have a significant and recognizable impact on the local population of people with head injuries and their families. The Headway branch needed to utilize this post effectively because the funding was for a limited period, and future funding would be dependent on the efficacy of the post. The area organizer was required to become a competent and confident practitioner as soon as possible to ensure that the post had a positive impact, with measurable outcomes that could be utilized as evidence for continued funding.

My mentee and I developed a program of learning to develop her knowledge of the needs of people with head injuries. This included visiting hospitals and community services to which she had access through the mentorship program, giving her quick access to locations that might otherwise have required lengthy negotiations.

As my mentee developed her knowledge of the needs of people with head injuries and their families, our agenda turned to redesigning the service and developing high-impact interventions. The needs of people with head injuries are unique and challenging; therefore, developing third sector service interventions through a single post required both my knowledge relating to people with head injuries and my mentee's knowledge of working in the third sector to be used in creative and resourceful ways. An example of this was that I knew that people with a head injury sometimes have difficulty with social and leisure activities, so my mentee developed a group leisure activity program to introduce people to, and support them in, a range of leisure activities. However, I also knew that, because of their cognitive impairments, people with head injuries sometimes have difficulty with initiating actions, remembering appointments, and organizing their time, and thus they may fail to attend the leisure program. My mentee took this issue to the branch members to identify how she could promote engagement. They co-created a solution, which was the development of a system to alert people in the morning, via text, that the program was happening that day and to send a further text an hour before the program commenced. This innovative intervention used my mentee's skills and time effectively and was specific to the needs of Headway members and so was well received by them.

It was challenging for me to mentor a member of staff outside my normal sphere of work and within an entirely different organization. However, this experience expanded my skills and knowledge in ways that are directly applicable and beneficial to my own team and organization. Mentoring is a valuable skill for developing staff, and I have found that having the chance to mentor someone I would not normally line manage has allowed me to step outside my manager's role and embrace the true nature of mentorship. This is a skill I intend to continue developing.

The experience also gave me a greater understanding of the needs of people with head injuries outside of statutory service provision, which has encouraged me to consider how mainstream services could better contribute to meeting these needs. My knowledge of the issues that people with brain injuries face after discharge from the hospital setting led me to develop a protocol to ensure that all people with a brain injury being discharged from the rehabilitation ward are offered a discharge appointment for them and their family with a member of occupational therapy staff. During this appointment, the occupational therapist identifies the relevant statutory and nonstatutory services available to the person and his or her family in their locality, describes the remaining physical or cognitive deficits and their impact on day-to-day functioning, and provides self-help strategies to rehabilitate or compensate for those deficits. The occupational therapist supplements the discussion with written information on these topics. This appointment enables people with a brain injury and their families to access and utilize relevant services and manage the expectations of the individuals' function on discharge, preparing them to self-manage their condition. The feedback from families in particular has been extremely positive, confirming that this service development meets the needs of this group.

A FUNDING OPPORTUNITY

Four years ago, the chair of another branch of Headway in the North East of England approached me, in my role as the manager of a neurosciences occupational therapy service, to discuss how best to spend funding that the charity had received through a successful bid to two local Primary Health Trusts. The Headway branch had identified that people with head injuries in their locality were not receiving help to meet their ongoing occupational therapy needs after hospital discharge because of a lack of specialist community occupational therapy provision from the NHS in that area. They wanted to use the money to fund an occupational therapy post that would help to promote social engagement and vocational activities for people with head injuries, and they were requesting my advice and assistance in this matter.

I knew that supporting this venture would involve an investment of my time, but I did not know exactly what that time demand would be. I discussed the request with my line manager, and we agreed that the time investment would be worthwhile because the outcome would be to support the development of services for people affected by head injury in the area local to the hospital and would facilitate a closer working relationship with Headway.

The chair of the Headway branch wanted to ensure that they received the best possible value for their limited funds, so we discussed various options that would help them to achieve their aims. The branch suggested employing an occupational therapy assistant to work with their members, with a view to gaining as many staff hours as possible for the available funding. I agreed that a member of occupational therapy staff would be appropriate to help them to meet their needs; however, when I explored the context of the role, I found that the post holder would not only be required to work independently, without supervision, but would be required to assess the occupational therapy needs of people with head injuries, create intervention plans, and deliver those interventions. I therefore asserted that a qualified occupational therapist should be appointed. The chair understood my reasoning about the grading of the post and, after discussion with the branch, decided that a qualified occupational therapist should be employed.

The chair and I then spent some time discussing how the post holder should be employed. That particular branch of Headway did not have any paid employees, only volunteers, so employing a paid member of staff was a new venture for them. Initially, the chair suggested that the occupational therapist should be employed directly by the branch; however, I reasoned that there could be a better solution for all concerned. I strongly recommended employing the occupational therapist through my own organization because I believed that this would enable the member of staff to provide better value for money for a variety of reasons: the occupational therapist would receive professional supervision from my team, would be able to utilize the Trust's documentation procedures, and would have access to office space. The post-holder would adhere to my organization's clinical governance structure and health and safety policies, ensuring that he or she would receive appropriate training and education, his or her interventions would be evidence based, and any risks relating to the post would be appropriately managed. These procedures would be more robust in a large NHS organization than they would be in a branch organization with only one employee. Although this method of employment would carry with it a nominal management premium to cover the costs to the NHS and would therefore be financially the more expensive option, the chair gained agreement from the branch to proceed.

I then wrote the job description and advertisement, which were checked and confirmed by the chair and regional officer of the local Headway branch. Together with another senior occupational therapist, I carried out the shortlisting following NHS protocol. An interview panel was drawn together, again following NHS protocol, consisting of two members of NHS staff and three members contributed by Headway. A skills-based interview, which is the usual interviewing procedure within my organization, took place, and the decision on appointment was unanimous.

The successful candidate was initially appointed for 15 hours (2 days) a week for a year. She was given office space and documentation storage facilities with the community neurosciences occupational therapy team members, who also provided supervision. Headway had decided that the post should serve not just branch members but also the local population of people with head injuries. Therefore, the post-holder was rapidly able to establish a caseload with referrals from both Headway and from NHS staff via previously established referral procedures. The occupational therapist's interventions were community based, so she mainly dealt with face-to-face contacts in either clients' homes or the relevant community setting, such as a shop, workplace, or educational facility.

Having already had the experience of working with Headway's agenda and priorities while mentoring one of their staff members, I understood the necessity of ensuring that all activity undertaken by the occupational therapist was rigorously recorded to create a clear picture of what the financial investment in this post was yielding for Headway members. Having the occupational therapist employed by a local NHS Trust meant that the post-holder was able to implement high-impact interventions swiftly and with the support of existing service structures, which the chair of the local branch and its members immediately appreciated.

The original funding for the part-time occupational therapy post was for 12 months, but through fundraising by the members, an additional 9 months were funded. Unfortunately, the timing of the need for continued funding for the post then coincided with the demise of Primary Care Trusts and the formation of Clinical Commissioning Groups. Clinical Commissioning Groups are clinically led NHS organizations that organize the commissioning and delivery of health care services within their boundaries. Inopportunely, while the local Clinical Commissioning Group was being formed, new bids for funding outside of mainstream services were rarely considered, and funding for the post was not provided. In reviewing the failed bids and analyzing bids that had been successful in receiving funding from the Clinical Commissioning Group, I discovered that the trend seemed to be toward the commissioning of targeted interventions for a set number of individuals in a particular client group, rather than funding staff posts. On reflection, I concluded that perhaps the bid would have yielded success if it had been composed around the provision of social integration for a certain number of people with head injuries.

Before the post-holder left, she gave feedback that being employed by a large occupational therapy service within a statutory organization and working into a third sector organization had been a hugely valuable experience. She had been able to develop an innovative and pioneering post while receiving the security of supervision and governance from a mainstream organization.

The post-holder was able to share with the rest of the neurosciences occupational therapy team both her experiences of working differently from NHS staff and the valuable perspective of Headway members regarding their needs, rather than the traditional patient perspective with which the team was familiar. The team members were then able to reflect on how they might implement changes to ensure that the needs of people affected by head injury are met throughout their journey. The post-holder had been able to access the national training program that Headway has developed for its staff without incurring additional costs. Again, she was able to cascade that learning to the rest of the occupational therapy team, and they benefited from receiving information and learning on topics specific to head injury that are usually difficult and expensive to access.

The time invested in this venture was substantial, but it was beneficial in many ways to me and to my service. Being the first point of contact for a third sector organization when it wanted to employ an occupational therapist confirmed that they respected and valued my input and wanted to work in partnership for the benefit of local people affected by head injury. Negotiating the need for an occupational therapist rather than an assistant grade of staff for this post challenged me to market what my profession can offer. In helping to guide the post-holder and influence the development of the role, I had to consider how another organization wanted to deliver occupational therapy intervention, to deliberate on that organization's priorities, and to ensure value for money for their members. I valued the opportunity to undertake these thought processes and actions because marketing occupational therapy services is, and will increasingly be, important as competition for funding escalates, even within mainstream services such as the NHS.

A COMMITTEE POSITION

In 2012, Headway wanted to set up a new branch in a local area that was not covered by the existing Headway network. The regional manager asked if I would assist in the new branch development process. Any person with a head injury in the area concerned who required inpatient intervention was referred to the hospital where my team worked, but community services were outside of the team's remit. People with head injuries in that area depended for community intervention on local services, and the Clinical Commissioning Group in that area did not provide specialist community occupational therapy for these people. The regional manager of Headway was aware that I was keen to improve community services for people affected by head injury throughout the region and urged me to get involved.

Once again, I had to think about whether this venture was worth the investment of an as-yet-unknown amount of time from my NHS post. I reasoned that although this venture was not directly part of my NHS work, I had a professional responsibility to assist in the development of services in areas into which I was discharging people. In that locality, there were no statutory specialist community services for people affected by head injury because the Clinical Commissioning Group had not commissioned specialist community head injury services and did not have plans to do so. As part of this venture I would therefore be helping to improve services for people with head injuries by developing third sector services in a location where statutory services were absent. I reasoned that the time investment would, in turn, enable me to experience working with people affected by head injury to develop services for themselves, thus gaining a new perspective on service development.

Having thought it through, I willingly accepted the offer to become involved. The initial planning committee for the new branch consisted of the regional manager, people affected by head injury, solicitors (who provided premises for the meetings), occupational therapists from independent services, and me. Each member of the committee contributed his or her own experience for the benefit of the branch development. I was able to make a major contribution to the planning process because I was the only member of the committee who was aware of the statutory service provision pathway in that locality, from acute surgical intervention to community provision. This meant that I was able to identify the typical journey of a person with a head injury from admission, through an acute neurosurgical unit, to his or her home destination. I also understood the occupational therapy needs of people after hospital discharge because I supervised community neuro-occupational therapy staff working in another area. This knowledge enabled me to advise the committee on where the gaps were in service provision for people with head injuries in that locality.

The immediate challenge was to find initial funding for premises and activities. The regional manager helped the committee to approach local funding sources, including the local Community Foundation, for start-up funding. Community Foundations are charitable trusts, established across the United Kingdom, that enable philanthropists to invest in their community by giving grants to organizations such as Headway to address specific local needs. The requests for funding were successful, and a small start-up fund was established. The committee then mounted a local media campaign as part of its continued awareness raising to reach as many people as possible affected by head injury in the locality. This included a local radio interview with the chairman of the branch, who described his own experience of life after a head injury, and articles in local and regional newspapers.

The committee decided that the new branch would initially offer two forms of support: a telephone help line manned by volunteers from the committee and monthly drop-in sessions, again supported by volunteers from the committee. Although I reasoned that I could justify the time involved to assist the branch to become established and to take a position on the committee, I decided not to volunteer to support the help line or the drop-in sessions because this would be a regular and considerable time commitment from my NHS post.

To date, the help line and drop-in sessions have been successful, and the number of members of the new branch continues to grow. The committee also wants to look toward employing a member of staff, which could either be a Headway area organizer or a Headway occupational therapist. I have had experience of working with post-holders in both of these positions and envision that, if funding is secured, my knowledge could be used to expedite the initiation, development, and direction of either post. In addition, the knowledge I have developed regarding bids to the Clinical Commissioning Group will be useful because the committee will have to be specific about the aim of the intervention and the number of members that the intervention is for, rather than simply applying for funding for a post.

I have found that working alongside people with head injuries to co-create a new service to meet their needs has challenged the way in which I normally approach service development and has been a valuable learning experience. Previously, I had striven to carry out consultation with service users when developing services within the NHS, offering them the opportunity to comment on planned developments, but the dynamic of power in that situation is weighted toward the health professional. Now I recognize that people affected by head injury and other neurological conditions should be involved from the generation of the strategic direction of services through to their operational delivery. I acknowledge that this will require a cultural and resource shift to support individuals to identify and articulate their needs and the services that they require to meet those needs. Through my involvement in this venture, I have observed how this cultural shift can be advantageous to all involved. Working collaboratively with people affected by head injury has demonstrated to me how this approach can promote their empowerment. The therapist's focus on what people require from services can enable them to develop effective self-management skills through consideration of available options for service provision or interventions, judgments about the efficacy of those options, and a partnership approach with service providers to ensure that their needs are met. Individuals who effectively self-manage have a better quality of life, remain independent, and utilize statutory services less (Department of Health, 2013), so investing time in developing this culture will result in a decreased demand on resources.

AN INTERVIEW PANEL

In 2013, the occupational therapy service that I manage received funding for an additional member of staff to work on the neurorehabilitation ward. Reflecting on my experience of the value of working on various ventures alongside Headway, I reasoned that involving this third sector organization in the selection of a new member of NHS staff would bring a different perspective and further develop the relationship between our organizations.

Within the NHS there are several national initiatives and drives to encourage patient involvement in the planning and provision of services. For example, clinical governance is a quality improvement framework utilized by the NHS that encourages the incorporation of the patient and carer perspective. Legislation, such as Creating a Patient-Led NHS 2005 (Department of Health, 2005) and Patient Choice 2005 (Department of Health, 2006), has moved the NHS toward becoming a service that responds to the requirements and requests of patients.

After this clinical governance initiative, I was able to approach the Headway regional manager to ask for a representative of Headway to join the interview panel. The regional manager immediately said that he would be happy to perform this task himself because, due to the short time frame for recruiting to this post, there would be inadequate time to prepare and support one of his members. I advertised and shortlisted for the post, following NHS protocol, and the regional manager contributed to planning the structure of the interview and the questions to be asked. During the interview, the regional manager was able to consider the perspective of the members of Headway and make a recommendation about the candidate to be appointed, based on consideration of his members' needs.

Through having input into the selection of a key member of staff for the neurorehabilitation ward, a third sector organization was enabled to contribute to the development of statutory services, thus promoting a cultural shift toward the co-creation of services. Previous time invested in establishing a sound relationship with this particular third sector organization meant that involving someone from Headway was a quick and simple process. However, although we were happy with the involvement of the Headway regional manager, in the future, time should be allowed for preparing and supporting a person affected by head injury to participate in the recruitment process.

People affected by head injury have diverse and complex needs, and additional time, effort, and resources would be required for them to become involved. This could be as straightforward as organizing the time of day or location of the shortlisting meetings or interviews to support a person's physical or fatigue requirements. Equally, it might require more thought about how written information is presented or the augmentation of interviewees' verbal responses with visual prompts to support memory. Certainly, all these adjustments could easily be accommodated, particularly by an occupational therapist committed to service user involvement. However, I would need to ensure that additional time for these preparations was allowed at all stages of the process, from the funding being released to when the appointee needs to be in post.

TIME TO REFLECT ON TIME INVESTED

Five years after the start of my relationship with Headway, I have reflected on the wisdom of investing so much of my time in the four ventures described in this chapter. In this section, I consider the outcomes of my engagement in all these ventures in their totality and summarize the benefits, as I perceive them, to me and to my service.

These ventures with Headway have offered me opportunities to develop, refine, and practice a range of skills that are directly applicable to my day-to-day work within the NHS. I have developed skills in mentoring, marketing, and service development. I have deepened my understanding of commissioning and of the priorities set by organizations outside the NHS, which has enabled me to consider service developments within my own organization from a different perspective.

One of the outcomes of this learning has been that, when creating business plans for new posts, I now consider a service package rather than a post because Clinical Commissioning Groups have moved away from funding particular posts. The current trend seems to be toward funding specific services for particular client groups, such as vocational rehabilitation for people affected by head injury. I have started to repackage the occupational therapy services to appeal to both statutory and nonstatutory organizations for funding. The first service to tackle was the community neuro-rehabilitation team, who wanted to improve the profile of their service among the health and social care professionals who could refer into it. I assisted the team to analyze a year of data to identify referrals, patient need, and interventions provided. This resulted in the team being able to establish and clearly articulate the specialist interventions they provided, which would differentiate them from the generalist rehabilitation services available in the community. The team was then able to relaunch its service, highlighting their specialist interventions, which included a service information leaflet for patients and staff. Referrals are now accurate and targeted, and patients' expectations and compliance have improved. The second part of this work is to carry out an economic analysis of each of the specialist interventions provided, which will mean that we can identify not only the specific contribution occupational therapists can make to the rehabilitation of people affected by head injuries but also the cost of each intervention.

Working with Headway has given me an insight into, and wider understanding of, the needs of people affected by head injury from an alternative perspective to my previous NHS experience. It may seem obvious to state that, in order to design and develop occupational therapy services so that they continue to meet the needs of the people who use them, it is crucial to elicit the views of these people. Within statutory services, pressure on time may mean that only token attention is given to service user and carer involvement.

Services need to provide value for money and engaging users in design, and monitoring can ensure that the services are targeted and effective and therefore economical. If the Headway area organizer whom I was mentoring had created a social and leisure program but had not consulted the members on how they could be encouraged to access it, then the service would not have represented value for money. The views of users are a precious resource that is generally underutilized by statutory services, but accessing this resource can be difficult. People affected by head injury, alongside many other patient groups, are typically a hard-to-reach community representing a diverse group of needs. The time I invested in working with Headway has meant that I can now access this previously hard-to-reach community quickly and efficiently.

The co-creation of services is the gold standard of user involvement (Bovaird, 2007; Needham & Carr, 2009), and although I agree that it is a worthy aim, I have found that true co-creation within statutory services is challenging from both the aspect of accessing people affected by head injury and that of negotiating change in established practice. There are currently no mandatory requirements to include service users in service planning and development in statutory services. A journey toward co-creation has already commenced, but moving this forward requires the development of a User Involvement Strategy to ensure that there is active involvement in as many aspects of service provision and evaluation as possible. The strategy should be developed within wider clinical areas and not just within occupational therapy. This will involve engaging with stakeholders and mapping existing user involvement activities to discover what is already in place. An involvement culture should be created and, most importantly, involvement champions created in each of the professions or clinical areas involved to tie all these elements of engagement into an approach that will promote active service user involvement in the planning, delivery, and organization of services.

Within my service, key aspects of cooperation should be reasonably straightforward to implement now that a relationship has been established with Headway. For example, users of the service I lead could be utilized to evaluate service provision through clinical audit. Users could assist in the design of an audit and relevant data collection tools and ensure that the audit is relevant and measures the elements of service provision that are important to them. Another example is that people affected by head injury could be involved in the design of service information leaflets. For example, they could advise on the layout and ensure that the language used is appropriate. My service has a range of service information leaflets that have all been approved via the governance structure within the hospital; however, although people affected by head injury suggested the design of some of the leaflets, their involvement in the future should be from inception to completion on any information outputs from my service. Users can also advise on when, how, and in what format information should be given to people affected by head injury. This advice is a valuable resource that can only come from people who have been in the situation themselves. I will continue to engage Headway members on interview panels for the recruitment of staff, but I hope also to find ways of using them throughout the recruitment process, from the development of bids, through deciding how funding could be utilized, to the design of advertisements and the selection process. I accept that additional time will be required for this but am now able to justify why the time investment will be worth the outcome.

Investing my time into these ventures with Headway required me to take a considered risk because that time may have been lost to patients without concomitant benefit to the service. However, I am able to reflect that the value gained from these ventures far outweighs the financial cost of my time. Engagement in each venture, with its individual merits and risks, was carefully reasoned, but the total worth to my service of engaging with this third sector organization is more than the sum of these individual parts. I have learned how to value and utilize service-user involvement in the planning of services and also how to market occupational therapy services to appeal to the commissioners of statutory services. These are practical and necessary skills that I have been able to utilize in my service directly. The impact on my own development and that of my service has been considerable and ultimately benefits the people affected by head injury using our occupational therapy service.

REFERENCES

Bovaird, T. (2007). Beyond engagement and participation: User and community co-production of public services. *Public Administration Review, 67*, 846-860.

Department of Health. (2005). *Creating a patient-led NHS: Delivering the NHS Improvement Plan*. London, England: Author.

Department of Health. (2006). *Our health, our care, our say: A new direction for community services*. London, England: Author. Retrieved from www.dh.gov.uk

Department of Health. (2013). *NHS mandate*. London, England: Author.

Needham, C., & Carr, S. (2009). *Co-production: An emerging evidence base for adult social care transformation* (SCIE Research briefing 31). London, England: Social Care Institute for Excellence. Retrieved from http://www.scie.org .uk/publications/briefings/briefing31

NHS Confederation. (2013). *Tough times, tough choices. Being open and honest about NHS finance*. London, England: Author. Retrieved from http://www.nhsconfed.org/~/media/Confederation/Files/Publications/Documents/Tough -times-open-honest-report.pdf

Spiritual and Ethical Reasoning
Interplay Between the Personal and the Professional in Decision Making

Sílvia Martins, MS, OT

This chapter addresses the process of reasoning and learning that I, as an occupational therapy lecturer, went through from 2007 to 2011 during my involvement in setting up the first occupational therapy education program in Mozambique, a Portuguese-speaking country in sub-Saharan Africa.

That experience has been one of the most rewarding professional challenges that I have faced since graduating as an occupational therapist in 1989. When the editors of this book invited me to reflect and write about the reasoning and learning that happened during those years, I realized that my professional decisions could not be isolated from the personal values and beliefs that were all the time influencing those decisions. The interplay of professional reasoning and personal beliefs has never been so clear to me in my practice as it became during this experience. Maybe the reasons for this are that my involvement in the education program in Mozambique obliged me to go completely beyond the limits of my comfort zone while, at the same time, I was dealing with a very painful life event, the death of my mother. Looking back, I can say for sure that those were years of immense personal growth.

The development of occupational therapy education in Mozambique was an initiative of a psychiatrist, the director of the National Mental Health Department. After being in contact with the work of some occupational therapists in Brazil, she suggested to the Instituto Superior de Ciências da Saúde (ISCISA), a public multiallied health professionals higher education institute, that a graduate program for occupational therapists should be integrated into the national health care plan to assist people with HIV/AIDS.

Finding this proposal meaningful and having no occupational therapists working in the country, ISCISA charged two of their teachers from other programs to develop an occupational therapy curriculum to present to the Ministry of Education for approval. After having the program approved, and enrolling 36 students, one director and an adviser of the institute went to Portugal intending to contact the President of the Portuguese Association of Occupational Therapists to assist with its implementation. This was the point at which I came into the project.

Cole, M. B., & Creek, J. (Eds.).
Global Perspectives in Professional Reasoning (pp. 57-75).
© 2016 Taylor & Francis Group.

In this chapter, I highlight the reasoning processes that were involved in making decisions about what actions to take and some of the lessons that I learned during the course of the project. These include the following:

- The influence of emotional factors on decision making and the need to balance them with practical considerations
- The importance of relationships and personal bonds in maintaining motivation
- The moral basis of reasoning, rooted in the principles of altruism and occupational justice
- The inescapability of the spiritual aspects of professional reasoning
- How to align personal values with the institutional mission
- The need to let go of preconceptions and expectations and to be open to change

This chapter is organized chronologically, beginning with an explanation of how I made the decision to become involved in the project. The planning process for developing the cooperation and the start of the occupational therapy program are described. Developments during the first 4 years of the program are discussed, followed by reflections on the lessons I learned during the entire process. The chapter finishes with my conclusions.

DECIDING TO BECOME INVOLVED

The first decision in relation to the education project in Mozambique was made when I first heard about it. I was at an allied health professionals' conference in Lisbon, presenting a paper on the European occupational therapy tuning project (TUNING, 2009). The tuning project was set up in response to the Bologna Declaration of June 1999, which called for the establishment of a coherent, compatible, and competitive European Higher Education Area, attractive for European students and for students and scholars from other continents (www.enothe.eu).

At the end of my presentation, two gentlemen approached me saying, "You are the right person to help us." Due to having a strong predisposition to help (the same willingness that made me choose a health profession as my career), I listened carefully to what those gentlemen had to say and had already decided to do anything I could to help, even without knowing what was the problem. From their physical appearance and accent I perceived that the two gentlemen had come from abroad, and this made me even more willing to help because of my fascination with different cultures. Reflecting on this fascination, I think that my curiosity came from the experience I had at the age of 9 years when I went abroad for the first time to France and was amazed by how different daily habits and lifestyles could be in other countries. After that first trip, I became eager to visit and to know more and more about other realities.

The Decision-Making Process

After finding that the help these gentlemen were asking for was to start an occupational therapy program in Mozambique, I felt quite excited and wanted to know more about why and how occupational therapists were going to be trained for the first time in their country. They told me that the coordinator of the national department of mental health from the Ministry of Health, Ministério da Saúde de Moçambique (MISAU), had approached their institution, ISCISA, asking for a training program in occupational therapy. This had come about because the country needed occupational therapists to work with the huge numbers of people experiencing the severe consequences of living with HIV/AIDS. During our conversation, I felt more and more excited; all the imagery I had in my mind about Africa was strongly supporting my decision to say, "Yes, I will go!" Also, I could perceive from the attitudes and nonverbal expressions of the two gentlemen that they were relieved to be speaking to an occupational therapist at last.

After my initial excitement, I tried to calm down and bring my professional reasoning to bear on the conversation. I began to ask questions about deadlines and was astonished to be told that the institution had already enrolled 36 students and wanted to start the program in 2 weeks. There were 2 weeks to go and Mozambique was a 10-hour flight from Portugal! When I reflect back on that moment, I can see that the main reason I did not quickly say it would not be possible to do it was because I am a person who has difficulty saying no to any challenge. In that moment, it was clear to me that it would be impossible to prepare for starting a program in such a limited time; my rational left brain was saying "Impossible to do it," but my emotional right brain was saying "You go for it!"

Saying no would mean losing an opportunity to take occupational therapy to a new country and to bring forward the profession, and that would have made me very sad. So I was already attracted to the idea of helping to develop occupational therapy in Mozambique and alert to finding a way of making it possible. Why?

Since discovering occupational therapy, I have always felt a responsibility to contribute to its development. When I realized that the field is often viewed as one of the less important health care professions, I became strongly committed to demonstrating how important our profession can be—being a wonderful way of bringing light to many persons who are struggling with difficulties in living a meaningful life. From that moment on, it became clear to me that I could play a role in the development of my profession in my own country, and, subsequently, I have tried never to lose an opportunity to do so. Sometimes this drive can put me in quite difficult situations because I always say yes to such opportunities, even when I do not have enough time. This same drive led me to become the head of the Portuguese Association of Occupational Therapists for 12 years and to collaborate in many European and world projects in the area of occupational therapy.

Another factor that had a strong influence on my decision was the romantic idea of being one of those Westerners who goes to Africa to help. I thought that I could, in some way, make a contribution to changing the world, helping to solve the terrible inequities between the Western world and developing countries.

In thinking about the process of making a decision, I can identify the strong influence of my values and beliefs on not saying no straight away. I would struggle with the idea of thinking of myself as someone who could say no to a request for help and deny myself an opportunity to learn so much from another culture. I also like the idea of being someone who is prepared to travel outside my comfort zone, which is something I have learned is an important contributor to my evolution as a human being. There is also the social belief I share with many Portuguese people that we should repair what our ancestors have done through the colonization process in Africa, which has played an important role in my decision making. I used to hear terrible stories from my cousins, who did their army service in Africa in the 1970s, fighting to maintain colonies under the power of the Portuguese government, and what they did made me feel both ashamed and responsible. There I was, being offered an opportunity to repair some of the damage my ancestors did many decades ago: How could I say no?

So my heart had already committed me to meeting the challenge, and I had to quickly put my mind to work on finding a way of making it possible. I had to move swiftly on from these romantic and emotionally driven thoughts to a more rational way of thinking—to find strategies to support my decision that I would go to Mozambique to support the development of their first occupational therapy education program.

At this point, a lot of questions came into my mind: What was the curriculum design and content of the program, and how had it been built? What kind of professionals and teachers did they have at the institute? What was their academic calendar? As I learned the answers to these questions during our conversation, light was dispelling the dark, and I could see a practical way in which I could contribute. It was clear to me that this was too huge a task to be accomplished by one person, and therefore I had to analyze the curriculum of the new program and find a way to involve the occupational therapy school where I had been working as a lecturer for more than

20 years. We needed to set up a meeting between these two gentlemen and the director of my institution, with the aim of agreeing on a memorandum of understanding.

By then, I had decided that I would do whatever was necessary to make the possibility a reality. In analyzing which factors had the strongest impact on my decision, I would say it was the emotional ones, although this was to be a professional commitment.

The Planning Process

My next decision was about how to present this project in an attractive way to the director of my institution. It was clear to me that this was a good opportunity for my school to develop international cooperation, but so far, that was not one of the institution's strengths. The project might be seen as an opportunity, but it might equally be seen as a threat. In my mind, the project still seemed like a dream, but I already felt strongly attached to it and would find it difficult to let the opportunity go if my institution decided that the project was not coherent in its mission. I had to think about that mission, and the values and the projects of my institution, and explore how this project would fit with them.

Aligning Personal Values With the Institutional Mission

My reasoning involved identifying similar past opportunities and thinking about how they had or had not been valued by the institution. For example, I had been involved in delivering some modules on new occupational therapy programs in Georgia and Romania, in the context of the European Network of Occupational Therapy in Higher Education (ENOTHE), and I used all my learning from those experiences in planning how to present this idea. I also did some reading and consulted with a colleague who has expertise in such projects. I was trying to control as many variables as I could before presenting the idea to the person who had the power to sanction this project.

I had to be able to show the decision makers of my institution the advantages of investing in such a project. My strategy was that, while I spoke to my line manager, the directors from the occupational therapy school in Mozambique would contact the director of my institution, giving some information on the project and asking for a formal meeting. So I started with the coordinator of the occupational therapy department, and after gaining her agreement, I asked for an interview with the director of the school.

Having done what I could to prepare for the visit of the directors from ISCISA, I then had to wait for their email requesting a meeting. For a few days, no email came, and I had to face the possibility that nothing was going to come of this fascinating overture. It was painful to face that situation because of the expectations I had created about it. But, finally, the email came, and I could present the project to my director.

During the discussion with my director about the project, I tried to identify verbal and non-verbal signs of his willingness to involve the institution in the project. I adapted my language and behavior to make clear the advantages to our school of becoming involved. I am aware that my motivation, enthusiasm, and energy can sometimes be a bit overwhelming for others and may even be seen as unprofessional; with that awareness, I tried to express myself rationally rather than emotionally when presenting the project.

To my surprise, the director quickly agreed that the project would be a good internationalization opportunity for our institution, and we planned the meeting with the directors of ISCISA. (Later I came to find out that he had emotional attachments to Mozambique because he had done his army service there.) Things were now becoming real, but after the formal meeting between the directors from both institutions, there was still a final step, which I was not aware of until then. This was the submission of the project to the main institution that owns our school: every project has to be approved by the main board of directors of the institution. Surprisingly, everything seemed to be happening at the right time, because two of the board members of that institution were aware of the health needs in Mozambique and one of them had been the World Bank representative in that country. Finally, we had a positive decision, and it seemed that now there was just a question of connecting the dots.

Pragmatic Considerations

The period between my first contact with the two gentlemen from Mozambique at the conference and the final decision to become involved in the project had been quite ambivalent for me. I could not stop myself from dreaming about the experience, but at the same time, I had to prepare myself for the likelihood of it all coming to nothing. It was therefore a happy moment for me when the positive decision finally came through: I could go and support the implementation of occupational therapy education in Mozambique. Again, in the euphoria of that moment, I had to move quickly on from that emotional response to the reasoning that would enable the planning of all that needed to be done against the clock: The program was due to start in 1 week.

Two other teachers from the occupational therapy department in my school also joined the project, being selected because of the specialist subjects they were teaching and because of their high motivation and commitment to going. Our first task was to revise the curriculum and to find some teachers from ISCISA who would be willing to learn about occupational therapy (distance learning) so that they could introduce occupational therapy to the students in the first semester. None of the Portuguese teachers would be able to go to Mozambique in the first semester because of our workload within the occupational therapy program of our institution.

After contacting the director and the coordinator of the occupational therapy course in Mozambique, a psychiatrist and a psychologist, respectively, we found that they would not have the time to take on this teaching, and no one else was available to do it. Finally, we had to agree that the first semester would run as planned by ISCISA, with lectures from other professionals on non-occupational therapy subjects. Only in August, at the beginning of the second semester, would the Portuguese teachers come to teach the first occupational therapy–specific subjects. The task of revising the curriculum would also have to wait until August so that it could be done jointly with the director and coordinator of the course. During those months from February to July, we would be in regular contact with the director and coordinator, trying to explain occupational therapy to them; learn about Mozambican culture and its social and health needs; discuss the aims, units, and contents of the program; and plan our first visit to the country.

The decision not to teach any specific occupational therapy subjects in the first semester was difficult to make. I strongly believe that the most important subjects to teach to first-year students are the occupational therapy–specific ones, such as the profession's history and philosophy. This approach gives them the opportunity to identify themselves with the profession, or not, and to decide whether they really want to become occupational therapists. I have a tendency to want things to be done the right, or even perfect, way, but because it was not possible for that teaching to take place in the first semester, I had to let go of my expectations. That would be the first of many situations in which I had to revise my preconceptions, accept things as they were, and quickly assess the real situation to see what best could be made of it.

At that time, I still had a romantic idea about the whole project, but I also felt responsible for the smooth running of the program. So, during those months before the first visit to Mozambique, my main tasks were to read and discuss with experts Mozambique's history, culture, and social and health needs to gain a more realistic view of the country. The drive to develop occupational therapy in Mozambique, and a strong belief that it could make a real difference to health and social needs, led my colleagues and me and kept our motivation high most of the time.

STARTING THE OCCUPATIONAL THERAPY PROGRAM

The occupational therapy program started, as planned by ISCISA, at the beginning of February, with lecturers from other departments of ISCISA teaching non–occupational therapy-specific subjects. During that first semester, we did not have much contact with the director and the coordinator of the occupational therapy program; many of our emails went unanswered, and we were unclear about what was happening. On our side, we continued to revise the curriculum and plan our first visit to Mozambique. We were a team of three staff members who were highly motivated to go and teach in Mozambique, and every task was a joy.

Setting the Program in Context

The occupational therapy curriculum that had been approved by MISAU contained the essential subjects but with many incongruities, because it had been put together by professionals who did not know much about occupational therapy and from the curricula of two different occupational therapy programs. To revise this curriculum, we had to become better acquainted with the reality of Mozambique, so we continued reading about the country's culture and health and social needs and speaking with some experts in African studies in Portugal. One of our contacts was the adviser to the director of ISCISA, a former Minister of Health in Mozambique, who had great knowledge of and influence on health developments in Mozambique. Through these means, we were gaining the knowledge to build a more accurate picture of the country.

Something else that helped us was having discussions with experienced occupational therapists from other countries about occupational therapy approaches in the social field and about occupational therapy interventions for people living with HIV/AIDS. These discussions were extremely important because, although Portugal and Mozambique share a common language, the culture and the physical reality are very different; some of the occupational therapy approaches used in Portugal would not be the most effective to implement in Mozambique.

Searching for information about Mozambique put me in contact with a lot of Portuguese people who had dreamed of going to Africa. I became aware that the drive I felt to go to Mozambique was related to this shared cultural feeling. After independence, almost all the Portuguese who were living in the former colonies returned to Portugal, often under terrible conditions, without any belongings and in a state of occupational deprivation; they felt segregated and stigmatized. Through their eyes, we could see how marvelous life had been and how terrible it was now, living with a few donated things in a cold country (compared with the African climate) where the majority of people were not keen to have them back. I had been fortunate enough to have contact at school with some of these children born in Africa, and I could still remember the stories they told about how beautiful and peaceful life was in Mozambique before independence, how people were living free and close to nature. The stories they told about running free and playing with other children, near wild animals, made it sound like living in paradise.

A Personal Dilemma

Three months before I was due to go to Mozambique for the first time, a huge and terrible challenge came into my personal life when my mother was diagnosed with a pancreatic tumor. According to the doctors, she had no more than 3 months to live. This turned my world upside down and made me question everything. It was strange to keep my life going while my mother was having her last months. I could not afford to stop working, but this dark cloud was always above my head. While I was working on the Mozambique project and my mind was dreaming about Mozambique, my heart was in pain as I prepared for the loss of my mother. All this time, I was dealing with these contradictory feelings: dreaming about Mozambique and wanting to prepare for the trip but also wanting to give my mother as much love, time, and presence as I could because every moment could be the last one.

By that time, I was questioning everything I had believed about life, love, and compassion. I was suffering greatly, but this helped me to become more mature and teach me about compassion. It was even making me more sensitive to everything I was reading about the health and social reality of Mozambique.

Until the moment when I got into the airplane, I was unsure whether I would be able to go to Mozambique because of my mother's health status. The final decision to go caused me great suffering. I was thinking of myself as an egoistic person for wanting to leave Portugal at this time, but the desire to be involved in the project, and to finally see the reality I had been reading about, was too strong: This was a huge conflict inside me. One factor that helped me in my decision was that I could see my mother's health was a bit more stable compared with the period when she was first diagnosed. The 3-month life expectancy the doctors had predicted was coming to an end, and she was quite stable. She was enjoying a good quality of life, and we believed that she would win the battle against cancer. However, there was always the possibility that something unexpected would happen, and I would not be by her side. The doctors helped me decide to go by saying that she was responding in an unexpectedly positive way to therapy and that her general health was good. Also, the social network around my mother made me feel that it was all right for me to go; she was living in a small neighborhood near her sisters and many familiar neighbors. With all these competing considerations, I experienced intense ambivalence during this period.

Finally, at the beginning of August, 7 months after I first dreamed of this project, the director of my institution and our team of three occupational therapists traveled to Maputo, the capital of Mozambique, where ISCISA was located.

THE FIRST TEACHING VISIT

We made the decision about how long to spend in Mozambique by thinking about the hours needed to teach the planned subjects and the budget allowed for this first visit. Through discussions among the ISCISA directors, the director of my institution, and the occupational therapy team, we agreed on 2 weeks. Classes were held from 1 p.m. until 7 p.m.; during the mornings, the team made visits to the main health institutions in the area and met with stakeholders.

For our director, and for the directors of our parent institution, the success of that first visit would be crucial to the decision of whether or not to invest in the project; this was mainly because of the lack of contact from the Mozambicans teachers involved in the program during their first semester. We knew that by the end of the visit, a decision would have to be made about going forward with this project because it involved a significant workload for the occupational therapy teachers and an expensive budget, mainly to cover the costs of travel. All this meant that, during our first stay in Mozambique, we had to address tasks and reasoning related to the teaching of occupational therapy to students who had never heard about it before while also dealing with tasks related to situational analysis and negotiations about the project.

Preparation

With regard to the teaching, we made a lot of decisions before going to Mozambique to prepare lectures and audiovisual materials because we wanted to show the students as much as we could about occupational therapy intervention. Decisions about the content of the lectures and about teaching methods were made on the basis of the extensive knowledge we had about occupational therapy, the small knowledge we had about Mozambique, and our previous experiences of similar situations. We were not sure about the cultural adequacy of our teaching and learning methods, but we believed we would have to be flexible and ready to change all our plans, if and when needed, to adapt to the culture and to the student group. An additional difficulty was created by our not knowing what the students had been taught during that first semester because of difficulties with our email communications. However, thanks to previous experiences I had had in such projects, when lecturing on the first occupational therapy programs in Romania and Georgia and working in ENOTHE, I was aware of the need to be as flexible possible and to always have a Plan B and a Plan C.

Our excitement was huge, and the preparations for lectures were intense. Within the occupational therapy team (we were three senior lecturers in different subject areas), and with support from occupational therapists who had expertise in setting up new programs, we decided on what to include in the first two modules: Introduction to Occupational Therapy and Foundations in Occupational Therapy.

A goal for the first visit was that the students should be able to understand and discuss the scope of occupational therapy and how it could be of benefit in meeting the needs of the population. They should also be aware of and discuss their important role in establishing and developing the profession in their country. We were aware that this was an ambitious goal. However, we knew that half the class was composed of mature students who had been recruited from MISAU employees across the 11 provinces of the country, and this made us confident that the goal was achievable because of their previous knowledge and experience of the health and social needs around the country.

I can still picture clearly in my mind our first contact with the students. When we came into the classroom, all the students were wearing bright, white uniforms that matched the light of their smiles. I felt "I am at home," and that feeling has never left me. Still today, when I land in Mozambique, I always have the feeling that I am returning home. This is something I cannot explain with my brain; I can only feel it in my heart.

Adaptation

Our first contact with the students was mainly to introduce ourselves, so we had a question and answer session. More than half of the class was male, which is the opposite of our classes in Portugal, and they behaved formally in front of us, even when having discussions between themselves. That first day progressed in a formal and quiet way with few questions, and it was difficult to generate a real discussion. The students were very ceremonious and did not seem comfortable about relaxing or daring to expose themselves. We could see and feel that they were not used to group discussions—and we had planned to have a lot of group discussions!

That evening, after the first teaching session, the occupational therapy team restructured our materials for the next day's classes. And the same thing happened almost every evening thereafter. Instead of using a lecture format, we involved the students in role-plays about the daily occupations and rituals of their villages. We needed them to be more at ease because they were the ones who could tell us about their occupations, routines, and rituals. It turned out that they had been expecting a course based on a biomedical model, so it was not easy for them to understand that much of occupational therapy is concerned with everyday activities.

One tradition that appeared in the discussions and in role-play was *lobolo*, mainly from the south of Mozambique. According to this tradition, when a man wants to marry a woman, his family should compensate her family for the loss that her leaving represents to the family. The students role-played the discussion between the families for the value of the *lobolo*. From this role-play, we learned about the diversity of traditions in Mozambique with the south, being a matrilineal society, very different from certain provinces in the north. The *lobolo* was still common in the south and valued by the young people; however, it did not make sense for some of the students from the north, and they saw it as an old-fashioned and nonsensical ritual. We also learned about the importance of women in Mozambican society: They are the ones who take care of the children and do all the housework and who also provide an income for the family. We could also see how, depending on the region, some men could help in those activities, whereas to others it would not make sense. Some of the female students from matrilineal societies were used to being the ones who did all the housework. This role-play and discussion was a great starting point for exploring the occupations of daily life in the different regions.

Despite initial difficulties, the students responded well to role-play, and we had an intense, enriching day. By the end, they were feeling more comfortable about discussing and sharing with us all their concerns about the program. For a whole semester, they had only had lectures on general subjects, without having any idea of what their future profession was like. Other students from the institution had been teasing them because they could not explain what kind of professionals they were going to be at the end of the program. We could sense their anxiety and expectations, as well as a lot of curiosity.

This visit tested our flexibility all the time, and the word for the day was *adapt*. The timetables were very different from Portugal: Our days started with a meeting at 7:30 a.m., followed by visits or interviews in the second half of the morning, classes from 1 p.m. until 7 p.m., and evenings spent restructuring classes and assignments for the next day. The hot and humid climate and the antimalaria medication had a sedative effect on us, and the smells, colors, and sounds were a constant invitation to distraction, even in the most formal situations. Each visit to an institution or interview with a stakeholder was an intense experience from which we could learn a lot about the reality of the country, but many times we felt that we were not at our best.

Motivation

Fortunately, our motivation and the joy of being there, finally meeting the reality we had been dreaming about, provided the energy to keep us going during those long working days. Between the three of us, and with the input of students and also of some staff members, we were able to restructure all our teaching materials in the evenings. We could tell from the responses of the students that the new materials and methods were more appropriate. For example, because the students had never had the opportunity to see occupational therapists at work, we found it was important to show them videos to promote discussion about occupational therapy approaches. Our classes were dedicated to sharing and discussing information about occupational therapy and about therapeutic approaches with different populations and within different contexts. We also talked about occupations and rituals from the students' own communities. These days of learning and sharing were demanding and fulfilling.

From past experiences, I had developed a strong belief in the importance of students feeling and acting as active partners in the whole educational process, committing themselves to the mission of bringing occupational therapy to their country. As mentioned earlier, half of the 36 students had many years of experience working as assistants within the national health system, and they were a vital resource in our discussions about how occupational therapy could contribute to meeting the health and social care needs of the country. The more they discovered about the profession, the more the students became enthusiastic and proud of being the pioneers of occupational therapy in Mozambique.

Evaluation

One of the assignments we gave the students was to visit, in small groups, a social or health care service and collect data (brief history, staffing, clients) to identify the potential need for occupational therapy. This was the kind of assignment that I had already used when lecturing on the first occupational therapy programs in other countries, and it had always worked well. The idea was that it would promote the profession more widely and give students an opportunity to see what kind of representation of occupational therapy they were formulating. Through feedback from staff of the institutions they visited, the students felt satisfied that the assignment was useful, and it gave them the confidence to keep investing in their future profession. They realized in an immediate way that there was a lot of potential for their new profession to take action in the future and that was a big source of motivation for them.

We also challenged the students to organize a party for the end of these 2 weeks, during which they would present a drama about occupational therapy history and paradigms to which all the board members and teachers of the institution were invited. The students organized everything: the food, the drama, and the invitations. This gave us another opportunity to learn about the local culture, and we found that even the students were surprised to discover that there were differences in daily occupations according to tribes and regions. The party was a good collective occupation that helped to create a stronger bond between us. From the drama, we saw how the students viewed the relationship between health professionals and clients; the person who played the health professional role showed by his posture and verbal communication that he put himself in a higher position than the client, and the student playing the client assumed a humble posture and passive role.

In the drama, it became clear how important traditional healers are in collective social representations of disease and cure. On the one hand, we could see how health professionals did not value the role of the traditional healer or even joked about it; on the other hand, we could see that, for clients, the advice of traditional healers was of central importance when making decisions about their health. Some of them said that they only came to the doctor when the traditional healer told them to. Even to me, who was not familiar with this reality and had never seen a traditional healer, it was clear that these healers held a position of power in the health care system. Students told us after the party that it is common for everyone to visit a traditional healer, either to consult on health problems or to ask for advice when making any important decision.

That party was the culmination of our visit and, by the end of our stay, we could see that the students were feeling proud of their future profession and committed to promoting occupational therapy in Mozambique. Their assignments showed that they already had a reasonable idea of what occupational therapy was about, and because of their years of experience as health assistants, they could see the potential of their future profession in their country.

DECIDING TO CONTINUE WITH THE PROJECT

During the visit to Mozambique, we carried out a situational analysis to support our decision about whether we, as an institution, were going to remain involved in the project and, if so, the conditions for our continued involvement. During the visit, we had to create the time and opportunities to collect and analyze all the information that should have been collected before the program started. This process involved collaboration between the team from my institution and the team from ISCISA, mainly the adviser of the director and the director and coordinator of the occupational therapy program. During the mornings, we had intensive meetings with ISCISA directors or visited institutions delivering health and social care in Mozambique, including hospitals, health centers, community centers, and nongovernmental organizations. In addition to looking at the buildings and the client population, we had opportunities to interview some of the staff.

The results of the situational assessment made it clear that there were a lot of positive reasons for us to engage in this project, including the policy context, the level of government support, and the commitment of our stakeholders.

Using community development theory to structure our thinking, we collected data about the legal and political environments and policies of the country and how they might influence the development of the program. We found that the legal and political contexts were favorable for Mozambican people wanting to undertake formal education, and many people were upgrading their studies. For example, 20 of our students were MISAU employees who had been given the opportunity to gain a professional qualification, in the context of a national call for candidates for higher education.

Through my involvement in organizations that represent occupational therapy at the European (ENOTHE and the Council of Occupational Therapists for the European Countries [COTEC]) and world levels (World Federation of Occupational Therapists [WFOT]), I was aware that there had been unsuccessful attempts to set up occupational therapy programs in some countries. We therefore wanted to find out whether there had been any previous attempts to set up an occupational therapy program in Mozambique and the reasons for their failure so that we could learn from them. However, we found that this was the first attempt to set up an occupational therapy program in the country.

Identifying Stakeholders

One important task was to identify clearly who the stakeholders in this project were, how they were thinking, and how they would work together. The main stakeholders were the ISCISA, the MISAU, and my institution, the Escola Superior de Saúde do Alcoitão (ESSA).

ISCISA is a public educational institute that was founded in 2004. When the occupational therapy program was first proposed, the institute was offering 11 allied health professions programs, including nursing, radiography, psychology, and technical surgical assistants. One of the board advisers was a visionary person who knew well the reality of the country, its history over more than 50 years, and the situation of the other countries bordering Mozambique.

MISAU, which was the main employer in the area of health care, wanted to place occupational therapists in all the main health care institutions in the country to promote the social inclusion of people with mental health problems, mostly associated with AIDS/HIV.

ESSA, which was the first institution to offer an occupational therapy program in Portugal, in 1957, had a long experience with offering occupational therapy programs. Our program was developed with the support of occupational therapy teachers from the United Kingdom and United States and has been recognized by the WFOT since 1964. The primary institution to which ESSA belongs is a 500-year-old social welfare institution that is responsible for the main social projects for deprived persons and groups in the region of Lisbon.

From the beginning, the strength and support of these stakeholders gave us confidence. Some of our partners were people at a high level in the political scene with good connections, including the director and the board adviser of ISCISA, who were both former health ministers. From MISAU, we had the involvement of the director of the National Mental Health Department, who facilitated the bureaucratic process and gave us an accurate picture of the health situation in the country. Although there was not much official information available about health needs or about the nongovernmental organizations operating in the country, our stakeholders had a privileged knowledge of the country's situation. It seemed to us that we had three strong and motivated partner organizations for our project; we just had to work out how they could work together.

Avoiding Power Struggles

From the first moment, we could see that ownership of the program was an issue. The Mozambican partners wanted us to own the project and to take responsibility for it because, as they said, they did not have any experience or knowledge of occupational therapy. However, for us it was clear that the ownership of the program should belong to Mozambique, with us being an important partner and providing the occupational therapy resources, including teaching and some materials and equipment. Our institution would also provide a person in Portugal to coordinate the project, including curriculum review.

It was agreed that ISCISA would own and be responsible for the program, as it had already enrolled 36 students. They would run the entire program and find teachers for the non–occupational-therapy-specific subjects, and ESSA would make it possible for its lecturers to come to Mozambique and teach the occupational therapy modules. A coordinator and a director for the occupational therapy program were already in place, so management of the project would be shared by a teacher from ESSA (at a distance) and the coordinator and the director from ISCISA. It was also agreed that MISAU would fund the students who were its employees and guarantee that they would be employed as occupational therapists when they finished their training. The responsibility of finding fieldwork places for the students was also taken on by MISAU.

For the Portuguese teaching staff, it was clear from the beginning that the program should meet the *WFOT Revised Minimum Standards for the Education of Occupational Therapists* (Hocking & Ness, 2002) and incorporate the ENOTHE/COTEC tuning competences (TUNING, 2009). We were familiar with these standards and thought that following them would ensure the institution provided a good occupational therapy program. In the beginning, our partners at ISCISA did not accept this because they were afraid that if the degree was recognized globally, the occupational therapists would leave the country to work abroad once they graduated, and Mozambique needed them very much. However, we explained to them the importance of WFOT recognition for the program for graduates to be accepted into postgraduate courses abroad, for their mobility in the future, and, of course, for the quality of their program. Eventually, we were able to come to an agreement. The trust that had been developed between the ISCISA staff and the ESSA staff during our visit made the process of decision making and planning quite easy.

By the end of the visit, and based on our situational analysis and the meetings we had together, the occupational therapy staff and directors of the Portuguese and the Mozambican schools made the decision that we were going to continue this project together. We were sure that all the population of Mozambique would benefit from having access to occupational therapy approaches, but three main areas for intervention were defined: HIV/AIDS, malaria sequelae for children and adults, and mental health problems. One of the reasons for choosing these areas was that many nongovernmental organizations and public institutions were already operating in them and could offer practice placements to students.

Reflecting on the process of making this big decision to go forward with the project, I can say for sure that the personal relationships developed between the lecturers and director from my institution and the board members from ISCISA were the most important influence. Also, my director had been in Mozambique during his military service and had positive memories from that time. Coming back after all these years was, for him, a key factor in his coming to a positive decision.

For me, even before going to Mozambique, I felt deeply involved in this project and wanted it to be successful. After meeting the students and hearing their histories, I realized that if the project failed, they would have lost a whole semester and have been far away from their families; this made me feel even more responsible. By the end of our visit, we could see how committed the students were to being the pioneers of a new profession in their country. Another tie binding me to the project was the huge bond I developed with the assessor from ISCISA. He was a visionary, born in Mozambique, who had graduated as a surgical doctor in Portugal more than 50 years earlier and was known worldwide. He had been and still was involved in the historical development of the health care scenario in Mozambique. I felt inspired by this person at our first meeting, and that made me feel that this was my life project. We felt that we were partners, both in the project and in the romantic vision of life we shared; a warm empathy developed between us.

The biggest impact on our decision came from the strong, positive emotions aroused in us by the people we met, the challenge we were facing, and the feeling that what we were doing was important. Of course, our positive feelings were reinforced by the positive data from the situational analysis, but I suspect that even if it seemed the project had a small chance of success, we would have decided to go ahead anyway: We were totally involved emotionally.

During that first stay in Mozambique, my mother's health was an additional challenge for me, because every evening when I called her I was anxious about what I would hear. Fortunately, everything went well, and my mother's health was stable throughout my time away. I came back to Portugal feeling enriched and grateful for all that I had experienced.

DEVELOPING THE PROGRAM

Three main issues had a big impact on the development on this project: the absence of any occupational therapist in Mozambique, the fieldwork component of the course, and the sustainability of the program.

Knowing that neither I as a coordinator of the project nor any of the lecturers from ESSA would be able to come back to Mozambique very often, we had to think about preparing a local person to become the bridge between the students and us. It was agreed that two occupational therapy lecturers would travel to Mozambique once or twice in each semester for 2 weeks, but this would not be enough to give some continuity to the lecturing. At first, we thought that the contact could be made by email, but after being there, we realized that this would not be possible. The board of the institution decided that the course coordinator, a psychologist, would be our link person, and she attended some of our classes. By the end of the first visit, we could see that this arrangement would not work because she was too busy to carry out the role. When we left Mozambique after the first visit, we were worried about the lack of a local contact, and that effectively continued to be a major issue in between our visits.

On our return to Portugal, we realized that the situation would be the same as before the visit, with contacts and communications between us continuing to be a problem, and no one answering our emails. But this time we knew that the students were there, and we needed to keep their motivation high. We tried to do this by email, but only one or two of them used email regularly. This was an ongoing, major problem that led to a lot of reflection and discussion.

When the board members of ISCISA visited our institution at the end of the year, we discussed the problem with them, and it was decided that there needed to be at least two occupational therapists permanently based in Maputo to give continuity to the lectures. Those professionals would be recruited from among Portuguese occupational therapists, but they would be employed by ISCISA, which committed to paying their salaries and providing lodging.

Finding Occupational Therapy Lecturers

We recruited two young graduates who each had 3 years of professional experience, one in mental health and the other in pediatrics, these being two of the main areas identified for our interventions in Mozambique. Our recruits did not have expertise in HIV/AIDS because not many Portuguese occupational therapists had experience with the disease at that time, but MISAU agreed to organize training for them once they arrived in Mozambique. Our main reasons for selecting these two therapists were the motivation and commitment they had shown as students, the fact that one of them was doing a postgraduate course in African studies, and that they were good friends and gave each other a lot of support. We thought that they would face many challenges in Mozambique, such as the different pace of life, the differences in cultural approaches to problem solving, the safety issues in the country due to the high crime rate, and their lack of teaching experience.

Arrangements were made for the two therapists to go to Mozambique, and we decided that they would travel 1 month before our next visit. That would give them time to identify what we needed to bring with us, and we would be able to help them solve any problems that had arisen in preparing their home. We were aware that there is a great deal of bureaucracy involved in getting a residence visa and permission to work in Mozambique. Requests for information from the Mozambican authorities kept changing, and we learned, as mentioned earlier, always to have a Plan B and C to cope with unexpected problems. In fact, things were quite difficult from the beginning, and those occupational therapists quit the project after 2 years due to burnout. The two main barriers that led them to quit the project were the hard task of trying to set up occupational therapy services that would provide fieldwork placements for students and also the cultural differences in planning and problem solving. This was a critical moment for the project because it would not be possible to run the program without any occupational therapists permanently based in ISCISA, and the project represented a large workload and significant financial cost for both institutions. ISCISA and MISAU had to cope with the many challenges of starting up a new profession in the country, and the financial costs were high due to paying for lodging for the two Portuguese therapists, which is one of the most costly expenses in Maputo. For ESSA, lecturers' travel costs were high, and, for the lecturers, the workload associated with assisting in the preparation of audiovisual materials and evaluation materials, with marking, on top of all of their normal work in ESSA, was demanding. Fortunately, the situation was resolved, and the project carried on. The first two occupational therapists were replaced by four new ones, who were more mature and had greater clinical expertise, and ISCISA made a commitment to be more involved in the course implementation, facilitating the work of those occupational therapists.

Looking back, I can say that this crisis led to positive change in the project, doubling the number of occupational therapists permanently based in Maputo and bringing different expertise. Reflecting on the factors that facilitated the resolution of the situation, I can say that the main one was the good personal relationships and bonds between the persons directly involved in the project at both institutions. My director instructed me that if things became difficult, we should end the project, but I could not bear to think of the students having to change to a different course after spending 2 years of their lives in the occupational therapy program. I thought of the persons in need of the occupational therapy services, and I could not bear to think of losing contact with all those wonderful people I had been working with in a country where I felt at home.

The same idea of ending the course was in the minds of the directors of ISCISA because of the burden it represented. Fortunately, the person in charge of funding and of the strategic development of the institution made the assumption that the project had to go on and that everything should be done to resolve the situation. Later, that person admitted that it was the bond we had developed and the fact that we were bringing a lot of positive feelings and joy to the institution, along with a new vision for health care, that motivated him to find more funding, new solutions, and the energy to keep the project going on.

Other crises occurred in the development of the project, but my attitude had changed; rather than resisting change, I trusted that problems would always be resolved and that something good would come of the process. In the hardest moments, what sustained us in working toward our vision was that we really liked to work together and felt that together we were strong and could solve any situation. We shared a common vision of the project and were determined to bring it to a successful completion.

The Fieldwork Component

The fieldwork component of the course was one of the major issues on this project. After curriculum revision, the design of the course included a fieldwork placement in the first year, but it was not easy to meet this requirement. First, there were no occupational therapists in Maputo, and when they finally arrived at the end of the first year, it was many months before they were ready to offer student placements. It took time for them to gain professional accreditation in Mozambique and to be able to work as occupational therapists. Then it was a slow process to integrate an occupational therapy approach into existing health and social care services. Only by the end of the second year were we able to offer the first fieldwork placement. Because of this delay, we had to prolong the course for an extra semester (nine in total).

We used the same model of fieldwork practice as in our institution in Portugal but with less variety of experience and less clinical supervisors. The four occupational therapists in Mozambique were responsible for setting up six student places. All of them met once a week to discuss and attempt to harmonize the tasks and level of demands of placements, as well the resources they were making available for students. The students were involved in the creation of the occupational services from the beginning, so they also gained competences to replicate that process in their own institutions once they finished the course. Each student undertook a placement with four populations during three semesters: children and adolescents, adults in the context of a physical rehabilitation department, adults in the context of a mental health service, and adults in the community.

At the end of their fieldwork placements, every student took a practical examination with a jury of three lecturers. They each had to write a report with a case study, present a practical session with the client, and finally discuss with the jury their approach to the case. I was present at all the examinations, and it was one of the most rewarding moments in the project: finally seeing the Mozambican students working in such different contexts and with such diverse populations. I still recall a session carried out with a child with cerebral malaria sequelae; the occupational therapy student was sitting on the floor, his body offering good positioning and warmth to the child who was playing with some toys, despite his spasticity and lack of coordination. And the child was smiling and trying his best. This was happening in a big room; in the corner was another child crying with pain because of the mobilization of his spastic legs and arms by a rehabilitation technician, who obviously was doing his best, according to what he had learned some years ago. In that moment, I felt that every difficulty, every crisis, every hard day in the project was worth it; it was such a joy seeing those occupational therapy students offering a human, effective, and creative approach to those children and adults in the context of the Mozambican health and social care systems.

There have been many rewarding moments like those during the project, and I would like to highlight three more. The first happened in the fourth year of the program when, as a final assignment, students had to do a piece of research. I had a wonderful surprise while reading one of those assignments.

To contextualize it, during our second visit to Mozambique, in the third semester of the course, we were at the main psychiatric hospital in the province of Maputo. We had been told that a program for homeless people was in action, and during that morning we would see the arrival of some homeless people who had been collected from the streets. Later on, we saw a van stopping and some men being forced to come out and enter the hospital. Once inside, the staff took one of them and started cutting off his long hair, until he had no hair at all. While the barber was doing this, the man's eyes stared at nothing. After this, they took him to another room and we have been told that they took off his clothes, washed and cleaned him, and gave him hospital clothes. Any belongings that he had were taken from him. The same was done to every man who had been in that van. We were told that the aim of this program was to take all the homeless people with mental health problems off the streets. For that purpose, a team, composed of a psychiatrist or a psychologist, a social worker, a nurse, and one or two guards, was going out into the streets very early in the morning, trying to convince people through words or physical means to get into the van that would bring them to the hospital. The plan was to integrate them back into their families later, but, for the moment, no action was being taken in that direction. I was shocked and embarrassed to see a human being treated like that and saddened that I was unable to do anything to change the situation. For many days, the image of what happened stayed in my mind, making me feel ashamed.

Jumping forward to the fourth year, reading one student's thesis could not have made me happier. The student used a case study to demonstrate the success of a social inclusion intervention with one of the homeless men who had been taken from the streets to the psychiatric hospital. With the team, the student helped to involve the man's family in the process so that he was successfully reintegrated; he regained his dignity and began projects to improve his life. While reading this account, I thought of the incident I had witnessed some years before and felt with joy that the new occupational therapists will really make a great contribution to the reality of health and social care in Mozambique.

Another great moment for the students and for everyone involved in the development of occupational therapy in Mozambique was their first celebration of World Occupational Therapy Day. The students and the occupational therapists permanently based in ISCISA involved many stakeholders in a big event to promote occupational therapy. Leaflets about the profession were distributed, and 150 people were invited to the event, including teachers, doctors, psychologists, nurses, students from ISCISA and other universities, clients, and the producer of a movie to fight discrimination about the struggle of four young persons with disabilities in their daily lives in Mozambique. The event appeared on television, and representatives from the Ministry of Health and from ISCISA were interviewed. Workshops were held with clients, their families, and the students to inform them about people with special needs. Students were actively involved in the whole event, and it resulted in greater cohesion among the students and a huge boost to their enthusiasm for their future profession. Feedback from all the participants was positive, and the occupational therapy course gained positive status among the other ISCISA students.

The third great moment I would like to share was the students' graduation on June 17, 2011. Of the 36 students who enrolled in the occupational therapy program in 2007, 28 earned bachelor's degrees with honors. Twenty-five of these students were from Mozambique and three from Equatorial Guinea. It was a happy moment to see their joy and the way their families invested in the party (some of them had traveled for days to be there), and there was a feeling of accomplishment.

Sustainability

The sustainability of the project was an important issue throughout the process. Two main goals were taken into consideration: The new graduates would be employed as occupational therapists in their previous institutions or in new ones, and there would be another intake of students for the occupational therapy program.

The first goal was negotiated with the Ministry of Health on our first visit and was accomplished within 6 months after the graduation of the first occupational therapists. All the new graduates were integrated into various health care services, spread across the provinces of Mozambique, and an occupational therapy job description was produced to create a career pathway in health care services under the Ministry of Health. The students acted as the pioneers of a new profession, which was important for the development of their competences for starting their own services once they graduated. They were involved in all the steps toward creating new occupational therapy services and in promoting occupational therapy nationally. Some of them returned to their previous institutions, and others went to different ones. One year after they started working as occupational therapists, I visited half of them at their workplaces and found that, in all the provinces visited, the representatives of the Ministry of Health and the Ministry of Social Care reported an urgent need for at least one occupational therapist per district (128), and the teams where occupational therapists were integrated expressed satisfaction with the new competences they brought.

Since we first negotiated that the project should be owned by ISCISA, with ESSA and the Portuguese lecturers as resources, it had also been agreed that the four best students would have the opportunity to do a placement in Portugal. This would be in our school and in clinical settings to prepare them to become the lecturers for a new intake of students. In their placement in Portugal, they developed their academic competences by assisting, planning, and giving lectures in occupational therapy–specific subjects, and each of them also did a clinical placement to develop their clinical competences.

A new intake of students was recruited, and the occupational therapy program began in February 2015. The coordinator of the program is one of the occupational therapists who gained a master's degree, and a group of six occupational therapists will lecture on occupational therapy-specific subjects. These young lecturers are preparing all the teaching materials with the assistance, at a distance, of senior lecturers from ESSA. For 2 weeks in each semester, a senior lecturer from ESSA will be present in Maputo.

It is important for the development of new programs that partnerships are formed with other occupational therapy programs in African countries, such as the Republic of South Africa. In the first course, some attempts were made to link with other universities, and lecturers from the University of Cape Town delivered a workshop on community intervention. In this new program, it is hoped that some formal partnership will be established for the development of academic and research projects.

Following their graduation, the Mozambican occupational therapists began the process of creating the Associação Moçambicana de Terapeutas Ocupacionais (Mozambican Association of Occupational Therapists), which is now a legally recognized body.

LESSONS LEARNED

When reflecting about what I have gained from this experience and trying to clarify what has been professional and what has been personal, things get confusing. Because of the great changes that I recognize in myself, I almost feel that I have lived two lives: one before and one after the period of setting up the program in Mozambique. If my personal life had been stable during the years of this project, I would say that the project changed the way I see and enjoy my life because it often obliged me to go out of my comfort zone, expanding my limits and gaining a different perspective of myself, both as a professional and as a person. However, this was also a time of grieving for my mother and for the responsibilities of my role as a daughter, particularly because my father had been dead for 4 years by that time. Another factor that I believe played an important role in all those experiences is maturity, as I turned 40 years old in the second year of the project. So I do believe that my learning and development were a product of the flow between the personal and the professional, described by Denshire (2002, p. 213) as a "personal–professional confluence." Reflecting on my experiences increased my sense of congruence: "the congruence we seek between our personal and professional identities" (Thibeault, 2000, p. 6).

Because of the impending loss of my mother, whose life expectancy was 3 months (she turned out to live for 11 months), and the suffering I encountered in Mozambique, I needed to find some significance or meaning for the pain and difficulties I had witnessed. I achieved this by exploring deeply my spirituality. I found many answers in the books and the dharma talks of the Zen Buddhist monk, poet, and peace activist Thich Nhat Hanh (1987, 1992, 2001) and in *The Tibetan Book of Living and Dying* (Sogyal Rinpoche, 2002). Using some of my professional resources, I also found great support in the books of Marie de Hennezel, a psychologist and expert in palliative care, and from a nonprofit association called Associação pela Dignidade na Vida e na Morte, which gives palliative care support. I learned that I could live my spirituality both within religion (Catholic, Buddhist, or any other that speaks about love and compassion) and outside religion, in my contact with nature and with other beings.

I can say that the greatest lesson I learned during this process was about compassion. The strong desire I had to see my mother free from suffering and the urge to take every action toward that goal came from the same motivation that made me want to train occupational therapists to reduce the suffering of children with HIV/AIDS, who were frequently abandoned by their families. It was the same will that I directed toward myself, wanting also to be free from suffering (self-compassion). To really free someone from suffering, we need to empathize with that person, to see the world through his or her eyes, and to identify and recognize what is causing the suffering, whether it is a child with HIV/AIDS in Mozambique (client), a woman dying from pancreatic cancer (mother), or an occupational therapist and daughter suffering from witnessing both situations. This compassion is not very different from the client-centered guidelines commonly used in our professional practice (Canadian Association of Occupational Therapists, 1991, 1993; World Federation of Occupational Therapists, 2002), according to which we should focus on the needs and desires of the client. However, by living through such painful situations, I came to embody this empathy, and it is no longer just a theoretical perspective that I try to understand intellectually. I feel as Thibeault (1997) did in her article about grieving her father's losses related to Parkinson disease. After having lived through such a situation, she was able to "uncover simple details that could make a world of difference for my clients" (p. 113).

During this process, I learned about the importance of being in the present and about mindfulness, the energy of being aware and awake to the present moment (Nhat Hanh, 1987, 1992, 2001). A couple of months before my mother died, the doctor told me that she could die at any moment, and that forced me to enjoy every moment with her as if it was the last one. I was able to use this experience to better understand Mozambican people and their way of being and enjoying life in a context of great vulnerability, brought about by extreme poverty or threats to safety from war and armed conflicts. This helped me to deal more effectively with the cultural differences that had a big impact on the development of the project, such as giving up any expectation of making detailed plans for the next semester in advance, because life was happening every day and changing all our plans. This new understanding allowed me to work in a way that made it possible to enjoy the process and not only the results. Having been used to working toward goals, I measured success by the outcomes—the final product—and often forgot to enjoy the present. Through this experience, I started to enjoy the process more and to value the gains that came out of this attitude.

Another lesson I learned was not to ignore my suffering and the suffering of others but, at the same time, not to forget to enjoy the wonders of life, for my own sake and for the benefit of others (de Hennezel, 2005, 2006; Nhat Hanh, 2001). This allowed me to enjoy every day with my mother and try to take the most out of it, rather than being unhappy and mourning all the time. I also believe that it allowed my mother to leave in a much more serene way, so that my close family members and I gained inner peace even when she left. The capacity of the occupational therapy staff to always try to bring joy and a positive attitude to our work, even during the greatest crisis, was and still is mentioned by our partners in ISCISA as a great contribution.

I also learned about letting go—of control and of expectations that reality should unfold the way I imagined it would. At the beginning of the project, those expectations prevented me from really seeing what was happening in the field and making the most of the conditions in the country. Many times, I had to deal with my frustration over feeling totally helpless to control the many variables interfering with our project. Slowly, I started letting go of that need for control, welcoming change and developing a strong trust in life and in the natural course of events. And it came as a relief to find that I did not need to be fighting all the time but could accept and embrace my and others' imperfections; that nothing bad came from it but, on the contrary, I could better invest my energy in the things that could be changed. In fact, the biggest crisis in the implementation of the project brought about a positive change in its development. Mozambican people have a great expression for this: *Nitaku yini*, which means "accept it if there is nothing you can do about it!"

CONCLUSION

Accepting the invitation to write a chapter about the interplay between the personal and professional in decision making has been a great challenge and a great opportunity to stop and reflect in a more structured way about thoughts and feelings that have been accompanying me in the past years, and I am grateful for that.

Having been in love with my profession for more than 25 years, I have always considered my work an opportunity for challenge, for flow, and for professional and personal growth, but where the personal had to be kept separate. In my training as an occupational therapist, and at the beginning of my career, I tried to make sense of the expectation that my professional dimension should be somehow separated from the personal one, and a lot of my energy was directed toward that goal. As I grew older, I started questioning why it should be like that, feeling that it was quite artificial trying to separate these aspects of myself. The period of my life that I reflect on in this chapter was intense in confronting me with my own vulnerability, due to the suffering and pain in my personal life and a big challenge in my professional life. This allowed me to be aware of and acknowledge the role of the personal dimension in my professional decision making.

Having experienced and reflected on it, it seems to me that using the personal dimension in my professional reasoning and decision making has helped me to grow as a person and as a professional as well. Theories about client-centered practice and about spirituality in health care, which have always held an important place in my professional practice, have gained another dimension. Empathy and compassion toward others' suffering are now experienced not only in my mind but mainly in my heart. And from my heart comes the genuine desire to free the person from suffering by looking deeply into what his or her needs really are and not at my idea of what those needs are.

Of course, it is important to be aware of the risks of incorporating the personal into the professional and not ignore them. There are moments when I stop and try to achieve a balance to prevent myself from acting solely on my emotions. The improved self-knowledge that I gain from this reflection, on what role the personal dimension plays in my professional reasoning and decision making, allows me to better recognize where I might fail to act professionally if my actions are based only on an emotional rationale.

This acknowledgment of the personal dimension and its use in professional practice has contributed to a greater feeling of congruence between my professional and personal identities and fostered a self-sense of coherence and well-being.

REFERENCES

Canadian Association of Occupational Therapists. (1991). *Guidelines for client-centred practice.* Ottawa, Canada: Author.

Canadian Association of Occupational Therapists. (1993). *Guidelines for client-centred mental health practice.* Ottawa, Canada: Author.

de Hennezel, M. (2005). *Diálogo com a morte.* Cruz Quebrada, Portugal: Casa das letras.

de Hennezel, M. (2006). *Morrer de olhos abertos.* Cruz Quebrada, Portugal: Casa das letras.

Denshire, S. (2002). Viewpoint: Reflections on the confluence of personal and professional. *Australian Occupational Therapy Journal, 49,* 212-216. Retrieved from http://ajot.aotapress.net/cgi/doi/10.5014/ajot.51.3.181

Hocking, C., & Ness, N. E. (2002). *WFOT revised minimum standards for the education of occupational therapists.* Sydney, Australia: World Federation of Occupational Therapists.

Nhat Hanh, T. (1987). *The miracle of mindfulness.* Boston, MA: Beacon Press.

Nhat Hanh, T. (1992). *Touching peace: Practicing the art of mindful living.* Berkeley, CA: Parallax Press.

Nhat Hanh, T. (2001). *Essential writings.* Maryknoll, NY: Orbis Books.

Sogyal Rinpoche. (2002). *The Tibetan book of living and dying.* New York, NY: HarperCollins.

Thibeault, R. (1997). A funeral for my father's mind: A therapist's attempt at grieving. *Canadian Journal of Occupational Therapy, 64,* 107-114.

Thibeault, R. (2000). Magnum miraculum est homo. *Canadian Journal of Occupational Therapy, 67,* 3-6.

TUNING. (2009). *Reference points for the design and delivery of degree programmes in occupational therapy.* Bilbao, Spain: Publicaciones de La Universidad de Deusto.

World Federation of Occupational Therapists. (2002). *Revised minimum standards for the education of occupational therapists.* Forrestfield, Australia: Author.

6

Political Reasoning for Disability Inclusion
Making Policies Practical

Theresa Lorenzo, BSc (Occupational Therapy) (Wits), HDipEdAd (Wits),
MSc (Community Disability Studies) (University of London),
PhD in Public Health (UCT), PgDip (Higher Education Studies) (UCT)

> *Powerful professions have the capacity to obtain leadership positions,*
> *advocate successfully in the policy arena, and*
> *secure the resources necessary to achieve their professional goals.*
>
> (Clark, 2010, p. 264)

Development practice is a relatively new field for occupational therapists, who are concerned with the community contexts and the social, economic, and political conditions in which individuals live and into which they are reintegrated after rehabilitation. The growth of occupational science has extended the profession's role in addressing the development and well-being of the broader population and not just those with impairments. Occupational therapists are able to think about the complexities of poverty reduction, the provision of equal education, and the achievement of health using their understanding related to the daily activities and roles in which individuals, families, and groups engage. This reasoning enables them to identify feasible solutions to the problems in underresourced areas, together with the people affected by them.

Development practice does require that we learn to work in interdisciplinary teams beyond the health care arena, together with public–private and nongovernmental sectors in the community. It involves local people playing an integral part in decision-making processes related to any projects that are identified and implemented in their community, so that development is more likely to be sustainable. The experience of research with women with disabilities is shared as an illustration of such engagement (Boxes 6-1 through 6-12; also see Lorenzo, 2010, for full description of workshop processes).

Rapid changes in development practice globally mean that both practitioners and academics need to acquire understanding and skills for interpreting policies that address the inequities in health, education, social development, and labor faced by persons with disabilities and their families. This need is evident as persons with disabilities still experience exclusion from the

Cole, M. B., & Creek, J. (Eds.).
Global Perspectives in Professional Reasoning (pp. 77-98).
© 2016 Taylor & Francis Group.

BOX 6-1. PARTICIPATORY ACTION RESEARCH WITH WOMEN WITH DISABILITIES FOR SOCIAL AND ECONOMIC DEVELOPMENT

Over a 3-year period, I cofacilitated a participatory action research project with a woman with disability, who was chairperson of the Disabled Women's Development Programme of Disabled People South Africa, and a young occupational therapist, both of whom spoke Xhosa. The facilitators met with women with disabilities once a month for a day's workshop. The focus of each workshop was identified through listening for generative themes (what participants felt strongly about and thought had relevance in their lives) to address issues that would facilitate women's participation in social and economic development. We worked with the Rehabilitation Project of the South African Christian Leadership Assembly Health Project, a primary health care nongovernment organization that had trained mothers of children with disabilities as community rehabilitation workers. The community rehabilitation workers invited women to a storytelling workshop in their area, and after running workshops in at least five communities, we met together with the women for narrative action reflection (NAR) workshops on a monthly basis. From their observations of what happened at the beginning and end of each NAR workshop, the research facilitators reflected back to the women the strength of their singing and dancing skills.

This story reflects the changes that Marjorie, the chairperson of the Disabled Women's Development Programme of Disabled People South Africa, experienced as a research cofacilitator.

As a disabled woman, I was very surprised and at the same time proud of being asked to be part of this participatory action research study with disabled women in Khayelitsha and Brown's Farm. We know that we as disabled people are always being researched. We just accept things brought to us by other people. But this time it was the women ourselves who contributed to the whole process. We are the ones who showed what we wanted from the research.

---

opportunities and resources needed to achieve education and employment. The rights of marginalized and vulnerable groups are still denied, even though there are numerous United Nations (UN) charters to address human rights and the discrimination faced by vulnerable groups, such as the *UN Convention on the Elimination of All Forms of Discrimination against Women* (UN, 1979) and the *UN Convention on the Rights of the Child* (UN, 1989). The UN requires that states report on their progress in the implementation of those conventions that they have ratified. Although professionals in public service contribute to the state's report, nongovernmental and civil society organizations are able to submit alternate or shadow reports to the relevant UN commissions. In this way, accountability and transparency are promoted. (Examples of reporting on equal opportunities for participation are shared in Lorenzo, 2004; Lorenzo & Cloete, 2004; Watson & Lagerdien, 2004).

A policy implementation gap exists because individuals and communities, as well as service providers, are not equipped with policy literacy—that is, an ability to interpret different concepts in policies so as to understand how to develop operational strategies and allocate necessary resources to make policies practical. Although many excellent policies have been developed, occupational therapists need to engage in understanding and interpreting policies so as to be able to implement aspects of the policies and/or monitor the process of implementation by other stakeholders. The professional reasoning of occupational therapists related to understanding human occupation has the potential to make a significant contribution to making policies practical for individuals and communities. For example, Lorenzo (2004) showed how the *UN Standard Rules*

Box 6-2. Action Learning Group 1: Abangane Choir

We are planning that all of us, as disabled women,
become part of a choir . . .
we wish to get a person who knows drama and music to help us.
We are going to practice to be good.

(Disabled woman in choir)

Through an action space that was created, the women decided to form a choir that would enable them to combine their cultural skills with raising awareness of disability issues and advocacy to challenge stereotypes related to disability. The women and community rehabilitation workers performed at various community events and celebrations, such as weddings, birthdays, and funerals. They began to take advantage of public events where they could market their skills, as well as develop links to disability awareness and advocacy campaigns.

The challenge of building group cohesion was difficult as some choir members attended sporadically because they were involved in other activities. The group also experienced difficulties in accessing resources needed to plan attitude-changing strategies. The women reported that they lived too far from each other and did not have telephones to communicate any changes to plans. The group also struggled with costs of transport to get to practices, which happened twice a week. Thus, there was a need to find focus to ensure commitment and accountability. They decided to have a constitution to guide membership. The members recognized the need for management and organizational development skills to build capacity to address the difficulties of working in a context of poverty.

---

on the *Equalization of Opportunities for Persons with Disabilities* (UN, 1993) was used as a framework for analyzing research data to identify how society and systems, including activities, services, information, and documentation, are made accessible to all.

This chapter focuses on the critical relevance of the professional reasoning of occupational therapists to enable the implementation of international policies and guidelines, as well as related national policies, to foster disability-inclusive programs, be it clinical practice in hospitals, development work in communities, corporate and business sector, or teaching, learning, and research in higher education. Expanding the boundaries of possibilities through policy implementation means addressing social inequalities to change the lives of individuals, families, and communities to become inclusive of persons with disabilities (as illustrated in Box 6-2).

In the next section, three key international policy frameworks are explored in terms of their relevance to disability-inclusive services and programs provided by occupational therapists. Service providers across different sectors require understanding and skills in disability inclusion to make policies operational at all levels of government, especially at the local, municipal level. The chapter also presents stories and vignettes of how occupational therapists develop professional reasoning to identify factors influencing policy implementation that ensures the participation of persons with disabilities.

Policies for Promoting Disability Inclusion

This section introduces three international policy and development frameworks that are intended to promote the social inclusion of persons with disabilities. The *UN Convention on the Rights of Persons with Disabilities* (UN, 2006), and the *Community-Based Rehabilitation (CBR)*

Guidelines (World Health Organization [WHO], 2010) provide relevant frameworks to ensure that the *Millennium Development Goals* (MDGs; UN, 2000) address the needs of people with disabilities across the lifespan.

Building on the *UN World Programme of Action Concerning Disabled Persons* in 1982 and the *UN Standard Rules on the Equalization of Opportunities for Persons with Disabilities* in 1993, the *UN Convention on the Rights of Persons with Disabilities* (CRPD) is an international human rights treaty intended to protect the rights and dignity of persons with disabilities (UN, 2006). The convention advocates for people to be seen as equal citizens with the same rights to opportunities for sustainable development as nondisabled persons. It adopts a social model of disability and defines disability as including:

> those who have long-term physical, mental, intellectual or sensory impairments which in interaction with various barriers may hinder their full and effective participation in society on an equal basis with others. (UN, 2006)

The first of 50 articles in the CRPD states that the purpose of the Convention is as follows:

> to promote, protect and ensure the full and equal enjoyment of all human rights and fundamental freedoms by all persons with disabilities, and to promote respect for their inherent dignity. (UN, 2006)

The principles underpinning both the CRPD and the *CBR Guidelines* (WHO, 2010) are protecting the dignity of the person, participation, respect, nondiscrimination, gender equality, and inclusion. Equal opportunities policies focus on ensuring that all services, activities, information, and documentation are available to all in society on an equal basis (UN, 1993). Universal design should be used when considering reasonable accommodation and accessibility of transport, information, and communication technology. Physical buildings and environment are seen as key strategies for ensuring the participation of persons with disabilities in everyday activities, with access to services and systems on an equal basis with others.

The MDGs were developed by the UN to focus attention and mobilize resources to address the major gaps in human development and poverty reduction. There are eight MDGs, each of which speaks to the right for equal opportunities for participation by persons with disabilities. Table 6-1 explains each MDG and suggests ways in which occupational therapists can contribute to its achievement. The WHO has also documented how CBR is a strategy to ensure the MDGs are disability inclusive (see www.who.int/disabilities/cbr).

The MDGs emphasize three areas in which improvements can be made to human capabilities and living standards:

1. Human capital related to education for children, nutrition, and access to health care for families

2. Infrastructure development, focusing on water and sanitation, energy and information and communication technology, food security, and transportation

3. Social, economic, and political rights, with a particular focus on empowering women, reducing violence, increasing political voice, ensuring equal access to public services, and increasing the security of property rights

The MDGs speak to many areas of occupation-based practice, yet these goals have not been monitored for the inclusion of persons with disabilities. A major inequity experienced by children and youth with disabilities, and those at risk, is high dropout rate from school (Lorenzo, Ned-Matiwane, Cois, & Nwanze, 2013). Occupational therapists have knowledge related to the principles and skills of universal design to ensure the accessibility of services, activities, information, and documentation for persons with different physical, sensory, and/or cognitive or psychosocial impairments. Occupational perspectives of health in relation to health-related MDGs have as yet not been sufficiently explored or articulated in the literature.

TABLE 6-1 **MAKING THE MILLENNIUM DEVELOPMENT GOALS** **RELEVANT TO OCCUPATIONAL THERAPISTS**	
MDG 1: Eradicate Extreme Poverty and Hunger	This goal seeks to make the right to development a reality for everyone and to free the majority of the world's population from want. Low human development is associated with poor health and limited education, both of which lead to the loss of power to choose what is best to improve well-being.

Occupational therapy's focus on work preparation and entrepreneurship development will lift many families out of poverty:

- Demonstrate the multidimensional concept of sustainable development
- Support the identification of people-centered initiatives to develop a range of skills that can lift them out of extreme poverty and promote participation in livelihood activities
- Describe practice that preserves the health and well-being of families and their communities
- Demonstrate innovative strategies for increasing sources of livelihood

MDG 2: Achieve Universal Primary Education	In sub-Saharan Africa, there are unacceptably high numbers of children who do not have the opportunity to start school or who drop out of school at some point. Occupational therapists can play a role in enabling all children, including children with disabilities and those considered at risk, to start and progress through school.

Occupational therapists work closely with children in early childhood development and school readiness. The health-promoting schools approach is a useful framework for occupational therapists to contribute to the goal of achieving universal primary school education. The occupational therapy role in school settings in one or more of the six action areas includes:

- Provide occupational therapy support to children's educational progress
- Develop healthy public policies (e.g., HIV/AIDS policy)
- Create supportive environments (e.g., teacher support and well-being programs)
- Develop personal skills (e.g., life skills for teenagers)
- Strengthen community action (e.g., involving community organizations in schools)
- Reorient school programs and related services (e.g., after-school leisure programs)

(continued)

TABLE 6-1 (CONTINUED)
MAKING THE MILLENNIUM DEVELOPMENT GOALS RELEVANT TO OCCUPATIONAL THERAPISTS

MDG 3: Promote Gender Equality and Empower Women	The focus is on eliminating gender disparities in primary and secondary education for girls as well as ensuring retention through to tertiary education. There is also a need to ensure the share of women in paid employment in the nonagricultural sector. The goal also calls for an increased proportion of seats in national government to be held by women.

Occupational therapy in Africa (and elsewhere) is increasingly embracing the need for a social vision of a more just society to address experiences of marginalization, deprivation, and isolation in different contexts. Occupational therapy scholars and practitioners are called on to be more politically conscious as human rights advocates in advancing social justice. Actions that call for social change relate to the following:

- Commit to eradicating disparities based on gender

- Empowerment of girls and women

- Safeguard the rights of girls and women

- Highlight the impact that women's economic advancement can have on the development of communities and society at large

MDG 4: Reduce Child Mortality MDG 5: Improve Maternal Health	These two goals are closely related to the health and reduction of deaths of children and their mothers. There is an important link between immunization and disability prevention. Environments that promote early development of children and their well-being are influenced by the degree of social participation. Children at risk of impairments because of birth trauma, premature birth, infectious diseases, and nervous system and sensory order impairments are also vulnerable. Improve maternal health by ensuring that professionals are skilled to manage pregnant women and to achieve access to reproductive health and family planning, especially for young women.

(continued)

TABLE 6-1 (CONTINUED)
MAKING THE MILLENNIUM DEVELOPMENT GOALS RELEVANT TO OCCUPATIONAL THERAPISTS

- Provide targeted occupation-based programs and partnerships between government and nongovernmental organizations to reduce child trauma and violence on children in families and households
- Create access to nutritional programs and food security
- Devise community-based rehabilitation and other community development strategies to improve access to health and social services, early intervention, livelihood opportunities, etc.
- Promote the well-being and reproductive rights of women
- Devise strategies to improve access to health care for pregnant women and children in different contexts

MDG 6: Combat HIV/AIDS, Malaria, and Other Diseases	Sub-Saharan Africa carries the heaviest burden of disease related to HIV, tuberculosis, and malaria.

Occupational therapy practitioners from different regions in Africa have developed innovative programs and strategies aimed at helping those infected or affected by HIV, tuberculosis, malaria, and other diseases to fulfill their occupational aspirations. Occupation-based interventions include the following:

- Focus on disability prevention and the promotion of well-being, enabling many individuals to resume their responsibilities and roles in everyday life and bringing satisfaction, following stroke, blindness, and amputations, often caused by hypertension and diabetes
- Make links among marginalization, occupational risk, and illness
- Seek networking opportunities to raise awareness about occupational perspectives and their contribution to lessening the burden of disease for individuals, groups, or populations
- Deliver programs to support caregivers
- Provide palliative care
- Provide early intervention, especially related to children with cerebral palsy, developmental delay, etc.

MDG 7: Ensure Environmental Sustainability	Ensure environmental sustainability by addressing sustainable development and management of resources (e.g., land, fish stock, water resources, and access to safe water and sanitation), with specific attention to urban settlements

(continued)

TABLE 6-1 (CONTINUED)	
MAKING THE MILLENNIUM DEVELOPMENT GOALS RELEVANT TO OCCUPATIONAL THERAPISTS	

Occupational therapy has an important role to play in promoting the integration of principles of sustainable development into policies and programs. The profession can ensure that such integration reduces the loss of environmental resources. We hold the potential to contribute because the occupations that people engage in are pivotal to the mitigation of climate change and food security. It is known that individuals, communities, and organizations have to adapt their occupations in anticipation of, or in response to, changing biodiversity (i.e., the variation of life forms within a given ecosystem or on the entire earth).

- Initiate or support efforts to bring drinking water and promote sanitation to underserviced communities
- Enable subsistence farming and agricultural work, including fishing
- Provide energy-saving devices for daily living
- Adapt environments

MDG 8: Develop a Global Partnership for Development	Partnership implies inclusion, which means everyone. International cooperation (partnerships) and development programs should be inclusive of and accessible to all marginalized groups. To achieve sustainable development, the active cooperation and participation of all members of the community is needed.

National and international organizations in the world community, disabled people's organizations (DPOs), and also occupational therapy associations and networks have an important role to play in promoting inclusive development. Occupational Therapy Africa Regional Group (OTARG), World Federation of Occupational Therapists (WFOT), Africa Network for Evidence into Action on Disability (AfriNEAD), and CBR Africa Network (CAN) are also of importance for the development of occupational therapy, especially in Africa where most occupational therapists work in isolation and in under-resourced settings, still having to convince others of the need for and importance of the profession.

- Look at how international networks (including African [inter]national networks) and funding organizations have supported specific projects/activities
- Focus on the development of occupational therapy and community services
- Create support systems for the development of occupational therapy (local, national, and international)
- Mainstream diversity issues in national policies
- Highlight good examples of the role of civil society and disabled people's organizations/parent organizations in the promotion of inclusive development

Reprinted with permission from the Scientific Committee, Occupational Therapy Africa Regional Group Congress, 2011.

Because these goals were expected to be achieved by 2015, discussion and debate have already begun on post-2015 sustainable development goals. Bates-Eamer and colleagues (2012) believe that there will be a recommitment to the unfinished MDG business with more ambitious targets, including minimum standards, with respect to poverty, education, health, and gender. This pursuit is likely to focus on inequality, improving food security, safe water and sanitation, the informal economy, and the transition to a green economy. The authors suggest that the post-2015 agenda is likely to include the dimensions of peace and security, civil and political rights, disaster resilience, connectivity, and governance. The aspirations of youth will be given particular focus, an aspect I return to later in the chapter. Many of these goals are relevant for persons with disabilities across the life span and achievable through inclusive policy and program development. The *CBR Guidelines* (WHO, 2010) provide the strategy for such inclusion.

The *CBR Guidelines*, produced by the WHO, UNESCO, International Labour Organization, and International Disability and Development Consortium in 2010, make an explicit link to the UN CRPD and the MDGs. CBR is a strategy within community development for the equalization of opportunities for persons with disabilities and their families by ensuring that all services and systems in the four components of Health, Education, Social, and Livelihood are accessible to all. The fifth component, empowerment of people with disabilities' organizations and the families of persons with disabilities through advocacy and communication, mobilization, and self-help groups, is the foundation of the CBR approach. The guidelines renew the call for a workforce that works intersectorally to achieve the aspirations of the CRPD and MDGs in ensuring the rights and inclusion of persons with disabilities in play, schooling, work, and all aspects of social and political life.

This section has provided a brief account of international policies that guide disability inclusion in human and environmental development. The next section discusses the professional reasoning of occupational therapists that will facilitate disability inclusion as it challenges the thinking and beliefs about impairments that exclude persons from assuming their rightful roles and responsibilities.

PROFESSIONAL REASONING FOR DISABILITY INCLUSION

So what do these international policies have to do with the professional reasoning of occupational therapists? The intentions behind policies have no significance if practitioners are not able to implement them. In an attempt to understand professional reasoning for disability inclusion, this section first demonstrates the link between equal opportunities and policy implementation that achieves the social inclusion of, and occupational justice for, persons with disabilities. Second, continuity of care is possible if we bridge the gap between hospital and community through liaising with individuals, families, and service providers across different sectors to manage transitions at different life stages, including schooling, work, and family life. Third, the relevance of universal design and environmental factors in enabling participation is described, particularly the need for accessible information and documentation for persons with sensory impairments—that is visual, hearing, and speech impairments. Last, the need to develop occupational outcome measures and indicators is an essential component for monitoring disability inclusion.

Link Between Equal Opportunities and Policy Implementation

The definition adopted by the CRPD, presented in the previous section, represents a strong call to see disability as more than a medical issue related to the impairments a person may have congenitally or have acquired. If we believe that all human beings are occupational beings and have the right to participate in all opportunities for their development, then it means that we need to ensure that disability is understood as an issue of equal rights and opportunities for participation. Social justice is evident through seeing persons with disabilities as citizens who make a contribution to the social, economic, and political development of their countries (Lorenzo, 2004; Lorenzo et al., 2013).

Occupational therapists have to shift from using clinical reasoning to employing professional reasoning that allows them to use occupational science in interpreting policies to promote social inclusion through action for change. Occupational science enables clinicians to explore and understand the underlying and diverse forces that shape human occupation. This understanding assists in making policies practical in everyday life because occupational therapists are able to identify the activities and roles of individuals, families, groups, and communities that enable them to translate policy into action. The benefits of occupational engagement by people in their everyday lives, related to social activities and relationships, productivity, learning, and self-care, can be monitored as they promote health, well-being, and quality of life across the life span.

Clinical reasoning is used to address aspects of performance related to functional abilities. For example, does a person have enough muscle strength, joint range, and balance after a lower limb amputation to be able to walk again? Professional reasoning encompasses our ability as occupational therapists to think about a person's potential by considering their abilities and resources and providing opportunities for them to engage in activities and events that hold meaning for them, so that a sense of belonging is nurtured. The environment and population are also considered as part of professional reasoning. Occupational therapists employ contextual analysis to identify the facilitators and barriers to participation in everyday activities. There are many possibilities for occupational therapists to work collaboratively in training community-based workers to assist the person and their family to access the services and resources they need (Chappell & Lorenzo, 2012; Lorenzo, Motau, & Chappell, 2012).

Our profession believes that human potential is fulfilled if a person is able to participate in everyday activities. We have the professional knowledge, skills, and values to support individuals and their families with managing life transitions, especially as a consequence of impairment due to a health condition and/or disability due to attitudinal and environmental barriers. The narrative action reflection (NAR) workshops with women with disabilities over a 2-year period illustrate how collective support can lead to transitions from ill health to healing and overall well-being (see Box 6-3; Lorenzo, 2005, 2010).

In most countries, health, education, and social development policies at local and national levels do not address disability needs in an inclusive manner. The current literature on social inclusion does not provide insights and guidance on how persons with disabilities, who are more often than not on the periphery of development opportunities in their communities, may be included. The experience of marginalization due to disability leads to shame experienced at both an individual and a family level. In the same way that Black people and women have advocated for social inclusion, occupational therapists should interpret policies with an occupational lens that would foster the participation and inclusion of persons with disabilities so that they can fulfill their life roles. Collective action by women with disabilities over many months showed their ability to make changes for themselves in their communities, as illustrated in Box 6-4.

Through professional reasoning, an occupational therapist is able to identify the values and beliefs behind a person's participation in daily living or his or her exclusion and isolation. The NAR workshops revealed to the women how they were undermining themselves, enabling them to recognize their abilities again and to assume previous roles or adapt to new roles, as shared values and beliefs about disability within themselves and their families changed (see Box 6-5).

In analyzing the women's stories after each workshop and sharing with them the themes that were generated, different action spaces were created that provided opportunities for further skills development (see Boxes 6-2 through 6-6). One of the key factors in facilitating action was the social support that the women gained from the group experience.

Occupational therapists are often faced with needing to understand and appreciate the different cultural values and beliefs that a person may hold and that may contribute to internalized oppression when they acquire an impairment. For example, stories told by women with disabilities in the NAR workshops revealed how impairment is seen as a punishment or curse, so that both the

---

BOX 6-3. MANAGING TRANSITIONS

One of the women shared the changes she had experienced after participating in monthly NAR workshops over an extended period:

After the first workshop where I told my story, I felt much stronger. I realized these workshops could really help other women in the same situation as me. Our rehabilitation did not help us return and settle back with our families or communities. Here I made a clay sculpture of a plate and two women to share how I changed from gaining knowledge of disability rights and advocacy skills. The workshops helped us to find knowledge and information for each other. We felt happier. We recognized the gains we've made in changing our living conditions. These skills have led to a better life together. I made myself using clay. I want to show you that before I became disabled, my body was thin. I was small before, and you can now see how big I am. So I want to share the good news so that others can be big like me. I must be the light, even in the community and preach about disability and how they can treat disabled people. I talk about disability. I became more confident and gained skills in being able to change things. I was used to speaking in church and sharing my testimony. Now I speak about disability.

BOX 6-4. SUPPORTING WOMEN'S ADVOCACY TO CHANGE STEREOTYPES AND STIGMA RELATED TO DISABILITY

The passion and energy for advocacy and spreading the message revealed an evangelical zeal. Bulelwa grew in confidence to speak about disability to other women as well as to wider community organizations. It inspired her self-development. She mobilized the women to rethink their images of disability and challenge public stereotypes. They acted collectively to raise awareness and advocate for change in attitudes toward disability.

One woman told how her children had found support from the workshops as well, as they also felt the pressure to change the stigma of disability. Gladys said:

I'm receiving a lot of support from my family. My two children always show interest in what I'm doing. At school they used to be laughed at by other children because of my disability. But they told them that with their mother, they can't see any disability, but they see a mother who is a role model and who can afford everything unlike [nondisabled] mothers who can't afford the basics.

---

person and/or parent and other family members may isolate themselves. Marjorie, as a cofacilitator, reflected on the inner and outer changes that occurred for each person, including the facilitators, at family and community levels by telling their stories and identifying actions they could take to change the situations they were in (see Box 6-7).

Bulelwa's story, presented here, represents the changes experienced by the women through participation in NAR workshops. Their deep spiritual beliefs gave them the confidence to mobilize collective action, as illustrated in Box 6-8.

The professional reasoning of occupational therapists in making policies practical, by creating opportunities for persons with disabilities to resume their roles and responsibilities in their families and communities, has been illustrated by stories of women with disabilities. Professional reasoning to manage the transitions after becoming disabled, by raising awareness and advocating

Box 6-5. Changing Values and Beliefs About Disability

One of the women shared how much she had been helped through participating in the NAR workshops:

I experienced deep changes about how I feel. I used to cry a lot, but since I met other women, I got new ideas. I joined the Nobantu group. When Lindiwe introduced me to the group, I was happy and I became one of them. I understand more about this impairment now. When I became disabled, I always undermined myself when I was with my friends. I always sat in one place. But when I met with the other women, I became stronger, and that thing of always feeling sorry for myself is gone. My in-laws did not love me, but today my house is always full. I'm strong. Today I'm not crying. Now no one can believe that I used crutches before. No one can say I'm disabled now. I identify myself with the sun because before it was dark and I didn't want to accept my disability. I couldn't even sit in the sun. Now I can do things with my hands and I got a certificate. After that I could do things for myself. Now I'm like a mother in the house even when the children are not there. I never used to be like that. I used to wait for them to come back from school. Now I feel that I can do anything.

Box 6-6. Action Learning Group 2: T-Shirts for Advocacy and Raising Awareness

One action space involved women in designing a T-shirt with messages to their families and the community about disability that they brainstormed to challenge stereotypes and raise awareness about their abilities and desires. Using symbols of identity from the stories women had told earlier, a graphic artist with disability assisted in designing a T-shirt, which was sold during the celebrations for National Women's Day in August, a public holiday in South Africa to celebrate women's contribution to the struggle to end apartheid. The sale of the T-shirts was also an income-generating opportunity because the money went to the group. There is the potential for T-shirts and similar strategies to be used more aggressively by disability organizations.

Box 6-7. Understanding Values and Beliefs About Disability

When we started the study with storytelling workshops, there were many women who were crying, who had nobody to talk to, nobody to cry with. But when we met once a month on our days, we talked about our stories, we talked about our pains, we talked about our joys. That made me gain as a disabled person; I realized that as a disabled woman I can listen. Maybe I didn't listen too much to disabled people before, but now I listen very well because I know their joys and pain. Sometimes a woman will withdraw because she doesn't want to say something, maybe especially to new people. When I say to her: "I've been there, I know what you're talking about, so come out with it even if it's going to hurt you," then that person opens up and talks about what has happened. The women also knew where I'm from as I used to be in the same position as them—looking for work as I had a family to support. I'm on a wheelchair.

Box 6-8. Spiritual Beliefs Fostering Collective Change

Bulelwa became the disability evangelist in the study. She was a vibrant entrepreneur and very hardworking while being very concerned for the well-being and growth of the other women. It was significant that the women began to recognize changes in each other over a period of time.

I see myself as a light for other disabled people and I'm not afraid. I know I'm able to talk. I'm usually shy, but since I've been here I am free. I used to worry a lot at home, but since I've been here I'm much better. When I see my neighbors quarrelling, I say to them, "Call your family and sort this out." Later they say to me, "Really we called them and we solved it." So that is why I'm saying, I'm a lamp. I see that even with the women there is change. I'm able to see how they were before and how they are now. Ever since they have been meeting in the groups, the load was taken away and everything has been lighter.

So I was not the only one who wanted to shine a light to change attitudes to disability ourselves, amongst our families and our neighbors. The workshops also helped us see how we could heal each other. The workshops gave us courage to be visible in our families and community again. I told a story from the Bible: I identify myself with the person who was next to the dam and people were coming and going not helping him. So Jesus asked him, "Do you want to be well?" "I want to, but I don't have a person who will help me and put me in this dam." Jesus said, "Take your mat and go, and by those words you are healed." So now I'm well, but it's sad when you see others having problems.

---

for changes in the values and beliefs related to disability, facilitates inward and outward changes that lead to collective action. The deep spiritual beliefs of individuals, families, and communities must be appreciated by the occupational therapist as a precursor to enabling the person to manage the various transitions.

Promoting Well-Being and Change Through Collective Action in Different Spaces and Places

The professional reasoning of occupational therapists in policy implementation seeks to bridge the gaps that occur between the spaces and places where people live, work, and play, especially when a person transitions from hospital to home and community.

By assisting individuals and groups to engage in roles and responsibilities relevant to their age group, occupational therapists can equip families and organizations with an understanding of how health and well-being can be promoted. The research story in Box 6-9 illustrates how the participatory action research project generated understanding of well-being through participation. Marjorie herself had disabilities, and her story reflects the changes she experienced in her role as research cofacilitator, as well as the changes identified in the women.

Occupational therapists can also provide guidance where women need to challenge members of community organizations about their need to participate in community activities or, as parents, they need to engage teachers about the participation of their child with disability in completing school. Participating in the NAR workshops and sharing their stories through creative activities that posed the problem to the group helped the women with disabilities to generate symbols of their struggles and the challenges they faced. Thus, they gained access to the listening ear of others in the group, which helped them to work out their own solutions to family problems and tensions regarding the needs of their children with disabilities or other family members (see Box 6-10).

Box 6-9. Fostering Well-Being Collectively

So now we are like sisters. We are not afraid to talk to one another about our problems. We are not afraid to talk about our pain. When we come together, we come to share. We started by sharing our stories, whether they were bad, whether they were good. We cried for each other, we cried with each other. At the same time we made it possible for each person to heal from whatever they had suffered. When we first talked with the women we saw that, although we were all disabled, we were also different.

Box 6-10. Collective Sharing for Finding Solutions

Marjorie reflected on the changes she had seen happen over the period of 2 years that we ran monthly workshops with the women and community rehabilitation workers.

As a facilitator, the other women saw someone who is disabled and who at the same time was capable of sharing with them and of knowing what we should do together. We have gained a lot from each other. I gained strength from them; I gained just from sitting down with them, even if we were just talking. We found a woman who was in a different position when she first came in, in a different state. But today we are talking to someone else who is so grown. Often the woman herself doesn't even realize it, but we saw how she came in and the difference today.

Transitions that the women faced within their families were often the most challenging, as families are our primary support system. Family members may need a space where they can share their concerns and hopes for the person with disability as well as their own needs. The stress of providing care may be compounded by the caregiver having to give up paid work, which can place additional strain on family relations. This was addressed through group support during workshop dialogues, as illustrated in Box 6-11.

Occupational therapists need to design spaces that are inclusive and enable participation to overcome self-imposed isolation or marginalization by others. Given that daily life occupations occur in neighborhoods and communities, occupational therapists focus on designing and creating inclusive spaces and processes that enable participation in occupations that are meaningful and purposeful to individuals, families, and groups. These spaces provide support for people to address the barriers they encounter in fulfilling the roles and responsibilities to which they aspire (see Box 6-12).

Occupational therapy practitioners and academics benefit from working collaboratively with community-based organizations (CBOs) and nongovernmental organizations (NGOs), which are rooted in communities. These organizations provide a base from which to facilitate disability inclusion in community based programs and events. CBOs and NGOs are also able to mobilize community members to advocate for accessible health and social development services. Marjorie's story about her involvement in a participatory research project with the occupational therapy department at a university illustrates the reciprocal benefits of collaboration (Box 6-13).

The professional reasoning of occupational therapists demonstrates how we: foster collective well-being; support family transitions by sharing stories and finding solutions collectively, and create inclusive spaces by adopting universal design principles to ensure accessibility to information, documentation, activities and services on an equal basis, no matter the nature of the impairment.

Box 6-11. Managing Family Transitions Collectively

Often, Marjorie recognized the need to facilitate a dialogue among the women from one workshop to the next, which was possible using the action reflection process, because some other women still experienced strain with family members. As a group, we learned how to respond to these feelings of struggle and problems that others still experienced. One woman cried as she spoke about how her mother still expected her to meet the family's financial needs with her disability grant.

I got sick and tired of my mother because whenever I phone her, she always nags me and asks me for money. "Do you have R100 [$6 USD] that you can bring me when you come to visit me?" I don't visit her and I'm not going to visit her anymore. I made that decision and I'm sick and tired of this whole thing.

Many women spoke at once: *But it is your duty to phone her. She is your mother and she will always be your mother, so you need to talk with her.*

Then MJ told us: *We hear you, sis, and I think we must listen to her and things are going to change as time goes on.*

Box 6-12. Social Support

We found that the workshops were a good space where we felt well looked after. One woman made a clay sculpture of a tree to symbolize the potential amongst us. The tree's roots represented the women growing as different people from different areas. We've made friends as we have been together in the workshops.

Box 6-13. Working Collectively With Disabled People's Organizations

I can be proud to say the project that we started is going to come to fruition. We are still continuing and there are still many, many women that are joining because they have heard what the others are gaining. I've learnt that research is not a 1-day or 1-month event. It is a stretch. We went a long way before we got what we wanted. We are saying that if we can do this again, we will do it with others. There are so many women out there who we would like to touch. Other researchers must include the disabled people as fellow facilitators of research. Disabled people must not be "the researched." We want to tell the researchers what we expect from them. The research was something that said: "Let's go forward, there's me in a wheelchair who's already there, let's follow, maybe we will reach where she is today."

In these ways, environmental barriers to the participation of persons with disabilities are overcome and policies are made practical through the implementation of strategies to ensure access to enable participation in programs and projects, followed by continuous monitoring of change.

Universal Design and Environmental Factors in Enabling Participation

The environmental factors that influence the participation of persons with disabilities provide occupational therapists with opportunities to work across interdisciplinary networks, involving engineers, economists, architects, and town planners, to name a few, to ensure a barrier-free environment. Clinicians, researchers, and academics need to know the relevant policy and use it to lobby and advocate for resources to improve access to services, activities, information, and documentation. For example, in many places, public transport and information and communication systems remain largely inaccessible, hindering equitable opportunities for participation.

Occupational therapists have the knowledge and skills to interpret policies that will promote inclusion, as we are able to address the environmental factors influencing a person's choices related to participation in daily occupations (Lorenzo, 2004). The WHO has classified five categories of environmental factors that lead to participation restriction: products and technology, natural environment, support and relationships, attitudes, and services, systems, and policies. Table 6-2 describes the barriers faced by youth with disabilities across the different public sector services in South Africa (Cramm, Nieboer, Finkenflügel, & Lorenzo, 2013a, 2013b).

Occupational therapists are able to provide appropriate assistive devices and products to support mobility, communication, and self-care. Information and guidance on how to make buildings accessible for people with mobility restrictions and sensory impairments are also areas of knowledge and expertise of our profession (Gcaza & Lorenzo, 2008).

Barriers related to the natural environment include seasonal changes; natural events, such as fires or flooding, that may necessitate disaster management; human events, such as violence and wars; and geographic location. Occupational therapists are in a position to support the reskilling of farm workers to be able to generate an income through work in the off-season. The occupational therapy response to disaster management is a growing field of practice (Habib, Uddin, Rahman, Jahan, & Akter, 2013; see www.wfot.org/Practice/DisasterPreparednessandResponseDPR.aspx).

Factors related to adequate support and relationships are closely linked to attitudes, which encompass values and beliefs about impairments that influence how we respond and behave in our interactions with persons with disabilities. Research with youth with disabilities showed that family and neighbors are a primary source of support, as well as local community organizations, especially religious groups and sports organizations (Cramm, Lorenzo, & Nieboer, 2013; Lorenzo & Cramm, 2012). Occupational therapists can make a critical contribution to providing opportunities for social interaction where friendships can be fostered, as we are able to advise on ways to remove environmental barriers to participation.

Services and systems are linked to the implementation and monitoring of policies to ensure delivery of and access to resources for people with disabilities. Education, financial services, information, communication, and transport systems were identified as barriers for youth with disabilities (Lorenzo et al., 2013). These are all issues that occupational therapists are able to address through facilitating collective action by persons with disabilities and community workers (Lorenzo, 2008a, 2008b). For example, solutions related to accessible public transport routes include an occupational therapist training community workers to teach drivers how a deaf or blind person would indicate where the bus or taxi needs to stop for him or her or how to transfer a person with a mobility impairment from his or her wheelchair to the seat of car or mini-bus (Lorenzo, van Pletzen, & Booyens, 2015).

Occupational therapists need to make sure that information is available in accessible formats for persons with communication and visual impairments. Often, the very people who are meant to benefit from these policies are excluded because information and documentation are inaccessible, particularly for persons with visual and hearing impairments (Lorenzo et al., 2015; van Pletzen, Booyens, & Lorenzo, 2014). A challenge for occupational therapists is being able to communicate in sign language to build a relationship with deaf persons. Innovative developments in information

TABLE 6-2

BARRIERS TO PARTICIPATION FOR DISABLED YOUTH IN SOUTH AFRICA: BELONGING AND PARTICIPATION

CATEGORY	SCHOOL	WORKING	SOCIAL SUPPORT	HEALTH SERVICES	AREA SERVICES	TRANSPORT	FREE TIME ACTIVITIES
Products and technology	Mobility Communication Self-care	Mobility Communication	Mobility Communication Self-care	Mobility Communication	Mobility Building	Communication Mobility Self-care	Mobility Communication Self-care
Natural environment	Geography Seasons Human events	Geography Seasons Natural events	Geography Seasons Human events	Geography Seasons Natural events	Geography Seasons Natural events	Geography Seasons Natural events	Geography Seasons Natural events
Support	Family Neighbors Strangers	Neighbors Family Assistant	Neighbors Family	Neighbors Family Assistant	Neighbors Strangers Friends	Neighbors Strangers Assistant	Neighbors Strangers Assistant Friends
Attitudes	Authority Family Friends	Authority Strangers	Authority Strangers Friends	Authority Family Beliefs	Authority Strangers Assistant Family	Strangers Authority Friends	Authority Strangers Friends
Services and systems	Funding Information Education	Education Funding	Education Funding	Funding Information Transport	Information Transport Funding	Funding Transport	Funding Safety Transport

Reprinted with permission from Lorenzo, T., Ned-Matiwane, L., Cois, A., & Nwanze, I. (2013). *Youth, disability and rural areas: Facing the challenges of change* (Disability Catalyst Africa: Series 3). Cape Town, South Africa: Disability Innovations Africa.

Box 6-14. Using T-Shirts for Knowledge Translation

The potential for engaging the women in advocacy and awareness raising using the medium of T-shirts seemed to be nonthreatening and to build their confidence, as family members and the community took an active interest in their experiences.

One person even said this [T-shirt] is teaching us a lot about you disabled people.

I wear it to the civic organization meetings and would sit to see whether they would give me a position. They would talk and at the end ask me if I want to say something. I would see that T-shirt forces them [to talk].

There are three people who have stopped me in [the city center] and read everything, even from the back. . . . Our children liked them as well.

I didn't know that what we were saying here [in workshops] could be written down on a T-shirt and have people reading it.

Even scholars usually stop me to ask who is selling the T-shirts.

The community rehabilitation workers from a rural area were even asking if they could sell them to men because they want them.

---

and communication technology systems make such communication easier because people can use computer programs to access information.

A strategy used by women with disabilities for disseminating research findings was printing T-shirts with a design using symbols and limited text to display the findings (see Box 6-6). Community responses suggested that the T-shirts were a strong advocacy tool, as well as an accessible way of disseminating research findings in the community (Box 6-14). People in the community engaged with the women when they were wearing the T-shirts and asked questions. Thus, it was found to be more effective in translating findings in a context where there were low literacy levels because it engaged people in conversation with the women more than the usual means of journal articles or research reports. The T-shirts encouraged interaction and dialogue, which helped to demystify the research process and actively engaged the women in sharing their experiences of the research.

The need has been recognized for universal design principles to be integral to the professional reasoning of occupational therapists because it can equip us with the skills to identify environmental facilitators and barriers. Such reasoning ensures both the participation of persons with disabilities and the social change that will generate greater inclusion in all activities, across the life span, that happen in families and in the communities where we live. The intended outcomes indicated in policies can be achieved through occupation-based practice.

Determining the Occupational Outcomes of Disability Inclusion

There is a need for our profession to develop occupational outcomes through which to monitor social action that contributes to achieving the MDGs. Articles 33 through 39 of the *Convention on the Rights of Persons with Disabilities* (UN, 2006) govern reporting and monitoring on its implementation by states that report to the UN bodies, which has relevance to occupational therapists when determining the outcomes of our practice. Table 6-3 illustrates the synergistic satisfiers used by women with disabilities to address the deprivations of their fundamental human needs and to strengthen their resources to achieve their potential.

TABLE 6-3

OCCUPATIONAL OUTCOMES RELATED TO SYNERGISTIC SATISFIERS OF FUNDAMENTAL HUMAN NEEDS OF DISABLED WOMEN

Identity: Confidence, self-esteem, sense of agency	Affection: Listening to stories, overcome isolation, foster reciprocity	Protection: Voice needs, community rehabilitation workers engage different sectors
Understanding: Community rehabilitation workers, optimize development goals, action spaces, skills development	Subsistence: Access to transport, resources, desire to work	Creation: Action spaces—choir, t-shirts, storytelling, drama
Participation: Present seminars, workshops, action spaces	Idleness: Reflective spaces, fosters reciprocity	Freedom: Voice needs, increased choices, action spaces

Reprinted with permission from Lorenzo, T. (2005). *We don't see ourselves as different: A web of possibilities for disabled women. How Black disabled women in poor communities equalise opportunities for human development and social change.* Unpublished PhD dissertation, Department of Public Health, University of Cape Town, South Africa.

Occupational outcomes to address the intentions of the five components of *CBR Guidelines* (WHO, 2010) to create an inclusive society would be aligned to the goals of participation in everyday living and the roles and responsibilities that a person aspires to resume after rehabilitation. Indicators of participation need to measure access to health services and maintaining well-being, the period of time children take to complete schooling, and transition to skills development for different forms of livelihood. There is also a need to collect information that monitors outcomes related to family life and belonging to a community. These outcomes and indicators contribute to knowing whether the desired change through occupationally focused interventions has addressed, on the one hand, the impairment needs of a person and, on the other hand, the removal of environmental barriers to his or her participation. The Campbell Collaboration (n.d.) has suggested that the outcomes of CBR vary depending on the targets of specific programs but could include improvement in social participation, clinical outcomes, and quality of life among persons with disabilities. Box 6-15 displays outcomes for CBR from the Campbell Collaboration, which are relevant for occupational therapy.

Designing programs linked to the various elements in each of the five components of CBR contributes to achieving disability inclusion in the MDGs, which would meet the fundamental human needs of people with disabilities. Table 6-4 suggests possible occupational outcomes that could be used to monitor disability-inclusive development in meeting the MDGs. Thus, our interventions and practice enhance, enable, and enrich being, doing, becoming, and belonging through meaningful and purposeful transactional endeavors by people with disabilities, individually and collectively.

This section has attempted to illustrate the richness, depth, and complexity of the professional reasoning of occupational therapists that enables us to contribute to systems development in health, education, livelihood, and social services to ensure the inclusion and participation of persons with disabilities and their families. Managing the transitions imposed by disability is possible. Professional reasoning is of critical relevance in facilitating disability-inclusive policy

> ## Box 6-15. Activities Related to the Different Components of Community-Based Rehabilitation
>
> - **Health:** training persons with disabilities in the use of assistive devices; providing information to persons with disabilities and their family or caregivers about time and location of activities for screening health conditions and impairments associated with disabilities
> - **Education:** providing education and training for families or caregivers of persons with disabilities; installing ramps in schools to make them accessible to persons with disabilities using wheelchairs
> - **Livelihood:** linking the job seeker with disability to existing support services; advocating before relevant public and private agencies to ensure accessible housing for persons with disabilities
> - **Social:** converting institutions for persons with disabilities in rehabilitation centers; providing information to persons with disabilities about sports opportunities available within the community
> - **Empowerment:** helping persons with disabilities to set up and run self-help groups; involving disabled people's organizations in project planning, implementation, and monitoring

implementation and monitoring outcomes to ensure such inclusion because occupational therapists are equipped to understand and address environmental factors through universal design that enables and supports participation.

Conclusion

Professional reasoning to make policies practical enables occupational therapists to interpret the relevance of international policies to our profession. Such reasoning enables us to promote disability inclusion as a significant contribution that we can make to social justice and health equity for oppressed and marginalized groups. The occupational therapy profession has a major contribution to make at all levels of policy processes in the public and private sectors to ensure that activities, services, information, and documentation are available to all. Then, and only then, will persons with disabilities and their families enjoy equal opportunities for participation in activities of everyday life. The strength of our profession is in our ability to recognize the creative potential of individuals who, when engaged collectively, have the power to move populations toward comprehensive health, well-being, and a sustainable quality of life.

References

Bates-Eamer, N., Carin, B., Lee, M. H., & Lim, W., with Kapila, M. (2012). *Post-2015 development agenda: Goals, targets and indicators.* Waterloo, Canada: The Centre for International Governance Innovation and the Korea Development Institute. Retrieved from https://www.cigionline.org/sites/default/files/mdg_post_2015v3.pdf

Campbell Collaboration. (n.d.). Retrieved from http://www.campbellcollaboration.org

Chappell, P., & Lorenzo, T. (2012). Exploring capacity for disability-inclusive development. In *Marrying community development and rehabilitation: Reality or aspiration for disabled people?* In T. Lorenzo (Ed.), *Disability Innovations Africa: Cape Town* (Disability Catalyst Africa: Series 2; pp. 5-35). Cape Town, South Africa: Disability Innovations Africa.

TABLE 6-4
POSSIBLE OCCUPATIONAL OUTCOMES LINKED TO THE MILLENNIUM DEVELOPMENT GOALS TO ENSURE DISABILITY-INCLUSIVE DEVELOPMENT

MILLENNIUM DEVELOPMENT GOAL	OCCUPATIONAL OUTCOMES
MDG 1: Eradicate Extreme Poverty and Hunger	Expose to choices and opportunities for livelihoods Skills development and continued professional/career development Decent employment through inclusive growth enhancement Placement of workers, goodness of fit to demands of job Accessible information about social grants and resources, consider occupational choices that grant makes possible Access and advocacy to financial institutions
MDG 2: Achieve Universal Primary Education	Engagement in appropriate play and schooling, retention in and completion of schooling
MDG 3: Promote Gender Equality and Empower Women	Create an understanding of the need and value of occupation across the life span (e.g., children in school, adults working, elders in creative social contributions) Address violence, refugees, consequence of marginalization and exclusion
MDG 4: Reduce Child Mortality	Community-based support to reduce trauma and violence experienced by children Improved nutritional programs Skills development to ensure food security in families
MDG 5: Improve Maternal Health	Support networks to promote well-being and participation Accessible information, resources, and services
MDG 6: Combat HIV/AIDS, Malaria, and Other Diseases	Early screening and identification Direct access to services Address contextual factors leading to stressful lifestyles
MDG 7: Ensure Environmental Sustainability	Land, agriculture, resources, and opportunities for development Adapt sustainable ecofriendly resources for participation in daily activities
MDG 8: Develop a Global Partnership for Development	Understand policy literacy and occupational engagement/participation Technical and economic assistance in program development, monitoring and evaluation, cost-benefit analysis, and effectiveness studies

Clark, F. A. (2010). Power and confidence in professions: Lessons for occupational therapy. *Canadian Journal of Occupational Therapy, 77,* 264-269.

Cramm, J. M., Lorenzo, T., & Nieboer, A. (2013, June 20). Comparing education, employment, social support and well-being among youth with disabilities and their peers in South Africa. *Applied Research in Quality of Life.* Advance online publication. doi:10.1007/s11482-013-9247-5

Cramm, J. M., Nieboer, A. P., Finkenflügel, H., & Lorenzo, T. (2013a). Comparison of barriers to employment among youth with and without disabilities in South Africa. *Work, 46,* 19-24.

Cramm, J. M., Nieboer, A. P., Finkenflügel, H., & Lorenzo, T. (2013b). Disabled youth in South Africa: Barriers to education. *International Journal of Disability and Human Development, 12,* 31-35.

Gcaza, S., & Lorenzo, T. (2008). Discovering the barriers that stop children from being children: "The right to the provision of mobility devices." *South African Journal of Occupational Therapy, 39,* 16-21.

Habib, M., Uddin, J., Rahman, S. U., Jahan, N., & Akter, S. (2013). Occupational therapy role in disaster management in Bangladesh. *WFOT Bulletin, 68,* 33.

Lorenzo, T. (2004). Equalising opportunities for occupational engagement: Disabled women's stories. In R. Watson & L. Swartz (Eds.), *Transformation through occupation: Human occupation in context* (pp. 85-102). London, England: Wiley.

Lorenzo, T. (2005). *We don't see ourselves as different: A web of possibilities for disabled women. How Black disabled women in poor communities equalise opportunities for human development and social change.* Unpublished PhD dissertation, Department of Public Health, University of Cape Town, South Africa.

Lorenzo, T. (2008a). Mobilizing action of disabled women in developing contexts to tackle poverty and development. In E. Crepeau (Ed.), *Willard and Spackman's occupational therapy* (11th ed.). Philadelphia, PA: Lippincott Williams & Wilkins.

Lorenzo, T. (2008b). "We are also travellers": An action story about disabled women mobilizing for an accessible public transport system in Khayelitsha and Nyanga, Cape Metropole, South Africa. *South American Journal of Occupational Therapy, 39,* 32-40.

Lorenzo, T. (2010). Listening spaces: Connecting diverse voices for social action and change. In M. Savin-Baden & C. H. Major (Eds.), *New approaches for qualitative research: Wisdom and uncertainty* (pp. 131-144). London, England: Routledge.

Lorenzo, T., & Cloete, L. (2004). Promoting occupations in rural communities. In R. Watson & L. Swartz (Eds.), *Transformation through occupation: Human occupation in context* (pp. 268-286). London, England: Wiley.

Lorenzo, T., & Cramm, J. M. (2012). Access to livelihood assets among youth with and without disabilities in South Africa: Implications for health professional education. *South African Medical Journal, 102,* 578-581.

Lorenzo, T., Motau, J., & Chappell, P. (2012). Community rehabilitation workers as catalysts for disability-inclusive youth development. In T. Lorenzo (Ed.), *Marrying community development and rehabilitation: Reality or aspiration for disabled people* (Disability Catalyst Africa: Series 2; pp. 36-49). Cape Town, South Africa: Disability Innovations Africa.

Lorenzo, T., Ned-Matiwane, L., Cois, A., & Nwanze, I. (2013). *Youth, disability and rural areas: Facing the challenges of change* (Disability Catalyst Africa: Series 3). Cape Town, South Africa: Disability Innovations Africa.

Lorenzo, T., van Pletzen, E., & Booyens, M. (2015). Determining the competences of community based workers for disability-inclusive development in rural areas of South Africa, Botswana and Malawi. *Rural and Remote Health, 15,* 2919. Available at www.rrh.org.au.

United Nations. (1979). *Convention on the elimination of all forms of discrimination against women.* General Assembly resolution 34/180 of 18 December 1979. Retrieved from http://www.ohchr.org/Documents/ProfessionalInterest /cedaw.pdf

United Nations. (1982). *World programme of action concerning disabled persons.* General Assembly resolution 37/52 of 3 December 1982.

United Nations. (1989). *Convention on the rights of the child.* General Assembly resolution 44/25 of 20 November 1989. Retrieved from http://www.ohchr.org/en/professionalinterest/pages/crc.aspx

United Nations. (1993). *Standard rules on the equalization of opportunities for persons with disabilities.* New York, NY: Author.

United Nations. (2000). *Millennium development goals.* New York, NY: Author.

United Nations. (2006). *Convention on the rights of persons with disabilities.* New York, NY: Author.

van Pletzen, E., Booyens, M., & Lorenzo, T. (2014). Community disability workers' potential to alleviate poverty and promote social inclusion of people with disabilities in three Southern African countries. *Disability and Society, 29,* 1524-1539. doi:10.1080/09687599.2014.958131

Watson, R., & Lagerdien, K. (2004). Women empowered through occupation: From deprivation to realized potential. In R. Watson & L. Swartz (Eds.), *Transformation through occupation: Human occupation in context* (pp. 102-122). London, England: Wiley.

World Health Organization. (2010). *Community-based rehabilitation guidelines.* Geneva, Switzerland: Author.

Collaborative Reasoning
Teaching and Learning to Facilitate Disability Inclusion in Policy and Practice

Theresa Lorenzo, BSc (Occupational Therapy) (Wits), HDipEdAd (Wits),
MSc (Community Disability Studies) (University of London),
PhD in Public Health (UCT), PgDip (Higher Education Studies) (UCT)

Occupational therapists need to find the courage of their convictions in occupational science to generate capacity for reciprocal learning among persons with disabilities, their families, and service providers. Creating an understanding of disability as a social justice issue rather than merely a medical concern shifts the focus to attitudinal and environmental barriers to participation. The experiences of discrimination and marginalization that a person with disability faces in everyday life require policy changes in all institutions and levels of government. Occupational therapy academics have opportunities to explore teaching and learning about disability inclusion in health, education, work, family life, and community living. Such knowledge will ensure that students and practitioners are equipped to create opportunities for the participation and inclusion of persons with disability on an equal basis with others so that occupational justice leads to greater social justice.

Occupational science offers a way of understanding the diverse dynamics and underlying forces that influence human occupation as it affects health and quality of life at individual and population levels. Townsend, Wicks, van Bruggen, and Wright-St Clair (2012, p. 43) described occupation as a central force in human existence and in the organization of societies. They identified four aspects of increasing occupational therapy consciousness that support our efforts to address daily life inequalities and sustain our energy for imagining and acting on the untapped potential of individuals, families, and communities.

1. They raised the question of how occupational therapists might build a culture of power, confidence, and the inclusion of those inside and outside clinical practice, without excluding innovators. Such exclusion can be seen as a form of invisible, unconscious, horizontal violence that is enacted through criticism of theory or the devaluing of those who are not engaged in clinical practice.

2. They viewed collaboration as a powerful, consensual way of working and questioned how occupational therapists might demonstrate leadership to coordinate services across education, housing, transportation, industry, child development, disability, unemployment, older people, and other systems, beyond the health care systems where the majority of occupational therapists practice, whether public or private. Studies by Duncan, Sherry, and Watson (2011),

Cole, M. B., & Creek, J. (Eds.).
Global Perspectives in Professional Reasoning (pp. 99-116).
© 2016 Taylor & Francis Group.

on disability, poverty, and occupation in remote rural development, and by Lorenzo, Ned-Matiwane, Cois, and Nwanze (2013), on disabled youth's livelihoods, highlight the urgent need for coordinated access to services. Lorenzo, van Pletzen, and Booyens (2015) illustrated how the training of community-based workers can provide an intersectional, coordinated system that could amplify the work of occupational therapists in addressing social action related to inequalities.

3. They suggested how occupational therapists might take proactive leadership as an essential approach to thinking and acting to advance equity of opportunity in occupational participation and social inclusion for all people. Proactivity is especially needed for the inclusion and participation of persons with disabilities.

4. They argued that, in pursuing a career beyond a job as a way of making a difference in local or global lives, occupational therapy regulatory power needs to be better oriented to include, not exclude, occupational therapists with job titles such as academic, advocacy coordinator, case manager, community developer, disaster relief manager, educator, executive director, or policy maker.

These four aspects of increasing consciousness indicate the largely hidden potential of the occupational therapy profession to contribute to disability inclusion in all policy processes and service delivery systems. Addressing the social inequities and discrimination faced by persons with disabilities and their families requires the transformation of beliefs and behavior toward persons with disabilities. Ramugondo (2012) identified the need for occupational consciousness in considering the intergenerational influences on the everyday activities that people engage in across the life span. The inclusion of persons with disabilities and their quality of life through participation in daily activities will be achieved if occupational therapists invest wholeheartedly in the potential of all human beings to take responsibility for their own health and well-being. Furthermore, the possibility of marrying research into policy and practice related to active inclusion strategies is enhanced. The adoption of health-promoting occupations has the potential to prevent impairments and consequent disability from noncommunicable diseases.

This chapter begins with a description of the elements of organizational capacity (Kaplan, 1999) as a theoretical framework for teaching disability inclusion. Paulo Freire's adult education approach (Hope & Timmel, 1995) and the action learning cycle (Community Development Research Association [CDRA], 2005; Taylor, Marais, & Kaplan, 1997) provide the principles and processes that enable reciprocal teaching and learning about disability inclusion through shared experiences. The Wheel of Opportunities for Participation (WOOP; Lorenzo & Sait, 2000) is presented as an example of a practical tool for translating policy into practice in a participatory way, which also enables teaching and monitoring of policy processes across different government sectors and facilitates the inclusion and participation of persons with disabilities in everyday activities. The chapter ends with an exploration of possible leadership approaches for facilitating social change for and with persons with disabilities and their families, with a focus on the value of intentional leadership.

Teaching Organizational Capacity to Facilitate Disability Inclusion in Policy and Practice

Organizational capacity is a term used to denote the ability of organizations to implement and manage projects. It includes the ability to deliver projects on time and in a cost-effective manner by building a sustainable organization that functions as a resilient, strategic, and autonomous entity (Kaplan, 1999). The first three elements of organizational capacity are intangible, which means they are difficult to identify and thus difficult to monitor. These are conceptual frameworks, organizational culture and attitude, and vision and strategy. The tangible elements are structures and systems, individual skills and abilities, and material resources, which are more visible and easy to measure. A description of each element follows, together with suggestions for assessment and intervention.

Conceptual Frameworks

The conceptual frameworks that inform the work of an organization enable it to make sense of the world around it, to locate itself within that world, and to make decisions in relation to the contexts within which it operates and by which it is influenced (Kaplan, 1999). These conceptual frameworks remain open to critique and modification as circumstances change. Kaplan asserted that an organization needs to have a competent, working understanding of its world, otherwise it is incapacitated, regardless of how many other skills and competencies it may have. A student needs to identify the model of disability that has informed the development of services and programs, such as the medical or individual model, social model, psychoanalytical model, human rights, or development approach. The internal policies of an organization also indicate the conceptual thinking and frameworks that have been adopted.

Organizational Attitude

Organizational attitude reflects the values and paradigms of power and control that inform the organization's fundamental understanding of the world. It reveals the organization's awareness of the realities faced in the districts or communities where services and programs are delivered. The underlying assumptions that inform the development of programs should be identified and made explicit to all those involved so that there is collective agreement. The values and paradigms inform the policies on disability inclusion, which should be influenced by national and international policy frameworks and mandates. Thus, an organization's attitude reveals how its members understand and accept responsibility for the social and physical conditions in which they operate, and how they see their role in responding to these conditions (Kaplan, 1999). In practice, this position leads to taking responsibility for making available the means to address problems that are related to the organization's vision and mission.

With this clear understanding of its values and how these influence intentions for action, the organization will be able to monitor its actions, what works, and what does not work, and then try new ways to give effect to its vision.

Vision and Strategy

The vision and strategies identified to achieve the vision need to be informed by Article 33 of the *United Nations (UN) Convention on the Rights of Persons with Disabilities* (CRPD; 2006), which affirms the requirement for people with disabilities to be involved and participate. Educators need to equip students with the skills to determine the aspirations of the disabled community they are working with and how they will achieve their vision and mission. The action learning cycle and the participatory approaches described later in this chapter provide the process and tools for incorporating the voices of persons with disabilities and their families.

Strategies include the use of media to communicate what is being done and what still needs to be done to achieve disability inclusion in services and development opportunities.

Postgraduate students may be set the task of analyzing their own organizations and programs to determine whether the strategies they are using will facilitate disability inclusion and where the barriers may be, whether conscious or unconscious. In understanding and determining the decision-making processes and who comprises the management of organizations, it is critical to question the nature of disability representation. Is the voice of the person with disability represented in the values of the organization?

Structures and Systems

This element of organizational capacity looks at the shape of the organizational administrative and management systems. According to Ubels, Baddoo, and Fowler (2010, p. 14),

> once organizational aims, strategy and culture are clear it becomes possible to structure the organization in such a way that roles and functions are clearly defined and differentiated, lines of communication and accountability untangled, and decision-making procedures transparent and functional.

Structure provides employees with an understanding of their responsibility and position within the organization. It also provides a shape for communication networks that determine who reports to whom and who interacts with or does not interact with whom. One of the key components of the organizational system relates to monitoring and evaluation, which are explored in more depth later in the chapter.

Acquisition of Individual Skills, Abilities, and Competences

The multisectorial and intersectorial nature of disability-inclusive development demands a workforce that takes responsibility for coordinating disability inclusion across the different services and programs provided by public, private, and/or nongovernmental organization (NGO) sectors. Most organizations have performance management systems for staff already in place, so the intention is to ensure that disability inclusion is a monitored component of staff performance. This integration will ensure that skills, abilities, and competencies are continually upgraded through postgraduate programs or continuing professional development programs as managers become aware of the gaps and areas of development needed in their team. The human resources on a program may also include volunteers as well as paid staff.

Material Resources

This element describes the nature of resources present, such as financial resources, stock, information and communication technology, and general equipment, and determines whether they are sufficient and appropriate for achieving the vision and mission of the organization.

Occupational therapists contribute to organizational capacity by making an occupational assessment of the competence, capacity, and assets of individuals linked to their roles, behavior and habits, and the six elements of organizational capacity (Table 7-1). The occupational therapy educator needs to teach students how to assess organizational capacity so that they are able to design interventions to address the identified gaps of specific elements.

To plan and implement sustainable interventions, students need to be able to identify the six elements of organizational capacity to facilitate disability inclusion in any practice learning placement by using the action learning cycle. This process enables students and practitioners to become competent in monitoring their own capacity as changes occur. Disability inclusion in policy processes is about relationships and the interconnections between the different stakeholders in the contexts where service delivery and development programs occur. The development of professional reasoning can be facilitated by using an action learning approach (CDRA, 2005; Taylor et al., 1997) to implement and monitor disability inclusion. This enables occupational therapists to make policies relevant in their work, be it clinical practice in hospitals, home visits, development work in communities, developing businesses, or teaching and learning in higher education.

TABLE 7-1
WAYS OF TEACHING THE ELEMENTS OF ORGANIZATIONAL CAPACITY FOR DISABILITY INCLUSION

ELEMENTS	ASSESSMENT DESIGN	POSSIBLE INTERVENTION
Conceptual framework	Approaches to disability Understanding international and national policies related to disability Primary health care and community-based rehabilitation	Workshops on disability theories and approaches Applied policy literacy Workshops on occupation-focused approach to disability inclusion and health promotion
Organizational attitude	Application of policies to your context and programs Looking at disability rights and equal opportunities in context Seeing disability as diversity	Complete Wheel of Opportunities for Participation Case studies Good practice case studies
Vision and strategy	Design vision and mission based on above two elements Use creative activities, such as clay work or drawing pictures, to develop a vision and strategy	Dialogues on strategy to address barriers and build on facilitators and assets Awareness campaigns in specific target areas Start projects to remove barriers
Structures and systems	Documentary analysis of minutes of meetings, progress reports, participant observation	Identify skills training needed in areas of administration, communication, report writing, financial management
Individual skills and abilities	Gap analysis linked to job description Aspects of three intangible elements can be assessed further at individual level	Address causes of burnout (e.g., care for the carers) Identify relevant workshops or short courses for individuals to attend Provided relevant readings or literature to inspire staff
Material resources	Participant observation, analysis of minutes of meetings Interviews or focus groups with staff	Fundraising and proposal writing Monitoring and writing good practice stories

ADULT EDUCATION PRINCIPLES AND THE
ACTION LEARNING CYCLE

To facilitate disability inclusion, there is a critical need for occupational therapy educators to make policies relevant and practical to students so that, as practitioners, they will be able to translate policies into everyday language and apply them in the lives of individuals, families, and community organizations. This strategy requires conscious awareness and critical analysis of the inequities faced by vulnerable and marginalized groups, such as persons with disability. Policy literacy teaches students and community groups the language and concepts embedded in policy and empowers them to hold their governments accountable by understanding what they are expected to deliver (Duncan et al., 2011). This skill is similar to learning to read and write in that it will foster political understanding and social inclusion. The teaching and learning of disability inclusion in policy processes may be guided by Paulo Freire's principles of adult education (see Hope & Timmel, 1995). Freire was a Brazilian educator who worked with communities that were seen as illiterate to raise their consciousness about their oppression and development. All these communities had spoken language and the power to change their social circumstances, even if they could not read or write.

DasGupta et al. (2006) revealed that, as the educator models this way of interaction for the student, so the student is able to engage the people who they are helping to share their knowledge and find solutions to the problems they are experiencing. The intention to find solutions collaboratively changes the educator–student relationship to one of mutual learning through interdependence. Educators purposely deprivilege their power and authority and make students conscious of their own power (DasGupta et al., 2006) so that, as future clinicians, they understand power relationships with their clients.

The creative adult education methods of Freire (Hope & Timmel, 1995) provide relevant tools for developing policy literacy in occupational therapy educators, researchers, students, and practitioners. Understanding the relevance of policy literacy in their work should facilitate the social inclusion of persons with disabilities and their families in the communities where they live. Using the principles of adult education outlined by Freire and the action learning cycle demonstrates for students how they should relate to and interact with their clients. The six principles are as follows:

1. Relevance
2. Problem posing
3. No education is ever neutral—banking approach vs. critical thinking
4. Mutual learning and critical dialogue
5. Action reflection
6. Radical transformation

The action learning cycle incorporates Freire's principles in a four-step process that can be used to teach policy processes in such a way that students engage with the practical nature of policies and their relevance to occupation-focused practice (Box 7-1).

Relevance

The principle of relevance generates consciousness and social awareness, which enable occupational therapists to invest time and resources in projects and programs. The art of listening to the everyday conversations of the target group, to identify what people feel strongly about, enables the occupational therapist to identify the problems and difficulties that people experience in their lives about which they will take action, as emotion is linked to motivation. Such engagement will make a difference in local communities, leading to ripple effects at national and international levels.

Box 7-1. Action Learning Cycle

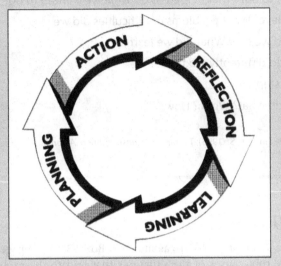

Reprinted with permission from the Community Development Research Association. (2005). *Action learning: A developmental approach to change.* Retrieved from http://www.cdra.org.za/articles-by-cdra-practitioners.html

Box 7-2. Examples of Codes to Present Generative Themes and Facilitate Dialogue

DATA TRIGGERS	FACILITATION TECHNIQUES	DATA-CAPTURING METHODS
Drawing	Buzz groups	Videotaping
Clay work	Pairing	Audiotaping
Singing	Small-group discussions (maximum of eight people in a group)	Scribing
Music		Field notes
Movement		Photographs
Drama	Plenary groups	
Critical incident stories	Brainstorming	
Writing songs		
Writing poems		

The topics participants feel strongly about are called *generative themes*. Once generative themes have been identified, the occupational therapist as facilitator needs to represent a group's thinking and feelings on a topic that is of current concern to them in a code. A *code* is a visual representation of the ideas, hopes, doubts, frustrations, and challenges that the group faces in everyday life. Any creative method may be used to represent and reflect their problems back to the group; some examples are given in Box 7-2.

Box 7-3. Six-Step Analysis of the Code or Trigger

1. What did we plan to do? What helped us do what we wanted to do?
2. What did we achieve? What problems or difficulties did we see?
3. What changes did we see? What did we learn?
4. What would we do differently next time?
5. What is our next step?
6. Who is going to do what? When? How?

Adapted from Hope, A., & Timmel, S. (1995). *Training for transformation: A handbook for community workers.* Gweru, Zimbabwe: Mambo Press.

Problem Posing

The facilitator asks a series of questions, as shown in Box 7-3, that engage participants in thinking critically about the root causes of the situations that lead to the problems and frustrations represented in the theme. This process of problem posing means that the educator encourages group members to ask themselves questions until a solution or action is found, and not simply to respond to the questions posed.

No Education Is Neutral

Raising consciousness about our own power and the contribution we can make in improving our own lives, and those of people who feel marginalized and oppressed, should be the purpose of teaching and learning. Occupational therapy educators need to recognize that everyone they interact with, at an individual or group level, comes with knowledge and prior experiences. Their approach should be one of critical engagement and not didactic teaching. The latter encapsulates Freire's notion of a *banking approach* in which educators deposit knowledge in the minds of the learners, with minimal interaction or questions and little regard for the prior knowledge and experience of students. Freire's alternative is to encourage critical thinking so that the learners ask questions about what is being taught.

Critical dialogue and critical thinking allow both educators and learners to challenge the assumptions and beliefs about theory and practice that inform our actions and reflections, so that occupational therapy remains relevant in addressing the social, political, and economic matters that practitioners encounter (Townsend et al., 2012).

Mutual Learning and Critical Dialogue

Mutual learning and critical dialogue between educators and students enable a person-centered focus to our practice, as power is shared with others through the recognition and appreciation of difference and diversity in all their complexity: We all have something to contribute despite our limitations and vulnerabilities. The process provides spaces in which everyone can share and explore so that each person is able to identify the actions he or she will take, individually or collectively, depending on the generative theme that was identified. A mutual intention of seeking and sharing knowledge will assist in changing the life situation of the individual and/or his or her family.

In this step of mutual learning and dialogue, students need to draw on existing theories that have relevance to their reflections or that will help them make sense of their reflections. Engaging

Box 7-4. Example of Action Reflection on a Policy Issue

Action: Ask students to choose one article from the *United Nations Convention on the Rights of Persons with Disabilities* that is relevant to a person in the community or patient in a hospital they have worked with during a practice or service learning placement. They then do some free writing about what they did with the person during a single session or over a period of sessions.

Reflection: Have students to write freely on what happened, what they felt while doing the session(s) with the person, what unspoken thoughts they had, what assumptions were made that were correct or incorrect, and what was significant in interaction with the person.

with different articles in UN policies or components of the *Community-Based Rehabilitation (CBR) Guidelines* (World Health Organization [WHO], 2010) is one possibility. The educator facilitates sense-making and has opportunities to give direct input on relevant theories and policies.

Action Reflection

The action reflection process is used to guide reasoning and identify the activities that people with disabilities are able to do. Action reflection focuses on getting participants to identify actions that they can take to address their own needs (e.g., participants need to read and reread a policy to become familiar with it so that they can highlight the action words in the policy). This step helps them make explicit links and connections between policy and practice as the intentions of the policy come alive. An example of action reflection on a policy issue is given in Box 7-4. Occupational therapists are action oriented so looking for the verbs and action words in policies can help to direct the planning and design of our interventions.

Radical Transformation

Students need to think about and identify possible actions that they can take in the next learning cycle to find further solutions to existing problems. Such planning needs to be linked to Freire's principle of radical transformation, which means that planned action needs to address the root causes of the problems identified in the generative themes. Chaffey, Unsworth, and Fossey (2010) commented that interaction and connection guide professional reasoning in practice. The principle of radical transformation elicits these connections through participants identifying and tackling the root causes of problems and not just the symptoms. There is no quick fix, but small steps taken by individuals and groups can lead to significant changes so that solutions can be sustained. A monitoring tool, such as the WOOP, is required to ensure sustained action toward equalizing opportunities for participation.

The Wheel of Opportunities for Participation

The translation of policy into practice can be facilitated by the generation of mutual understandings of environmental factors that influence disability inclusion. In Chapter 6, I argued that disability inclusion is the responsibility of all professions and sectors of government, as well as private and corporate organizations and nongovernmental organizations. Thus, all faculties in higher education institutions should strive to integrate disability thinking and critique into their curricula and research. To achieve the full participation and inclusion of people with disabilities

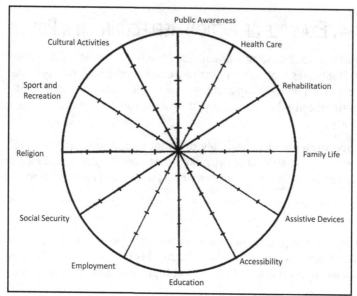

Figure 7-1. The Wheel of Opportunities for Participation.

in development, it is important to identify and overcome the social, legal, economic, political, and environmental conditions that create barriers to their full exercise and enjoyment of rights. There have been several conceptualizations of participation and inclusion. For example, the WHO *CBR Guidelines* (2010), which promote inclusive development and service delivery for persons with disabilities across the life span, are based on five principles: inclusion, participation, sustainability, and self-advocacy, all underpinned by empowerment.

Rifkin and Kagere (2002) developed a spider web as a participatory tool to measure community participation, by identifying five elements: organization, leadership, management, resource mobilization, and needs assessment. Lorenzo adapted the spider web into a WOOP to develop a tool for teaching and monitoring the *UN Standard Rules on the Equalization of Opportunities for Persons with Disabilities* (Figure 7-1).

A Teaching and Monitoring Tool

The WOOP is an innovative participatory tool, based on the *UN Standard Rules on the Equalization of Opportunities for Persons with Disabilities* (UN, 1993) for exploring opportunities and obstacles to persons with disabilities participating in everyday activities and accessing services in their communities. The WOOP also makes it possible to gather information related to the experiences of persons with disabilities regarding the provision of services outlined in the Articles of the UN CRPD and the components of CBR. It can be used in classrooms or workshops to help individuals or groups to determine the level of participation by persons with disability in target areas. South Africa ratified the UN CRPD in 2007, meaning that this framework can only be implemented through domestication of these principles into national policies and programs of action that are then implemented at a local district level. Occupational therapy educators need to be in tune with the debates around these operational plans at provincial and district levels in the different government departments of health, education, social development, housing, transport, environmental affairs, agriculture, and so on, so that students are equipped to contribute meaningfully to the occupational nature of persons accessing the services. Monitoring opportunities for participation and development cannot be isolated from the broader principles of management, accountability, and justification of resources.

The WOOP consists of a circle with 12 spokes representing a wheel. Four of the spokes represent the *preconditions for equal participation* (Rules 1 through 4): awareness raising (public awareness); medical (health) care; rehabilitation, and support systems (assistive devices and equipment). The other eight spokes represent the *target areas for equal participation*: accessibility; education (schooling from early education through to tertiary provision); employment; social security and income maintenance; family life and personal integrity (relationships and sexuality); culture (arts, film, acting, theatre, libraries, and the media); sport and recreation; and religion. To accommodate different levels of literacy, the target areas can be depicted in symbols rather than words.

The WOOP provides a process for different stakeholders, such as students, practitioners from different sectors, disabled people's organizations, and family members, to identify and analyze those factors that may facilitate or hinder individuals and their families in accessing resources, information, and services that promote their well-being and development. It is a participatory method for different stakeholders to appraise the equity of access to services, activities, information, and documentation to ensure equal opportunities for development. The tool can be completed individually, or a large group can be divided into smaller groups of 8 to 10 students or participants. In this way, everyone who has had some exposure to or experience of disability is involved in identifying the barriers and enablers to participation for persons with disabilities and their families.

A spoke is graded from the hub of the wheel (low) to the outside (high). With the WOOP in the middle of the group, each spoke is discussed in turn. Participants decide where they will place a marker that indicates if participation in that target area is low, average, or high. Reasons for placing the marker in a particular position are discussed. The group then identifies actions, individually or collectively, that they can take to change areas of low and average participation to high participation.

A Participatory Research Tool

The translation of policy into practice can be facilitated by the generation of mutual understandings of the environmental factors that influence disability inclusion. Lorenzo and Joubert (2011) described the experience of occupational therapy academics and postgraduate students from the Disability Studies Master's Program at the University of Cape Town, some of whom are persons with disabilities, doing collaborative research focused on the participation of disabled youth in social and economic development in South Africa (Box 7-5). The main benefit of the collaboration was reciprocal capacity development, as persons with disabilities and community workers shared their in-depth knowledge of the complexities of participating in development opportunities that deepened their understanding of the policy implementation process. Likewise, occupational therapy academics were able to share theoretical frameworks that could provide an understanding of the principles that foster community development and occupational outcomes for individuals, families, and different community groups.

Implementation strategies can then be identified by the group to tackle barriers to participation by using the 10 implementation strategies in the *UN Standard Rules on the Equalization of Opportunities for Persons with Disabilities* as discussion starters, as shown in Box 7-6.

Box 7-5. Identifying the Livelihood Assets and Opportunities of Disabled Youth

The WOOP was adapted to explore opportunities and obstacles for youth with disabilities, their vulnerability, and their livelihoods by investigating their human, social, physical, and financial capitals through a focus group. A local school for children with disabilities offered their hall for a day, which provided accessible facilities within reasonable distance of the homes of the participants. The focus group was facilitated by a community worker, who was a research assistant, and an occupational therapy lecturer, who was a coinvestigator and kept field notes. After a warm-up exercise, the community worker led the discussion using the WOOP to allow expression in the home language of each participant. Participants were asked to rate their participation in services, activities, and events, represented by each of the 12 spokes on the wheel, as low, average, or high in terms of meeting their needs. Available information or documentation from service providers, facilities, and stakeholders was rated simultaneously. Participants had to discuss the rating with each other and come to agreement on it. If consensus could not be reached, then two ratings could be given. The reasons for differences in response related to experiences were recorded. All the discussions were audiorecorded. See Figure 7-2 for the WOOP completed by the group of disabled youth.

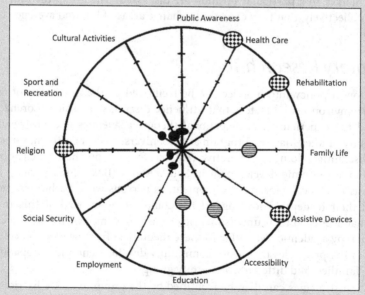

Figure 7-2. Measures of participation by disabled youth in the Hammanskraal.

BOX 7-6. IMPLEMENTATION STRATEGIES TO EQUALIZE OPPORTUNITIES THROUGH OCCUPATION

Information and research: carry out occupational studies into the living conditions of persons with disabilities and the impact on family and community living. Outcome measures related to functional independence and participation can be used in quality-of-life studies. Occupational therapists should be involved in national surveys and censuses to ensure there are relevant questions to identify occupation-focused inequalities and discriminations. Data analysis would also identify occupational inequalities that would inform evidence-based advocacy, that is, campaigns for rights of persons with disabilities based on research that demonstrates changes in level of participation and access to services and life opportunities.

Policy making and planning: write policy briefs focused on interventions by specific government departments and ministries. These can include measures to address environmental barriers and facilitators.

Legislation: include the teaching of legislation in undergraduate and postgraduate curricula as well as continuing professional development programs. Sessions at national and international conferences should focus on the influence occupational therapists have in addressing personal and social inequities, as well as contributing to reports on implementation of national and international legislation.

Economic policies: analyze government budgets through cost–benefit studies, using an occupation-focused lens, and then advocate for the allocation of financial resources to ensure that economic policies address the needs of persons with disabilities (e.g., provision of assistive devices and technology to facilitate learning and employability).

Coordination of work: train community-based workers, as frontline staff, to act as coordinators for persons with disabilities and their families, to access services and information about resources and programs, and to ensure continuity of care. These workers could also join community forums, hospital boards, and school governing bodies to advocate for the allocation of resources for specific programs.

Disabled people's organizations: build reciprocal capacity through the adult education approach described earlier.

Personnel training: capacitate human resource managers to understand the importance of matching people's skills and abilities to their jobs. Carry out activity analysis and provide advice on adaptations to the job or the environment, where necessary.

National monitoring and evaluation: assume roles and responsibilities related to occupational interests, present at conferences, and monitor policy implementation from an occupational perspective.

Technical and economic cooperation: contribute skills development, environmental adaptations, strategies for job creation, and inclusive employment options.

International cooperation: network, through regional occupational therapy groups on each continent, on different Articles in the Convention and on Sustainable Development Goals, and promulgate these to the relevant international bodies through the World Federation of Occupational Therapists. Link these networks with the CBR networks in Africa, Asia, and South America. Submit reports to the special rapporteur on the CRPD.

LEARNING HOW TO SELECT INDICATORS TO MONITOR DISABILITY INCLUSION

Monitoring disability inclusion to ensure the accessibility of activities, services, information, and documentation for persons with disabilities is part of the conceptual framework of an organization as well as of its structures and systems. In an earlier chapter on disability inclusion, occupational outcomes were suggested. These outcomes can inform the type of indicators chosen to monitor changes that lead to inclusive services and programs.

The ability to select indicators to monitor disability inclusion in services and programs can be enhanced through the establishment of collaborative partnerships with the different stakeholders involved in service delivery.

An action learning approach, as described earlier, provides a system for selecting outcome measures that are meaningful and authentic, and for continuous monitoring and reporting on activities and programs that are carried out on a daily, weekly, quarterly, and annual basis. The collation and analysis of these reports means that deep learning can occur as the patterns, habits, and achievements of the organization are identified. The action learning process contributes to developing a reliable disability information management system for each district, in departments of health, social development, labor, and education. The disability information management system needs to incorporate how information is communicated to all relevant role-players in the system, including families and community organizations, so that a comprehensive picture of a person with disability in the community is possible. For example, communication and transport systems are essential elements of an organization's capacity to achieve disability-inclusive service delivery.

Educators need to foster students' ability to learn how to select indicators so that relevant information is collected and properly managed. These indicators would be aligned to a specific program that corresponds to the elements of one or more of the five components of CBR that the organization has chosen to focus on. The unique contribution that occupational therapy practitioners and researchers make to social inclusion is through identification of those meaningful and purposeful occupations in which a person has potential to participate and that would lead to improved quality of life and fulfillment. The challenge is to determine indicators that can measure these occupational outcomes. An example of relevant indicators for one CBR component on inclusive education is shared in Box 7-7.

Agency is the capacity of an individual to make choices individually or to act collectively and purposefully to change a social structure. Courageous leadership for social change reflects the agency of individuals, groups, and communities that leads to sustained development. It involves the ability to make decisions that determine the path one intends to take in life, although societal structures may limit the choices of individuals and groups. Agency involves reflexivity regarding one's intentions.

INTENTIONAL LEADERSHIP: A THEORY FOR SOCIAL CHANGE

In Chapter 6, on professional reasoning for disability inclusion, I identified the need for occupational therapists to work collaboratively with different professionals in various sectors. In this section, relevant leadership approaches are described for occupational therapists to apply when promoting disability inclusion and the notion of intentional leadership in teaching, research, and practice. The five elements of radical collaboration (Tamm & Luyet, 2004) that may help occupational therapists build successful relationships are as follows:

BOX 7-7. POSSIBLE INDICATORS TO MONITOR THE EDUCATION COMPONENT OF COMMUNITY-BASED REHABILITATION PROGRAMS

- Increased social interaction of the person with disability and his or her family in community activities.
- Increased participation in decision making by parents of children with disabilities and persons with disabilities themselves. This could be measured by deciding on a percentage of children with disabilities who are part of screening and early identification programs.
- Determine percentage of children accessing early childhood development programs.
- Increased access and retention through primary and secondary education to completion for children with disabilities.
- The number of teachers trained to address barriers to learning for children with disabilities, including teachers with disabilities in mainstream or special schools.
- Use of universal design to make learning materials accessible for children with disabilities.
- Increased collaboration and coordination of services between health, education, social development, and other sectors through employment of community-based workers.
- Reassessment of children annually to evaluate progress and effectiveness of the program.

---

1. Identify the intention to collaborate
2. Build trustworthiness and openness
3. Create safe spaces where we can resolve conflicts, respond emotionally, and share vulnerabilities
4. Seek deeper self-awareness and awareness of others
5. Foster self-accountability and acceptance of responsibility for the choices we make and for learning skills and strategies for negotiating and solving problems

Box 7-8 illustrates how these elements guided the development of a collaborative research project on disabled youth's strategies for sustainable livelihoods, which involved academics, disabled people's organizations, and community organizations (Lorenzo & Joubert, 2011). The study found that each participant inspired and benefited from individual and collective participation.

Radical collaborative relationship building calls for active citizenship to hold the government and other stakeholders to account. Such collaboration is deepened by raising awareness and affirming conscious decision making and action that addresses the social injustices experienced by those who feel powerless. Mamphela Ramphele, a stalwart of the apartheid struggle in South Africa, has campaigned for active citizenship and transformational leadership following the country's transition to democracy (Ramphele, 2008), with the current challenges of addressing inequities in health and education, as well as social and economic development (Ramphele, 2012, 2013). Her approach of *Letsema circles* for healing the psychological and emotional scars of oppression and marginalization complements the professional reasoning of occupational therapists. The process encourages us to create spaces for dialogue involving persons with disabilities, their families, and other service providers in accessing resources and programs for social and economic development.

While transformational leadership calls for change, there is a need to be more focused and explicit in addressing policy imperatives for disability equity. For this reason, *intentional*

> ## Box 7-8. Learning How to Sustain Collaborative Relationships
>
> In a study exploring how youth with disabilities achieved sustainable livelihoods in South Africa, occupational therapy staff from six universities formed a research team, together with those community organizations where undergraduate students undertook their service learning placements and with disabled people's organizations in five provinces. Research workshops were held twice a year for 3 days, during which reciprocal capacity building occurred as safe spaces were established for mutual learning and the sharing of knowledge and experiences related to community-based research. At the end of a 3-year process, community workers were confident in participating in all stages of the research and referred to themselves as community academics. See Lorenzo and Joubert (2011) for details of the research process.

leadership is a conscious choice of action that draws the ideals of collaboration, proactivity, and transformation into a focused, purposeful direction. Occupational therapists may expect to carry out an action without any conscious idea of what the outcome will be. If, on the other hand, practitioners identify their intentions regarding the actions to be taken, they will think more deeply about the intended change. The reflective and reflexive practice of occupational therapists brings to consciousness the intended outcomes of an intervention, be it clinical practice, community-based occupational development, education, or research, but there is also a need to be aware of unintended consequences, which are the unplanned outcomes of action. Mistakes and failures are recognized and integrated with new learning and the shadow side of practice is related to how one's power as a profession may exclude or discriminate against a group.

In thinking about intentional leadership, occupational therapists draw on many factors as they need to hold together the various environmental and personal factors that influence participation when considering a plan of action or reflecting on what is happening and what needs to be done next. Chaffey and colleagues (2010) remind us that both intrinsic and extrinsic factors influence our reasoning. There needs to be continual reflection and communication of thoughts and ideas, and how decisions on what needs to be done are made. The CRPD (UN, 2006) and CBR Guidelines (WHO, 2010) call for the involvement of persons with disability in decision making.

Intentional leadership has the purpose of working collaboratively for sustained social change. Occupational therapy educators need to be intentional in their teaching of students and clinicians in undergraduate, postgraduate, and continuing professional development programs. This means that there is a deliberate, planned focus on addressing barriers to policy implementation and on monitoring disability inclusion. The intention of educators is also to instill in students and clinicians a conscious awareness of their power in relation to persons with disability and their families and of the need to work collaboratively with them. Together, they are able to make sense of the intentions and aspirations of policies from the different sectors that will ensure the implementation of disability-inclusive programs. As educators, we work primarily with students and clinicians who are adults, and so our pedagogy and methods of teaching and learning are informed by principles of adult education that enable practitioners to promote social justice in their practice.

CONCLUSION

The call for occupational therapists to be courageous in providing leadership related to disability inclusion is a thread throughout this chapter. Teaching organizational capacity as a theoretical framework consisting of six elements provides a means to generate a baseline on disability inclusion in services and programs of various organizations. This assessment enables monitoring of participation and access to activities, services, information, and documentation by persons with disabilities and their families.

Adult education principles and the action learning cycle assist educators, students, and practitioners to be conscious and raise awareness of the dynamics of disability inclusion. Curiosity and occupation-focused solutions draw on the intuitive nature of occupational therapists that strengthen reciprocal learning and agency for social change.

The WOOP provides an innovative teaching and monitoring tool for disability inclusion. The process fosters reciprocal learning and builds the capacity of stakeholders to strengthen efforts to remove barriers to participation. Learning how to identify outcomes to monitor progress in achieving disability inclusion will ensure the accountability of all stakeholders to each other.

The chapter ends with a call to intentional leadership in teaching and learning about disability inclusion so that educators remain focused on equipping all practitioners and researchers with sufficient capacity to achieve inclusive services and sustained development.

REFERENCES

Chaffey, L., Unsworth, C., & Fossey. E. (2010). A grounded theory of intuition among occupational therapists in mental health practice. *British Journal of Occupational Therapy, 73*, 300-308. doi:10.4276/030802210X12759925544308

Community Development Research Association. (2005). *Action learning: A developmental approach to change.* Retrieved from http://www.cdra.org.za/articles-by-cdra-practitioners.html

DasGupta, S., Fornari, A., Geer, K., Hahn, L., Kumar, V., Lee, H. J., et al. (2006). Medical education for social justice: Paulo Freire revisited. *Journal of Medical Humanities, 27*, 245-251. doi:10.1007/s10912-006-9021-x

Duncan, M., Sherry, K., & Watson, R. (2011). Disability and rurality. In T. Lorenzo (Ed.), *Intentions, pillars and players* (Disability Catalyst Africa, Series 1). Cape Town, South Africa: Disability Innovations Africa, Disability Studies Program, School of Health and Rehabilitation Sciences, University of Cape Town.

Hope, A., & Timmel, S. (1995). *Training for transformation: A handbook for community workers.* Gweru, Zimbabwe: Mambo Press.

Kaplan, A. (1999). *Organizational capacity.* Cape Town, South Africa: Community Development Resource Association. Retrieved from http://www.cdra.org.za

Lorenzo, T., & Joubert, R. (2011). Reciprocal capacity building for collaborative disability research between disabled people's organizations, communities and higher education institutions. *Scandinavian Journal of Occupational Therapy, 18*, 254-264.

Lorenzo, T., Ned-Matiwane, L., Cois, A., & Nwanze, I. (2013). *Youth, disability and rural area: Facing the challenges of change* (Disability Catalyst Africa: Series 3). Cape Town, South Africa: Disability Innovations Africa, Disability Studies Program, School of Health and Rehabilitation Sciences, University of Cape Town.

Lorenzo, T., & Sait, W. (2000, February). *Creating partners in disability: Lighting the candle of social human rights development* (Technical report for SCF Global Review of Community based rehabilitation). Commissioned by SCF Swaziland.

Lorenzo, T., van Pletzen, E., & Booyens, M. G. (2015). Determining the competencies of community based workers for disability-inclusive development in rural areas of South Africa, Botswana and Malawi. *International Journal of Remote and Rural Health, 15*, 2919.

Ramphele, M. (2008). *Laying ghosts to rest: Dilemmas of the transformation in South Africa.* Cape Town, South Africa: Tafelberg.

Ramphele, M. (2012). *Conversations with my sons and daughters.* Johannesburg, South Africa: Penguin.

Ramphele, M. (2013). *A passion for freedom.* Cape Town, South Africa: Tafelberg.

Ramugondo, E. L. (2012). Intergenerational play within family: The case for occupational consciousness. *Journal of Occupational Science, 19*, 326-340. doi:10.1080/14427591.2012.710166

Rifkin, S., & Kagere, M. (2002). What is participation? In S. Hartley (Ed.), *CBR: A participatory strategy in Africa*. London, England: University College London, Centre for International Child Health. Available on http:/afri-can. org

Tamm, J. W., & Luyet, R. J. (2004). *Radical collaboration: Five essential skills to overcome defensiveness and build successful relationships*. New York, NY: Harper Business.

Taylor, J., Marais, D., & Kaplan, A. (1997). *Action learning for development: Use your experience to improve your effectiveness*. Cape Town, South Africa: Juta.

Townsend, E., Wicks, A., van Bruggen, H., & Wright-St Clair, V. (2012). Imagining occupational therapy. *British Journal of Occupational Therapy, 75*, 42-44. doi:10.4276/030802212X13261082051490

Ubels, J. N., Baddoo, N.-A.-A., & Fowler, A. (Eds.). (2010). *Capacity development in practice*. London, England: Earth Scan. Available at http://www.capacity.org or http://www.snvworld.org/en/Pages/CapacityDevelopment.aspx

United Nations. (1993). *Standard rules on the equalization of opportunities for persons with disabilities*. New York, NY: Author.

United Nations. (2006). *Convention on the rights of persons with disabilities*. New York, NY: Author.

World Health Organization. (2010). *Community-based rehabilitation guidelines*. Geneva, Switzerland: Author.

8

Narrative Reasoning in Disability-Themed Films

Anne Hiller Scott, PhD, FAOTA, OTR/L and Richard Scott

> In our art
> We touch,
> If only for a moment,
> The realness of each other.
>
> (Anne Cronin Mosey, 1981)

Using the humanities where art serves as metaphor for life experiences is a staple in health care education (Darbyshire & Baker, 2012; Garden, 2010; Haller, 2012; Literature, Arts and Medicine Database NYU, 2014; Peloquin, 1996b). Films and documentaries portraying the disability experience serve as case studies for developing greater fluency with professional reasoning strategies (Garcia Sánchez & Garcia Sánchez, 2006; Garden, 2010; Hull, 2013). Exploring several types of illness narratives (Frank, 1995, 2013) revealed in disability films and documentaries presents a unique vehicle for enhancing competency in professional reasoning. In 1983, Rogers challenged therapists to critically use clinical reasoning within the ethics, art, and science of practice, blending humanistic and scientific elements. However, 30 years later, clinicians still struggle with effective application of professional reasoning (Reason, 2013).

Narrative reasoning is recognized as a centerpiece of practice (Burke & Kern, 1996; Clark, Ennevor, & Richardson, 1996; Mattingly, 1991, 1998, 2010). Mattingly and Fleming (1994) explored how therapists used two kinds of stories, storytelling and story making, as a vehicle to understand their clients' experience of illness and to project how treatment and future outcomes might evolve. Case studies are a basic staple of pedagogy to teach clinical reasoning (Kassirer, 2010). For physical therapy students learning clinical reasoning, the most valuable teaching tools were case studies and videos of actual patients (Babyar et al., 2003). Powerful disability narratives in film convey intense and vivid images with a sense of immediacy and potential for compelling learning experiences.

In everyday exchanges with clients, their narratives are not presented as closed captions superimposed on film, nor does occupational history emerge as chapter/scene headings. With film, one can replay the scene and revisit one's thinking to probe deeper into the complexity of working with

Cole, M. B., & Creek, J. (Eds.).
Global Perspectives in Professional Reasoning (pp. 117-143).
© 2016 Taylor & Francis Group.

people with disability (Burke, 2010; Giles, Carson, Breland, Coker-Bolt, & Bowman, 2014; Smith & Sparkes, 2011). It is incumbent on therapists to learn to read between the lines to reinterpret dialogue and plot. Empathetic understanding of the client's experience of the past and present, while forming a strong therapeutic relationship, supports the purpose and meaning the client values for his or her future narrative (Abreu, 2011; McColl, 2011g; Peloquin, 1996a). Through the process of story making and emplotment (discussed later in the chapter), therapists help clients to bridge the gap of present loss projecting toward future gains to create healing narratives (Clark, 1993; Mattingly, 1991; Mattingly & Fleming, 1994).

This chapter illustrates how exceptional films and documentaries about disability serve as illness narratives rendering poignant images of effective professional reasoning and facilitating a nuanced dialogue on practice. The ability to visualize the reasoning process is a powerful learning tool when it can be modeled and analyzed in real time, frame by frame. Being able to step back and stop action rarely happens in the clinical setting, and yet this can be a critical technique in clarifying how one interprets and reinterprets clinical information (Burke, 2010; Smith & Sparkes, 2011).

The first part of this chapter reviews the illness narrative literature as a premise for professional reasoning. To apply narrative reasoning in practice, the fundamentals are introduced: types of illness narratives, narrative analysis and methodology, ethical perspectives on professional interactions in various narrative domains with a client-centered focus, and how narratives resonate with meaning and spirituality. Lastly, the vital qualities of positive therapeutic interactions in occupational therapy (Abreu, 2011; Burke, 2010), therapeutic use of self and empathy (Abreu, 2011; Frank, 2013; Peloquin, 1995, 1996a, 1996b), are examined. With this knowledge we better understand the illness perspective supporting personal meaning and spirituality. These conceptual methodologies set the stage to view disability films using several learning experiences in the analysis of narratives and the reflective use of therapeutic relationships to plumb the depths of loss, isolation, stigma, pain, suffering, and courage. Through collaborative engagement in the artful use of the narrative process, we come to nurture therapeutic triumphs of the human spirit.

In the second section of the chapter, narrative reasoning is superimposed on disability films as a template for interpreting challenges in professional reasoning. Viewing films about people with serious illness or disability can enhance our appreciation of illness narratives (Garcia Sánchez & Garcia Sánchez, 2006; Pérez, 2013).

TYPES OF ILLNESS NARRATIVES

The moral imperative of narrative ethics is perpetual self-reflection on the sort of person that one's story is shaping one into, entailing the requirement to change that self-story if the wrong self is being shaped. The awareness of the general type of narrative one is telling or responding to—restitution, chaos or quest—is a crucial beginning. (Frank, 2013, p. 158)

Researchers from sociology, medicine, the humanities, and anthropology have examined the illness experience in film and literature (Darbyshire & Baker, 2012; Frank, 1995; Garden, 2010; Mattingly, 1998; Pérez, 2013) exploring how illness narratives portray patients' perspectives giving "voice" to their unique experiences (Frank, 1995, 2013; Literature, Arts and Medicine Database NYU, 2014). The three major types of illness narratives are restitution, chaos, and quest (Frank, 1995, 2013). These narratives have distinctive types of plots (biomedical or restitution), settings (hospital and rehabilitation centers), events (illness and disability), characters (patients, caregivers, and health care providers), emotional themes (that relate to all the characters), goals, and predictable as well as unforeseen outcomes or unknown endings. Frank also explored ethical dimensions and imperatives for sensitivity in practice reflecting a client-centered approach to interactions often critical of traditional biomedical protocol.

Restitution Illness Narratives

Frank likens the restitution scenario to a television commercial for a popular remedy product (Frank, 2013, pp. 79-80). The plot begins with a person coming down with an illness (e.g., a cold), which will interrupt or cancel an important event. In Scene 2, the character takes the remedy and shortly thereafter in the finale, health is restored and important activities are joyfully resumed. The restitution narrative focuses on restoring the body and resuming one's lifestyle. The hero is either the medical caregiver or the remedy, with the patient portraying the passive recipient of care.

Chaos Illness Narratives

The chaos narrative is seen as the opposite of restitution in which the illness and symptoms dominate. These stories are difficult to listen to because they generate anxiety for lack of immediate improvement. They are contrary to the typical (and preferred) sequence of remedy, progress, and resolution, which breaks down to reveal "vulnerability, futility, and impotence. If the restitution narrative promises the possibilities of outdistancing or outwitting suffering, the chaos narrative tells how easily any of us could be sucked under" (Frank, 2013, p. 97). In a chaos narrative, time perspective is lost in a never-ending present dominated by chaos with pain and disintegration dominating as the self becomes swept away. The experience of pain, uncertainty, and loss of control in chemotherapy is often described as a chaos narrative.

Kaethe Weingarten (2001), affiliated with the Dulwich Center of Narrative Therapy, authored an illness narrative illustrating her experience with Frank's chaos narrative:

> The chaos narrative [is] named for its obvious feature: its plot is chaotic. This illness narrative feels like being in a kayak in a class five rapid. While you are going through the rapids, time and place shift so rapidly, up and down, right and left transpose so often, that one truly feels inside a vortex, the way out of which is entirely unknown in any one moment. (Weingarten, 2001, para. 27)

Quest Illness Narratives

"Restitution stories attempt to outdistance mortality by rendering illness transitory. Chaos stories are sucked into the undertow of illness and the disasters that attend it" (Frank, 2013, p. 115). Now we consider the third type of narrative: "Quest stories meet suffering head on; they accept illness and seek to *use* it. Illness is the occasion of a journey that becomes a quest" (p. 115). Christopher Reeve personifies a compelling quest narrative in the aftermath of a horse-riding fall, which left him quadriplegic. After his tragic accident, Reeve had to reimagine his life. During an initial period of chaos, he considered suicide, but ultimately his mission became to find a cure for spinal cord injury, vowing he would walk again. "I have always been a crusader for causes I believe in. This time, the cause found me" (Christopher Reeve Foundation, 2014, para. 12).

Reeve's resolve turned from rehabilitation to research and fortified "with his conviction that 'nothing is impossible,' Christopher initiated a sea of change. Through his leadership . . . the Christopher & Dana Reeve Foundation was born and grew exponentially re-shaping the world of spinal repair research" (Christopher Reeve Foundation, 2014, para. 12). His quest narrative epitomizes the widespread and influential movement generated through his illness experience.

Illness Narrative Ethics

Frank referred to three aspects of ethics in the self-story: ethic of recollection, ethic of solidarity and commitment, and ethic of inspiration. In the telling and sharing of the self-story, "it becomes a self/*other* story" (2013, p. 132), available for others to identify with and experience a sense of belonging, of inspiration:

Ill people need to be regarded by themselves, by their caregivers and by our culture as heroes in their own stories . . . heroism is not perseverance but *doing*. . . . Quest stories as they are told, and chaos stories when they are honored, call for a shift from the hero as Hercules to the hero as Bodhisattva; from the hero of force to the hero of perseverance through suffering. The story is the means for the perseverance to become active, reaching out to others, asserting its own ethic. (Frank, 2013, p. 158)

Rather than serve simply as material for clinical analysis, the foundation of narrative ethics is to "think with [the] stories," immersing ourselves in the tale, with a "goal [of] empathy. . . . The other's self-story does not become my own, but I develop sufficient resonance with that story so that I can feel its nuances and anticipate changes in plot" (Frank, 2013, p. 158).

A challenge for health care providers is to listen to and to support clients in the midst of chaos narratives, which can trigger therapists' anxiety and fear of failure leading to denial of the storyteller's experience of reality. Health care professionals can

steer patients toward medical versions of liberation: treatment plans, rehabilitation, functional normality, lifestyle counseling, and remission. These phrases and many others like them reinstitute the restitution narrative . . . [however] life sometimes is horrible. The attendant denial of chaos only makes its horror worse. (Frank, 2013, p. 112)

It is a moral imperative to honor those in the midst of a chaos narrative; otherwise, we do not recognize their reality. "People whose reality is denied can remain recipients of treatments and services, but they cannot be recipients in empathic relations of care" (Frank, 2013, p. 109).

Narrative Reasoning in Occupational Therapy

With an unfolding illness story . . .
the meaning of life . . .
must be remade in the face of serious illness . . .
which does not merely damage a body but a whole life.

(Mattingly, 1998, p. 21)

The lives of our clients are often revealed in vignettes shared about critical personal events. As sensitive guides, therapists endeavor to understand clients' use of narratives, listening attentively to the story that gradually evolves within the clinical sessions. It is essential for therapists to facilitate client participation in the exploration of these events to help support and coauthor "healing dramas" (Mattingly, 1998). As clients use narratives, they can begin to articulate where they are in their illness journey, especially as they traverse periods of crisis and transition.

Mattingly's Ethnography

Mattingly (1991) observed therapist–client interaction within the dynamics of inpatient rehabilitation sessions. This ethnography "attends specifically to narrative as a structure of [occupational therapy] . . . practice" (Mattingly, 1998, p. 19). The narrative analysis process supported reflecting on practice rendered in syncopation with the client's evolving illness narrative. To focus on the client's illness experience was the core of clinical reasoning, rather than concentrating primarily on procedural treatment elements. Therapists were encouraged to create new stories for and with the client using a narrative feature called *emplotment*.

In team meetings, documentation, and informal discussions, therapists were observed engaging in two lines of reasoning. Using Bruner's model of cognitive thinking, the two forms of thought processes were identified as either paradigmatic or narrative (Bruner, 1986, 1990). Paradigmatic thinking is considered propositional referring to cognitive processes based on the use of reasoning and abstract principles, whereas the narrative mode is represented through storytelling. Telling stories is a universal way of sharing our life experiences.

In *chart talk*, therapists gave formal clinical case reports (assessment, findings, goals, intervention, and response), reflecting propositional or scientific principles (Mattingly, 1991, p. 999). In contrast, *storytelling* described the client and family members' participation as an unfolding personal story with emotional challenges reflecting the illness experience. Therapists' roles were to advance the client's story and to personalize therapy, engaging the patient in relevant activities that would link to rehabilitation objectives. Sometimes client resistance or obstacles in therapy were the springboard for developing a new "short story" (Mattingly, 1991, p. 1000) within this chapter of the client's narrative to gain his or her commitment to the hard work of therapy. The essence of this therapy-driven narrative was devising "powerful experiences of successfully met challenges . . . [and] the generation of therapeutic experiences along the way, in which clients developed increasing confidence and commitment to take on challenge" (Mattingly, 1991, p. 1002).

Keeping a Client-Centered Focus

Therapists were cautioned not to lose sight of the bigger picture; procedural reasoning and technical interventions can dominate the client–therapist interface and forestall real human needs. Intrinsic to therapists' problem solving is the recognition of how the illness is experienced by the individuals they are treating.

> [Therapists] often appeared unaware themselves of the profound human problems they were addressing. When they reduced their practice to helping someone feed himself, viewed as a kind of low-level technical task, they neglected the immense implications of their work and their patients' struggles, the level of shame and despair, which accompanies loss of the simple skills of everyday life. But when therapists recognized the subterranean phenomenological waters beneath a humdrum task like relearning to dress oneself, their practice was directed more to the illness experience than to the disease. (Mattingly, 1998, p. 21)

Mattingly maintained that through therapeutic emplotment, a dialogue is developed that sets the stage for narrative analysis that is client-centered. The therapist can help create a new story with ongoing discourse with the client regarding the impact of the illness on the meaning and purpose of his or her life and what the future may hold in stories yet untold.

An example of creating a new story line using therapeutic emplotment and expanding clients' narrative related to a group therapy called the Upper Extremity Group (Mattingly, 1991, pp. 1003-1004) that had a focus on exercising with equipment. Many of the patients were disengaged and rarely attended because this treatment approach did not speak to their narratives. The new group therapist in this New England facility drew from the clients' New York geographic roots to create a scene for the first session in which the therapy room became a New York City subway station, with her as the conductor. Therapeutic activities were embedded in this context by creating graffiti while using treatment equipment (weights, adapted drawing tools, etc.) to support treatment goals. Clients were quickly immersed in drawing or writing messages that depicted their frustrations and longings, engaging the body, mind, and emotions. They renamed the group the New York Gang. This new story line illustrated the "individualization of treatment goals" (Mattingly, 1991, p. 1003) that were person-centered and scaffolded by the primacy of sound professional reasoning, rather than following a standard clinical protocol that did not resonate with the patient's unique narrative (Rogers, 1983; Rogers & Kielhofner, 1985). To ensure patients move forward with a personalized narrative, the therapist needs to ask each new patient, "What story am I in?" (Mattingly, 1991, p. 1001).

Mattingly described a variation of emplotment with another category of narrative known as *borrowed stories* (2010), which occur when elements of well-known cultural stories/media heroes are incorporated into the client's unfolding treatment narrative. Fairy tales and popular film heroes are readily accessible to children. She tells of a young child who had been severely burned and was fitted for yet another uncomfortable pressure garment to prevent facial scarring. The therapist commented on how the facial mask looked like Spiderman. With this "borrowed story," the child began to more actively embrace difficult therapeutic challenges as the masked hero, supporting a "healing drama" (Mattingly, 2010, p. 181). Mattingly noted that "media manufactured dreams can offer a cultural resource for countering the waking nightmares that serious illness or disability provokes" (Mattingly, 2010, p. 180). These borrowed media-based stories offer greater flexibility than other illness narrative formats for ongoing variations through emplotment and co-construction (Frank, 2013).

NARRATIVE ANALYSIS AND THERAPEUTIC RESPONSES

To restore the human subject at the center—
the suffering, afflicted, fighting, human subject—
we must deepen a case history to a narrative or tale;
only then do we have a "who" as well as a "what," a real person,
a patient, in relation to disease—in relation to the physical.

(Sacks, 1987, p. viii)

Empathy

Frank urges clinicians to first be aware of the story the client is trying to convey and to be vigilant to the modulating flow of the narrative trajectory:

> The first lesson of thinking with stories is not to move on once the story has been heard, but to continue to live in the story, *becoming* in it, reflecting on who one is becoming, and gradually modifying the story. The problem is truly to *listen* to one's own story, just as the problem is truly to listen to others' stories. (Frank, 2013, p. 159)

Frank sees empathy as the medium to moderate and traverse difficult narratives being a sounding board with a true sense of "resonance" (Halpern, 1993).

It is especially difficult to hear chaos stories, and providers may distance themselves from the narratives' raw emotions and discordance rather than call on empathy resonating with the patient's experience (Smith & Sparkes, 2011). Frank (2013) suggested that medical staff may shift to "labeling" the patient as "depressed," a condition for which an effective treatment can be rendered. "When chaos is thus redefined as a treatable condition, the restitution narrative is restored" (p. 110). Chaos is an ever-present force that must be reckoned with; to ignore it is to deny the reality of the patient. In recent research, first-year physical therapy students were more open to hearing chaos stories, but third-year students preferred the more idealized restitution or quest story (Soundy, Smith, Cressy, & Webb, 2010). This is contrary to Frank's perspective: "What is needed, specifically in clinical work and more generally in any interpersonal relations, is an enhanced tolerance for chaos as part of a life story" (2013, pp. 110-111). This study recommended more emphasis on empathy in student training.

Empathic interpersonal relationships have been identified as a basic tenet of practice (Abreu, 2011; Peloquin, 1995; Taylor & van Puymbroeck, 2013). The question remains, however, of how skillful are therapists in projecting empathic resonance with their client's narratives. Qualitative research on a brain injury unit examining an interdisciplinary rehabilitation team's meetings and client interactions noted that the "clients were like ghosts... interdisciplinary team members did not empathetically interact with clients" (Abreu, 2011, p. 630). This finding was a "humbling experience" that highlighted the need to "improve and humanize our interactions with clients" (p. 630).

Abreu (2011), in *Accentuate the Positive: Reflections on Empathic Interpersonal Interactions*, identified six *positive interactions* to support empathy. Resonant with Frank (2013) and Mattingly's (1998) approaches of accessing the patient's narrative, Abreu (2011) took the position of "willingness to enter into the other person's emotional state and perspective" (p. 628). In doing this, she "sought a positive answer to the client's guiding question, *Are you sure you want to enter into my world?*" (p. 628). These *positive empathic interactions* supported client engagement. The first approach involved sharing "resilience stories" (p. 627) to kindle "inspiration and motivation" shedding light on "how do others like me cope and adapt" (p. 628). This example of using narratives and borrowed stories supports Frank's premise that the self/story becomes the self/*other* story through the "ethic of recollection, . . . the ethic of solidarity and commitment, . . . and the ethic of inspiration" (2013, pp. 132-133), honoring the illness experience as it is shared.

Another element of therapeutic relationships is appreciating the "pedagogy of suffering" (Frank, 2013, p. 145). How can therapists genuinely engage in healing dramas, which include pain, suffering, and uncertain or even terminal outcomes? Particularly if they assume the subtext for rehabilitation stories is the biomedical model with a predictable course of restoration/restitution versus the possibility of a chaos narrative. Paying honor to the "pedagogy of suffering" speaks to a social ethic of recognizing the vulnerability of the person and stories that are told "*through* a wounded body" (Frank, 2013, p. 2).

Many authors have noted the link between suffering and the meaning of life, and it is particularly relevant in life-threatening illnesses like cancer, where "suffering is experienced as 'total pain'—in relation to physical, psychological and existential distress" (Lethborg, Aranda, & Kissane, 2008, p. 68). The healing effect of narratives is recognized in cancer care literature (Lethborg et al., 2008) and can be beneficial in "enabling the expression of existential pain and suffering, cognitive processing of a life that has been disrupted, and enhancing the dignity by enabling the patient to share who he or she is as a unique person" (p. 63).

This cancer care model highlighted three primary domains: suffering, meaning, and coping. "Suffering exposes the limitations of one's existence, bringing about a greater awareness of the meaning in life" (Lethborg et al., 2008, p. 62). A critical role for therapists is to acknowledge the patient's pain and courage providing comfort and support in the context of meaningful occupations. These researchers proposed care addressing four goals: "encouraging meaning and purpose, acknowledging suffering, strengthening connections with others, and optimal palliative care" (Lethborg et al., 2008, p. 61). This approach appears relevant for many of our clients experiencing the "shame and despair" (Mattingly, 1998, p. 21) of serious disability.

Lastly, Frank (2004a) explored the quality of generosity in the therapeutic exchange. Mattingly commented that "generosity and small attentions are not the stuff of the medical chart" (1998, p. 22). Frank (2004b) described a "paradigm of consolation" (p. 2) and suggested that there is a real need for consolation to be extended with warmth and generosity similar to that of an attentive hostess. "The next level of generosity redefines health, illness, and death" (Frank, 2004b, p. 68), and "medical hospitality" (p. 3) serves to reduce the stigma and isolation of the illness experience.

Meaning

"Meaning in life is experienced as a total life orientation including a person's global beliefs, spiritual beliefs and a motivation to meaning" (Lethborg et al., 2008, p. 68). Meaning is one of the words most commonly associated with discussions of spirituality (McColl, 2011e). Drawing from Thibodaux (1998), McColl wrote: "meaning can derive from personal attributions, social or cultural values, or it can derive from the opportunity to see universal truths, and to see one's life in relation to the grander scheme of things" (2011d, p. 64). The exploration of the impact of patients' illness on their spiritual well-being intersects with their view of what gives purpose to their life and is also directly related to Frank's (2013) recognition of helping people "live a good life while being ill" (p. 156). Meaning is also emphasized in cancer care transcending the pain and struggle with this disease. Meaning is

> described as a commitment to making the most of the time left and awareness of what has been significant in life, with a determination to value these.... Also reflected in relating to others, deep understanding of inner strengths, a sense of personal significance, cherished moments of beauty, peace and intimacy with loved ones, a feeling of awe about human connectedness and a union with nature. (Lethborg et al., 2008, p. 68)

Lethborg et al. (2008) discovered that the use of narratives with people in cancer care provided them with the opportunity to explore their personal meanings and for staff to support and embrace the individual's spirituality in the process. As therapists, we need to consider our own emotional responses and potential biases, along with recognition of spirituality and meaning for the client in order to embody our therapeutic use of self with empathy (Abreu, 2011; Peloquin, 1995), "generosity of spirit," and a "paradigm of consolation" (Frank, 2013).

Spirituality

"It is necessary to understand spirituality from the perspective of people in the midst of spiritual change, growth, recovery or loss" (McColl, 2011f, p. 39). Views of disability often intersect with spiritual perspectives, such as the illness as a reflection of a greater power or the "will of God," as punishment, the redemptive value of suffering, as a source of sustenance, or part of the course of life (McColl, 2011e). As therapists, we bear both a personal and professional relationships to the topic of spirituality. To support client-centered spiritual values, we must maintain an appropriate stance, appreciating and respecting individual beliefs and diversity.

Since spirituality was introduced in the Canadian Model of Occupational Performance more than three decades ago (Canadian Association of Occupational Therapists and Department of National Health and Welfare, 1983), it has generated much discourse. Unruh, Versnel, and Kerr (2002) maintained that spirituality encompasses three dimensions—religious, sacred, and secular—representing a continuum from religious faith and practice, to the sacred, which holds "a force beyond human understanding, but not necessarily aligned with a specific religion or faith tradition" (McColl, 2011b, p. 55), to a secular, nonreligious perspective of the universe and humans (Unruh et al., 2002). Inquiry about clients' spiritual history (Rousseau, 2000) should help establish their values on this spirituality continuum. Puchalski and colleagues (2009) described several effective clinical history models for a spiritual history "to understand spiritual needs and resources" (p. 893).

A survey of Canadian therapists on spirituality revealed limited resonance between the professional emphasis on spirituality and its evidence in practice (McColl, 2011e). Most of the therapists acknowledged having sought additional "informal preparation" (McColl, 2011e, p. 50) for addressing religion or spirituality through independent study and personal development.

Addressing the role of pain, suffering, and self-exploration speaks to the client's spiritual views and responses. However, McColl (2011a) noted that therapists are generally more comfortable with *doing* rather than *being* (p. 272). "Spirituality requires stillness, reflection and the absence of *doing*" (p. 272). In regard to using spirituality in practice, other potential barriers are (McColl, 2011a, pp. 271-274) concern about the "personal–professional barrier," treating spirituality like a procedural modality, and the ongoing difficulty of language and definition of spirituality. For therapists working with clients in the midst of a painful chaos narrative, it can be a challenge to listen and to offer support and consolation with a spirit of generosity. Beyond physical and mental rehabilitation, we should bring sensitivity to concerns related to spirituality and emotional adaptation. This may require an adjustment of the therapist's view of therapeutic use of self and use of these processes to engage as coauthor in the personalization of the client's narrative with emplotment of individualized and meaningful goals in the spiritual realm (Mattingly, 1991).

Are there qualities of occupation that resonate with spirituality? McColl (2011c) recommends that occupation can serve as a "doorway to spirit" (p. 93). Occupations nurturing spirituality have these qualities: "familiar, expressive, purposeful, temporal and meaningful" (p. 93). Furthermore, these occupations serve as a bridge to "connect with self, others, the world and divine with a view of the persons' past, present and future" (p. 93). Spiritual health interventions (Pulchalski et al., 2009, p. 895) can address therapeutic communication skills, therapy, and self-care interventions with occupations such as "breathing practices, progressive relaxation, yoga, tai chi, art therapy (music, art, dance), journaling and use of storytelling." Rousseau (2000, p. 2002) offered guidelines on spiritual evaluation and intervention, including life review, religious expression, reframing goals, meditation, and guided imagery.

NARRATIVE REASONING IN FILM ANALYSIS

Through arts, therapists can learn about life from a number of scenes and characters.
They can step into experiences with illness, disability, and occupation,
using the realities of fiction as opportunities for observation,
reflection, and understanding.

(Peloquin, 1996a, p. 660)

Peloquin (1996a) heralded the "arts' use of metaphor to describe meaning" (p. 659), and disability films can yield many insights. "I came to see therapists in a role very much akin to that of a director of a film," Burke (2010, p. 860) related in *What's Going on Here? Deconstructing the Interactive Encounter.* "Therapists need to conceive and know the possibilities that a therapeutic interaction can produce and, like directors" (Burke, 2010, p. 860), they can benefit from "possess[ing] experience in the production process and have a strong sense of story development" (Osgood & Hinshaw, 2009, p. 6).

Burke (2010) analyzed films of occupational therapy pediatric assessment to better understand the "therapeutic juncture [which offers a time and place] to discover how therapists create therapeutic interaction, manage information, and direct action during therapy session" (p. 860). Using the technique of *microanalysis*, Burke analyzed assessment videotapes with each frame slowed down to one thirtieth of a second, offering an exquisitely detailed opportunity to review verbal and nonverbal content in context. Other processes used included line drawings of participants in frames and "conversation and movement convention" (p. 866) analyzing the complexity of the therapist's interactions with parents, children, and the environment. Analysis revealed patterns of therapeutic interactions among therapists and participants as well as missed opportunities for connections.

Abreu (2011) referred to the literature in social neuroscience on the development of empathy. Empathy has been identified as part of the mirror-neuron system and the insula and limbic systems (Berntson et al., 2011), along with other areas of the brain that support emotion and social cognition (Kramer, Mohammadi, Donamayor, Samii, & Munte, 2010). Through the mechanism of the mirror system, empathy is refined through

the perception of self and other as well as its facilitation, imitation, and communication.... Through imitation and the simulation of emotions and postures, we verbally and nonverbally communicate, make inferences from visible actions of personal and emotional states. This process enables us to respond in a more empathic manner to other people. (Abreu, 2011, p. 626)

This phenomenon explains in part how viewers of film can develop their own social cognition through empathizing with the film's characters, whether real or fictional. Reflection on this process can also inform our ability to reason in therapeutic encounters.

Approaches to Film Analysis

As novices of film analysis, we will use more traditional approaches, viewing film scenes with guiding analytic questions to "observe, analyze and deconstruct" (Burke, 2010, p. 860) film segments. Like Burke, our goal is to not only discover and describe characteristics and patterns of therapeutic interaction, but also to refine and critique practice. Watching others with effective or ineffective interactions, we can begin to emulate more empathic and healing responses.

To prepare for analyzing disability narratives, we first review primary types of illness narratives with integration of professional reasoning and therapeutic use of self. The *Occupational Therapy Practice Framework* (American Occupational Therapy Association [AOTA], 2014) includes narrative reasoning in the description of therapeutic use of self, which "allows occupational therapy practitioners to develop and manage their therapeutic relationship with clients by using narrative and clinical reasoning; empathy; and a client-centered, collaborative approach to service delivery" (AOTA, 2014, p. S120; Taylor & van Puymbroeck, 2013). Narrative reasoning (AOTA, 2014) is implicit in our therapeutic interactions and problem solving. Abreu (2011) and Peloquin (1995) have emphasized the importance of empathy as an essential quality of therapeutic use of self for "ensuring that practitioners connect with clients at an emotional level to assist them with their current life situation" (AOTA, 2014, p. S12; Taylor & van Puymbroeck, 2013).

The therapeutic relationship should also convey qualities valued in the illness narrative literature (Frank, 1995, 2013; Mattingly & Garro, 2000; Smith & Sparkes, 2011), recognizing the patients' suffering, "encouraging meaning and purpose, strengthening connections with others" (Lethborg et al., 2008, p. 68), and offering empathy and compassionate caring with generosity (Frank, 2004b, 2013). The ultimate consideration is the path the patients value for their changing life story as they reorient and reconnect their past, present, and future, embracing the essence of their spirituality and the people, passions, and pursuits that are most meaningful to them (McColl, 2011c).

DISABILITY FILMS AND THERAPEUTIC INTERACTIONS

Viewing disability films and therapeutic encounters can provide us with a unique opportunity for self-reflection and modeling of therapeutic interactions to expand our capacity for empathy. Comparable to case-based learning, the disability film viewing experience allows us to unobtrusively visit and replay how we would use professional reasoning within the illness narrative. Kassirer (2010) proposed that case-based learning affords the opportunity for immediate feedback and to review errors with an experienced coach/mentor reinforcing mastery of the reasoning process. In occupational therapy, the use of reflective video analysis for student assessments with simulated patients was a valuable approach, providing opportunity for faculty feedback and self-critique (Giles et al., 2014).

Smith and Sparkes (2011) examined responses to a chaos narrative and recommended for enhanced learning the use of "videotaping digital technology and the subsequent microanalysis of frame-to-frame records of embodied action" (p. 49). Similar to Burke's microanalysis, this allows exploration of verbal exchanges as well as silences. Abreu (2011) also sought other cues to "attend at a deep level" (p. 629) to the client's experience, by "read[ing] the client's actions, language patterns, variations and prosody," appreciating not only "what is said . . . but how [they] say it" (p. 629). Dialogue in film and in real life includes verbal exchanges, but we should also attend to what is left unsaid "to the multiple meanings of silence" and to appreciate the "various ways in which the body via its movement, postures and gestures is used to communicate meanings and inform responses that, even though they are beyond words, are central to the manifestation of the telling and listening self" (Smith & Sparkes, 2011, p. 52).

PROFESSIONAL REASONING IN DISABILITY FILM NARRATIVES

Clients' occupational narratives reveal the overall meaning of life events,
signifying their place in a plot that integrates past, present and future.
(Goldstein, Kielhofner, & Ward, 2004, p. 119)

In anticipation of firsthand experience applying narrative analysis, we will use illness narratives from disability films. This gives us an opportunity to view the human condition through a cinematic lens, reviewing or replaying scenes from clients' lives to further understanding narrative analysis and professional reasoning. We can consciously identify clients' narrative honoring their voice connecting on an empathetic level while nurturing a healing relationship and discourse. As therapists, we coauthor narratives, reflecting client-centered meaning using occupations that engage body, mind, and spirituality.

In movies, narrative sometimes unfolds in real time, as in a documentary or in a film with a creatively edited series of scenes that shifts among past, present, and future in nonsequential patterns. However, the profound experience of viewing a client's changing condition in real time in an uncertain course of treatment can be a daunting process for all involved. Therapists should avoid engaging reflexively in the restitution/rehabilitation model of narrative analysis. Sensitive therapists are more likely to recognize and address the illness experience rather than the disability in isolation (Mattingly, 1991). Staying in the moment helps therapists respond to the client in an emotionally interactive process, engaging him or her in "real time," as it were.

To analyze the film-based cases for several disability films, a synopsis of the films is provided, followed by the Film Analysis Learning Experience to synthesize the readers' experience with concepts of narrative reasoning, therapeutic use of self, empathy, and spirituality. Table 8-1 provides a variety of resources for the film analysis.

Through narrative reasoning, the client's experience of his or her life story and the challenges of his or her illness may be confronted and transformed to reach desired goals through occupation; while reframing his or her identity from "dependent victim to . . . purposive agent" (Polkinghorne, 1996, p. 303).

FILM ANALYSIS LEARNING EXPERIENCES

Four film viewing experiences are offered in this section. Each has a different focus, with guided questions and topics for writing and reflection. The reader is advised to begin by reviewing from the text and Glossary, the definitions and components of narrative reasoning based on Frank (1995, 2013) and Mattingly (1991), therapeutic interaction characteristics (empathy, compassion, etc.), and qualities of meaning and spirituality.

How to View the Films

To participate in this learning experience, you will need to view the films, but rather than viewing them in one sitting, view small segments to systematically analyze the plot, the narratives, interactions, and the clinical course. It is helpful to jot down brief notes, questions, and reactions, which can help organize your observations, reflections, and learning. It is natural to want to see the story in one viewing. However, this is often at the loss of details important for the overall perspective of evaluating the professional reasoning process.

TABLE 8-1	
DISABILITY FILMS FOR NARRATIVE ANALYSIS	
FILM	**WEBSITE AND RESOURCES**
Awakenings (Parkes, Lasker, & Marshall, 1990). Based on Sacks (1963).	*Awakenings.* (1990). Quotes. Retrieved from www.imdb.com/title/tt0099077/quotes Article on original events from *Awakenings*: Jiménez Serranía (2007)
Silver Linings Playbook (Giglotti, Cohen, & Gordon, 2012). Based on Quick (2008).	Trailer: www.imdb.com/title/tt1045658/ Article online (president of American Psychiatric Association Jeffrey Lieberman; trailer interview with director/screenwriter David O. Russell): www.cnn.com/2013/01/30/health/lieberman-mental-illness-movie/ *Silver Linings Playbook* (2012) Quotes—selections of extensive dialogue from major scenes: www.moviequotes andmore.com/silver-linings-playbook-quotes.html#1
Alive Day Memories: Home From Iraq (Gandolfini, Alpert, & Kent Goosenberg, 2004).	HBO Alive Day official website: Trailer and biographies of soldiers: www.hbo.com/documentaries/alive-day-memories-home-from-iraq/index.html# View on YouTube: Part 1: www.youtube.com/watch?v=L4yCdblq1tk Part 2: www.youtube.com/watch?v=CswHis8T3FA Part 3: www.youtube.com/watch?v=2SLaNy9wWhl Part 4: www.youtube.com/watch?v=LEoEYOmPpBE
Voice/Over (Barry, Bonilla, & Garoian, 2004).	View on YouTube: *Voice/Over*, second part of trilogy *Whole—A Trinity of Being*: https://www.youtube.com/watch?v=0Ubl_Rl2i2w Article: Hiadki (2008)

I. WATCHING A MASTER CLINICIAN—*AWAKENINGS*

A unique way to observe the intricacies of the professional reasoning process is to see the evolution of an illness narrative through the eyes of an experienced researcher. Dr. Oliver Sacks, through his illness narratives, is acknowledged for "rewrite[ing] the art and science of medicine" (Hull, 2013). *Awakenings* (Parkes, Lasker, & Marshall, 1990), scripted from Sacks' book (1963), chronicles his work with patients with dementia and other chronic mental illnesses at Beth Abraham Hospital in Bronx, New York.

As you screen the film, complete the exercises in the Film Analysis Learning Experience to document how you observe and identify the professional reasoning process at work. Table 8-1 has another resource, a medical article about the actual patients and events (Jiménez Serranía, 2007). The film synopsis provides a brief overview of the plot (refer to Table 8-2).

TABLE 8-2

AWAKENINGS: FILM DESCRIPTION AND SYNOPSIS

SETTING

The movie set is Beth Abraham Hospital in Bronx, New York. In the film, Robin Williams plays Dr. Sacks, a trained neuroscientist who has accepted a position as a clinical physician in this hospital for the chronic mentally ill, some of whom have been institutionalized for decades.

PRIMARY CHARACTERS AND CAST

Dr. Malcolm Sayer: Robin Williams

Nurse Eleanor Costello: Julie Kavner

Leonard Lowe (patient): Robert DeNiro

Mrs. Lowe (Leonard's mother): Ruth Velso

Lucy Fishman (patient): Alice Drummond

Dr. Kaufman (supervising MD/administrator): John Heard

DR. SAYER'S ROLE

Dr. Sayer enters the setting filled with good intentions and research experience, but he is not a mental health practitioner. He overcomes this obstacle with compassion and a strong desire to help the patients awaken from what seems like a permanent slumber. He brings to bear all of his insights as a scientist to find the key that unlocks the door that seems to be blocking the patients from escaping the catatonic state in which they are imprisoned. By bonding with the patients, he gains their trust, discovering that they are more aware of reality than they appear to be. With compassion and scientific exploration, he penetrates the thick fog of dementia to find the humanity and individuality that has been suppressed by the illness. Dr. Sayer reasons that L-Dopa, a drug used to treat Parkinson disease, might have a beneficial effect on the patients. Using the drug with one of them, a seemingly miraculous result takes place. The patient is able to communicate and respond in a way that had been dormant for 20 years. Eventually the drug is used with all the patients, with varied but mostly positive outcomes. Unfortunately, these results are short lived and the patients return to their previous conditions.

CLOSE-UP OF LEONARD

Through flashbacks, we see one of the patients, Leonard, struggling as a child to keep up with the other children, with little success. No longer able to move or speak, he eventually had to be cared for at home by his mother. Talking to Leonard's mother helped Dr. Sayer gain a better understanding of the situation. Her ability to communicate with her son and to feel that he was responding to her was an indication that

(continued)

Table 8-2 (continued)
Awakenings: Film Description and Synopsis

Leonard was more "awake" than previously assumed. During a test of Leonard's brain waves, Dr. Sayer discovered that saying the patient's name produced brain-wave activity. Later, in an attempt to get Leonard to spell his name on a Ouija board, Leonard instead spells the name of a poem and its author. The poem was "The Panther" by Rainer Marie Rilke (1902). Upon reading it, Dr. Sayer knew he was plunging head-first down the rabbit hole into the very place that Leonard and perhaps the other patients dwelled. The brilliant metaphors of the poem were a touchstone and a road map to navigating the landscape of this illness from the inside looking out.

The Panther
(Poem by Rainer Marie Rilke)
His vision, from the constantly passing bars,
has grown so weary that it cannot hold
anything else. It seems to him there are
a thousand bars; and behind the bars, no world.
As he paces in cramped circles, over and over,
the movement of his powerful soft strides
is like a ritual dance around a center
in which a mighty will stands paralyzed.
Only at times, the curtain of the pupils
lifts, quietly—. An image enters in,
rushes down through the tensed, arrested muscles,
plunges into the heart and is gone.

Through his experiences with Lucy and Leonard, Dr. Sayer believes that there is hope that these patients can be helped. He reasons that L-Dopa might be beneficial. He gains permission to use the drug with Leonard, and after several days there is a dramatic improvement. The panther is no longer pacing behind bars, his will no longer paralyzed. The curtain of the pupils lifts to allow images heretofore unseen or received. The panther is alive and awake.

Film Analysis Learning Experience I—Awakenings

The purpose of this learning experience is to sensitize you to the types and use of professional reasoning in illness narratives, appropriate therapeutic use of self, and recognition of meaning and spirituality applied to practice as portrayed in the film. The first step is becoming more familiar with the concepts through seeing them on film. A unique aspect of film is to be able to view scenes from multiple perspectives (different staff members, patients, and caregivers) and to revisit scenes for reflection and clarification.

If you would like more clinical information on the actual medical story of *Awakenings*, refer to the article by Jiménez Serranía (2007), which is available online in English and Spanish. After viewing the film, answer these questions.

Types of Illness Narratives

Use the outline below to identify three scenes illustrating various types of illness narratives. Each scene should include one of the major characters: Leonard, Leonard's mother, Lucy, or someone else. For each scene/narrative, describe the typical themes associated with the illness narrative and the therapeutic response of the health care provider.

a. Brief scene description:

b. Character:

c. List type of illness narrative:

d. Identify examples of emotions/plot and activities/themes typically associated with this type of narrative and what you observed in the scene:

e. Does the character experience stigma and loss? Discuss.

f. Describe what has meaning and spiritual relevance for the character:

g. Provide examples of therapeutic response to emotions expressed (empathy, compassion, being with the patient in his or her story, etc.):

h. Give examples of narrative analysis (addressing the illness experience, storytelling, emplotment, etc.).

Therapeutic Interactive Approaches

Review Frank (1995, 2013), Mattingly (1991), Abreu (2011), and Burke (2010) and consider appropriate therapeutic interactive responses to the characters.

a. List two or three therapeutic interactions used in specific scenes by Dr. Sayer or Nurse Costello and include the film scene:

CHARACTER	FILM SCENE	THERAPEUTIC INTERACTIVE APPROACHES

b. Chose three scenes and give two or three examples of therapeutic interactions that you could display relating to the character if you were employed in the setting in the designated scenes.

CHARACTER	FILM SCENE	THERAPEUTIC INTERACTIVE APPROACHES

Summary

In terms of knowledge of professional reasoning, as you review the responses on the Film Analysis Learning Experience—*Awakenings*, comment on your insights and expanded understanding of the application of these concepts.

For a synopsis and description of the main characters in *Awakenings*, please refer to Table 8-2.

II. Exploring the Theme of Mental Illness: *Silver Linings Playbook*

The second disability film analysis is of a contemporary film also relating to the theme of mental illness, *Silver Linings Playbook* (Gigliotti, Cohen, Gordon, & Russell, 2012). The film's director, David O. Russell, also wrote the screenplay, adapted from the book by Michael Quick (2008). After reviewing the film and the synopsis in Table 8-3, proceed with the Film Analysis Learning Experience and refer to Table 8-1 for resources.

Film Analysis Learning Experience II—Silver Linings Playbook

The focus of this film analysis will include application of principles of narrative analysis and therapeutic interactive approaches. Review these concepts from the chapter before starting this exercise. Table 8-1, which provides film quotes and other resources, offers extensive dialogue from film scenes, which will be helpful for this learning experience. You can also refer to Table 8-3 for the synopsis.

Narrative Analysis: Chart Talk and Storytelling

Mattingly (1991) referred to *chart talk* as the official dialogue that therapists use in medical reports and storytelling as their perspective on the personal story of the patient. In this film, Pat's symptoms are revealed as the plot develops. As therapists, we can also transcribe the symptoms to chart talk by acknowledging how they fit in the diagnostic criteria. Then, going back to the story and through storytelling, we can see how they have an impact on Pat's life. Use the Fifth Edition of the *Diagnostic and Statistical Manual of Mental Disorders* (DSM-5; American Psychiatric Association, 2013) to list the major criteria of symptoms for the diagnosis of bipolar disorder (Pat's diagnosis). Document symptoms as they occur in the film and comment on how they influence Pat's emotions and behavior.

a. List the film scene, corresponding symptom(s), and narrative impact:

FILM SCENE	CHART TALK: DSM-5 SYMPTOM	STORYTELLING: PAT'S IMPACT ON OTHERS

b. How has this exercise affected your view of diagnostic symptoms, chart talk, and storytelling?

TABLE 8-3
SILVER LININGS PLAYBOOK: FILM DESCRIPTION AND SYNOPSIS

SETTINGS

The Philadelphia home of the Solitano family and the neighboring community and Eagles football team and stadium.

PRIMARY CHARACTERS AND CAST

Pat: Bradley Cooper

Tiffany: Jennifer Lawrence

Pat's father, Pat Sr.: Robert DeNiro

Pat's mother: Jackie Weaver

Pat's friend, Danny: Chris Tucker

Pat's best friend and Tiffany's brother-in-law, Ronnie: John Ortiz

Dr. Patel: Anupam Kher

Pat Solitano, who has bipolar disorder, is released from Karel Psychiatric Facility into the care of his parents after 8 months of treatment. This is a forensic facility where patients are committed for behavior that is considered criminally insane. Pat is determined to reunite with his estranged wife, Nikki, who obtained a restraining order against him because of his violent behavior. Against medical advice, he stops taking his medication and embarks on a mission to reinvent himself.

Upon entering the reception area of Pat's court-appointed psychiatrist, he hears Stevie Wonder's song "My Cherie Amour" (1969) playing over the speakers and goes into a rage. After calming down, he confronts Dr. Patel about the song and is told that it was played intentionally to see if it was still a trigger. Apparently, Pat had come home early from work one day and discovered Nikki having sex with another man, as Pat and Nikki's wedding song, "My Cherie Amour," played in the background. Overcome with rage, he nearly beat the man to death. Dr. Patel uses Pat's violent reaction to the song in the waiting room to illustrate that discontinuing medication is not an option. Pat tries to downplay the reaction and also asserts that the crime that got him committed was "just one incident." Dr. Patel replied that "one incident can change a lifetime."

At dinner with his friend Ronnie, Pat meets Ronnie's sister-in-law, Tiffany Maxwell, a recently widowed young woman who also just lost her job and is suffering with depression. Pat and Tiffany develop an odd friendship through their shared mental illness, and Tiffany asks Pat to be her partner in a dance competition. He reluctantly agrees, and the two begin a practice regimen over the following weeks. The dancing seems to be a cathartic and therapeutic bonding experience for both of them.

Narrative Reasoning and Therapeutic Interactive Approaches

This question draws from Mattingly (1991) and Frank's (2013) narrative analysis and concepts of therapeutic interaction from Abreu (2011) and Burke (2010). In the outline that follows, describe two or three therapeutic approaches used by Dr. Patel to treat Pat and the type of narrative.

FILM SCENE	TYPE OF NARRATIVE	THERAPEUTIC INTERACTIVE APPROACHES

a. How effective were Dr. Patel's approaches? Would you modify them? Why? How?

b. How has this exercise affected your view of therapeutic interactive resources?

Illness Experience and Creating New Chapters in the Narrative

This film provides multiple perspectives on how an illness is viewed. Considering the illness experience in Mattingly's discussion of narrative analysis, we can gain a deeper appreciation of Pat's struggle to move on with his life and goals, and how his sense of meaning and spirituality are transformed in the process. We also witness how others (family, friends, and doctor) try to coauthor new chapters for Pat's recovery.

Describe briefly the narrative of Pat's illness from varying perspectives. Consider changes in perspective at the beginning and middle of the narrative before the dance contest. Also consider the family dynamics and the role of stigma and loss. Describe the illness experience from the perspective of each character.

ILLNESS NARRATIVE AND THEMES (E.G., FAMILY DYNAMICS, LOSS, STIGMA)		
CHARACTER	BEGINNING OF STORY	MIDDLE OF STORY
Pat		
Pat's mother		
Pat's father		
Dr. Patel		
Tiffany		

Using Frank's categories of narratives (restitution, chaos, and quest), classify each of the foregoing narratives (choosing a specific scene) and the characteristic emotions, experiences, and responses associated with them.

Narrative Reasoning

a. Consider Pat and how his narrative changed when he was released from the institution and what challenges existed.

b. What strategies and occupational pursuits supported or undermined him?

c. What role does meaningful activity and spirituality play in his narrative?

Occupational Narrative

a. Give an example of an occupational narrative from Tiffany's perspective.

b. What role does meaningful activity and spirituality play in her narrative?

Summary

How has your understanding of illness narratives, emotional themes, and narrative reasoning evolved?

For a synopsis and description of the main characters in *Silver Linings Playbook*, refer to Table 8-3.

III. Chaos Narratives in Disability Films and Documentaries: *Alive Day Memories: Home From Iraq*

Chaos narratives can temporarily or permanently derail a client's life story. Disability films and documentaries offer an extended temporal dimension before, during, and after a disabling condition with the evolving narrative played in real time. Documentaries transcend temporal boundaries revealing a perspective that a therapist would rarely, if ever, have. *Alive Day Memories; Home From Iraq* (Gandolfini, Alpert, & Kent Goosenberg, 2004) is a powerful example offering narrative snapshots of 10 severely injured US Iraq War veterans. The term *alive day* refers to the date of injury and the concept that this is the first day of their "new" life postinjury.

This project, produced and narrated by James Gandolfini, bears witness to the tumultuous impact on the lives of survivors, whose injuries are massive, including multiple amputations, disfigurement, loss of vision or hearing, traumatic brain injury, and posttraumatic stress disorder. Some stories include videos of the person's lifestyle and valued occupations before injury, poignantly conveying the trauma of the injury, loss, and tortuous journey back to a more functional place. For some, the journey is foreclosed; for others, emotional scars and psychological devastation plunge even deeper than physical scars. The narratives of these survivors project indelible images that barely scratch the surface of how difficult, if not impossible, it is to understand their illness experience. Such films provide a unique introduction to a perspective most resonant with chaos narratives. After viewing the film, complete the Film Analysis Learning Experience. Table 8-1 lists resources to access the film, trailer, and biographies.

Film Analysis Learning Experience III—Alive Day Memories

As the filmed interviews with individual veterans are very brief, only several minutes each, the film analysis for *Alive Day Memories: Home From Iraq* is structured differently. For additional information, you can refer to the film, the trailers, and to the biographies on the HBO *Alive Day Memories: Home From Iraq* website in Table 8-1.

Questions

View two stories from the film and review the corresponding biographies from the website. These stories vividly bring to life Mattingly's (1991) illness experience and Frank's (1995, 2013) chaos narratives. For each of the veteran's stories, respond to the following:

a. Describe the type of narrative(s), and discuss the relevant themes portrayed (loss, pain, suffering, feeling alone, courage, stigma, etc.) and note if they changed over time.

b. Comment on the role of meaning and spirituality in their lives and how or if it changed.

c. Comment on how you would like to see the client/patient/caregivers proceed with therapy and with their lives. What would be their therapeutic story if you were creating a new chapter of their narrative?

d. What are your personal and emotional responses to the client/patient and the family/caregivers?

e. How would your personal and emotional responses affect your future interactions with the client/patient?

f. What would be difficult for you about working with this client/patient, that is, "being" with the patient in his or her story?

g. How would you construct the therapist's response demonstrating sensitivity to the patient's suffering with use of empathy, compassion, hospitality, etc.?

h. What you have learned about the illness experience and chaos narrative from these veterans?

i. Discuss the emotional impact you experienced in response to these stories.

IV. DISABILITY ADVOCACY IN INDEPENDENT FILMS: *VOICE/OVER*

Films made by independent filmmakers can be very useful in our understanding of people with disabilities because they do not have to function within the narrow parameters of commercial mainstream movies. They can offer unique perspectives in a much more individualized and personal way. To help people with disabilities relating with empathy, a therapist must understand their struggles. *Voice/Over*, an independent film by Shelly Barry (Barry, Bonilla, & Garoian, 2004), is a powerful tool that aids our understanding of the disability experience from a firsthand perspective. In this emotionally gripping film, Ms. Barry talks about a shooting that almost killed her and how it changed her life in profound and unexpected ways.

This is a compelling story about a young woman who wears her scars as medals of victory and celebrates her existence through art and the triumph of creativity over adversity. She is more than a survivor; she is the heroine of her own life. She wants us to know that she is here and she wants to leave behind her words and films when she is gone so that her inspiring message can live on. Table 8-1 includes resources for completing the Film Analysis Learning Experience.

Voice/Over is part of an award-winning trilogy, *Whole: A Trinity of Being* (Barry, 2004). The work of the author speaks to the role of advocacy by people living with disability (Hiadki, 2008). Shelley Barry is a South African woman of color and now a disability advocate, who saw her life shattered in a second as her spine was severed by a bullet. In her journey, rescued by the healing power of occupation, she became a filmmaker narrating her own journey. What better way to understand a disability narrative? In a discussion of her award-winning, autobiographical film, she relates, "Unless we as people with disabilities, as women, as Black people, as lesbians, become the makers of our own images, our lives will constantly be depicted on the basis of assumptions that others hold about who we are, how we live, and how we love" (Barry, 2006, p. 66). In the capacity of promoting positive media images, Barry went on to serve in President Nelson Mandela's administration as the Media Officer in the Office of the Status of Disabled Persons.

Films that depict disabilities can serve as metaphors and/or as sources of meaningful information about the day-to-day aspects of life experiences. That being said, it is also important to use a critical eye when viewing disability films. Just as it is counterproductive to stereotype patients (Garden, 2010) in general, it is also a mistake to stereotype all disability films. Some are more realistic than others, but every film of this type has lessons that can be gleaned and elements that can be rejected. As with art of any kind, these films are inherently subjective and open to varying interpretations.

Film Analysis Learning Experience IV—Voice/Over

Disability Film: Meaning and Spirituality

Resources for this film are listed in Table 8-1, including the video file available on YouTube. This film portrays the profound impact of a disability on a person's life and his or her spirituality. It also bears testimony to film as a metaphor for the lived disability experience with vivid, haunting images and rich symbolism.

Questions

a. Outline the main plot points and themes for the illness narrative.

b. Describe the presence of Frank's narrative(s) and discussion of themes (loss, pain, suffering, feeling alone, courage, stigma, etc.) that are relevant and note whether they changed over time.

c. Consider the perspective of the victim, her family, and lover in response to her illness/disability. What were your emotional responses?

d. Comment on two ways the filmmaker has used symbolism or metaphor as a way to portray her illness experience (refer to the article in Table 8-1 by Hiadki, 2008).

e. Comment on the role of meaning and spirituality in her life.

f. What you have learned about the illness and disability experience from this filmmaker?

g. Discuss the emotional impact you experienced in response to this story.

ADVOCACY AND EMPOWERMENT IN DISABILITY FILM NARRATIVES

One of the few guarantees in life is that it will never turn out the way we expect.
But, rather than let the events in our lives define who we are,
we can make the decision to define the possibilities in our lives.

(Ellison, n.d.)

People with disability are a major voice for advocacy. Shelley Barry's participation in many regional and international disability film festivals has given her a platform to deliver this message. Therapists and advocacy groups can cosponsor local film festivals to promote greater understanding of the disability experience and to support mutual agendas (Snyder & Mitchell, 2008). Our challenge as advocates becomes how to use professional reasoning to empower and transform images of disability in film to real-life narratives empowering clients' authentic self with full community participation.

Figure 8-1. Logo of the Brooklyn International Disability Film Festival. (Copyright © Anne Scott.)

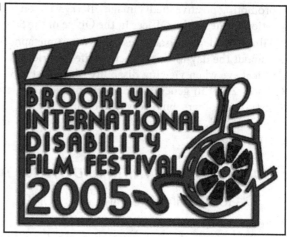

To commemorate the 15th anniversary of the passage of the American's With Disabilities Act, for my (Anne's) sabbatical project at Long Island University, my husband and coauthor, Richard, and I brought together several disability advocacy groups to sponsor The Brooklyn International Disability Film Festival and Wellness Expo (2005; Dewees, 2005; Gorenstein, 2005; Figure 8-1).

Support from external grants included funding from the Christopher & Dana Reeve Quality of Life Grants (2014). Among the 35 disability-themed films, the feature film was directed by Christopher Reeve, *The Brooke Ellison Story* (Cairo & Reeve, 2004), based on Ellison's autobiography, penned with her mother (Ellison & Ellison, 2002). Ellison, who became quadriplegic after a childhood accident, continued her academic career after her injury, spurred by her passion for learning and her family's unwavering support. She was the first person with quadriplegia to graduate from Harvard (completing bachelor's and master's degrees) and recently obtained a doctoral degree from SUNY Stony Brook. Ellison has run for political office, holds the rank of assistant professor, and is an advocate who passionately promotes a disability and social justice agenda (www.brookeellison.com).

Perceptions of disability are changing, and people with handicapping conditions are seeking to become mainstreamed rather than marginalized. Views have evolved from the medical model using an illness paradigm with disability as condition to be corrected versus disability as a social construction and complex phenomenon, encompassing social, cultural, and environmental contexts as chronicled in the historical documentary of the disability rights movement "Lives Worth Living" (Gilkey & Neudel, 2011).

Life imitates art. Using film as a metaphor, health professionals can trace the arc of patients' development. We can rewind the narrative and seek truths about the beginning of the patient's problem, or we can fast forward our questions to project what kind of outcome is possible. Films that depict disabilities can serve as metaphors or as sources of practical information about the day-to-day aspects of their experience. They can also open the doors to new areas of concern, such as wellness for people with disabilities (Kilty, 2000).

Wellness provides common ground for forging partnerships with advocacy groups (Salem et al., 2011; Scaffa, Reitz, & Pizzi, 2010; Scott, 1999), particularly for those with disabilities, who have much greater risks for secondary conditions (National Center on Health and Physical Activity and Disability, 2014; Rao, 2014). *OTs Walk With NAMI* (2008) is an example of a collaborative project linking occupational therapists and people with mental illness to reduce stigma and enhance wellness, including a website with health promotion resource material. The wellness agenda for this initiative was documented in a film produced with the local chapter of the National Alliance for the Mentally Ill (NAMI). The video *OTs Walk With NAMI* (Doyle & LaMourie, 2008), available online, was coproduced by an occupational therapy student, Eileen LaMourie, as a community health promotion project. It featured consumers of the local NAMI chapter, who related personal experiences with occupations to focus on wellness and community participation (Doyle & LaMourie, 2008). To support healing and wellness for the disabled, Kilty (2000) who experiences crippling arthritis, has spoken of the therapeutic value of engaging in writing and sharing illness narratives:

> It is no longer enough for others to interpret or analyze what they think our illness experience is; rather there is a real need for them to accept our stories in their totality. Only when the whole story is honored will we truly be heard. Seeing the whole person allows for a deeper healing into wellness where the mind, body and spirit can move on to the next chapter in the living story. (Kilty, 2000, p. 18)

CONCLUSION

Narratives well known propensity to offer an emotionally charged,
symbolically provocative rendering of experience has been
routinely linked to its power to illuminate the
personal experiences of illness and healing.

(Mattingly, 1998, p. 14)

Movies mirror life in a myriad of ways. They have the ability to appeal to our emotions and stimulate us intellectually by tracing the arc of individual characters as they traverse from one point in their lives to another. There is an adage that movies can make us laugh and/or cry. This is attributed to the fact that film is essentially a medium based on reaching the inner emotional core of the viewer by portraying relatable characters in a primal way. Using professional reasoning to analyze movie narratives about differently abled people can help us move occupational therapy into the future where a new landscape of holistic thinking can blossom. Occupational therapists have always been pioneers and should continue that tradition so that they may truly address the needs of their clients in newer and more productive ways, beyond the science and the data and into the hearts and minds of humankind.

In the movie *Awakenings* (Parkes, Lasker, & Marshall, 1990) one of the patients (Leonard Lowe) says:

> People have forgotten what life is all about. They've forgotten what it is to be alive. They need to be reminded. They need to be reminded of what they have and what they can lose. What I feel is the joy of life, the gift of life, the freedom of life, the wonderment of life!

Occupational therapy should be in the forefront of reminding clients of life's wonderment.

It is essential for therapists to understand the therapeutic value of storytelling and the need for each individual to be the narrator in his or her own "movie." We should endeavor to spark their imaginations. When John Lennon wrote his song "Imagine," it is evident he was challenging us to be bold and reject cynicism. I believe he wanted us to open our hearts and our minds so that we might embrace the art of the possible. This art and the hope its message inspires are often displayed in disability films.

As more and more filmmakers, some of whom have disabilities themselves, present the themes we have discussed here, it becomes clear that occupational therapists need to harness this creative energy to reconnect with life narratives and illness dramas through the study and analysis of disability films.

For some clients, spirituality is primarily centered on their religious beliefs, and we need to understand how that plays a role in their treatment; for others, the meaning of that word might also apply to yoga, music, or anything else they are passionate about and that gives their lives meaning. Personally, we feel that spirituality in any form is the light that exists in our lives and in the stories we tell about ourselves. For some of clients, the light has been dimmed or extinguished. Carl Jung reflected, "As far as we can discern, the sole purpose of human existence is to kindle a light in the darkness of mere being" (1965, p. 326). As occupational therapists, we can use disability-themed films to help us kindle a light in those we serve.

ACKNOWLEDGMENTS

This chapter is dedicated to our newly wedded son, Jake, and daughter-in-law, Tanya, who share our love of cinema and the desire to help others.

REFERENCES

Abreu, B. (2011). Accentuate the positive: Reflections on empathic interpersonal interactions. Eleanor Clarke Slagle Lecture. *American Journal of Occupational Therapy, 65,* 623-634. doi:10.5014/ajot.2011.656002

American Occupational Therapy Association. (2014). Occupational therapy practice framework: Domain and process (3rd ed.). *American Journal of Occupational Therapy, 68*(Suppl. 1), S1-S41. doi:10.5014/ajot.2014.682006

American Psychiatric Association. (2013). *Diagnostic and statistical manual of mental disorders* (5th ed.). Arlington, VA: Author.

Awakenings. (1990). Quotes. Retrieved from http://www.imdb.com/title/tt0099077/quotes

Babyar, S. R., Rosen, E., Sliwinski, M. M., Krasilovsky, G., Holland, T., & Lipovac, M. (2003). Physical therapy students' self-reports of development of clinical reasoning. *Journal of Allied Health, 32,* 227-239.

Barry, S. (2004). *Voice/over.* (Second part of *Whole: A Trinity of Being)* [Video file]. Retrieved from youtube.com/watch ?v=OUbl_Rl2i2w_voice/over

Barry, S. (2006). Disability and desire: Journey of a filmmaker. *Feminist Africa, 6,* 65-67. Retrieved from http://www .agi.ac.za/sites/agi.ac.za/files/fa_6_standpoint_1.pdf

Barry, S., Bonilla, M., & Garoian, S. (Producers), & Barry, S. (Director). (2004). *Whole: A Trinity of Being* [Motion picture]. South Africa: Two Spinning Wheels Productions.

Berntson, G. G., Norman, G. J., Bechara, A., Bruss, J., Tranel, D., & Cacioppo, J. T. (2011). The insula and evaluative processes. *Psychological Science, 22,* 80-86. doi:10.1177/0956797610391097

Brooklyn International Disability Film Festival and Wellness Expo. (2005). Retrieved from http://www2.brooklyn.liu .edu/CommunityConnections/Enriching%20The%20Community/BIDFF.html

Bruner, J. (1986). *Actual minds, possible worlds.* Cambridge, MA: Harvard University Press.

Bruner, J. (1990). *Acts of meaning.* Cambridge, MA: Harvard University Press.

Burke, J. P. (2010). What's going on here: Deconstructing the interactive encounter. Eleanor Clarke Slagle Lecture. *American Journal of Occupational Therapy, 64,* 855-868. doi:10.5014/ajot.2010.64604

Burke, J. P., & Kern, S. B. (1996). The issue is—Is the use of life history and narrative in practice reimbursable? Is it occupational therapy? *American Journal of Occupational Therapy, 50*(5), 389-392.

Cairo, J. (Producer), & Reeve, C. (Director). (2004). *The Brooke Ellison story* [TV movie]. United States: A&E Television Networks.

Canadian Association of Occupational Therapists and Department of National Health and Welfare. (1983). *Guidelines for the client-centered practice of occupational therapy* (H39-33/1983E). Ottawa, Canada: Department of National Health and Welfare.

Christopher Reeve Foundation. (2014). *About us: The history of the Reeve Foundation.* Retrieved from http://www .christopherreeve.org/site/c.ddJFKRNoFiG/b.4431493/k.7265/The_History_of_the_Reeve_Foundation.htm

Clark, F. (1993). Occupation embedded in real life: Interweaving occupational science and occupational therapy. *American Journal of Occupational Therapy, 47*(12), 1067-1078.

Clark, F., Ennevor, B. L., & Richardson, P. L. (1996). Grounded theory of techniques for occupational therapy storytelling and story making. In R. Zemke & F. Clark (Eds.), *Occupational science: The evolving discipline* (pp. 373-392). Philadelphia, PA: F. A. Davis.

Darbyshire, D., & Baker, P. (2012). A systematic review and thematic analysis of cinema in medical education. *Medical Humanities, 38,* 28-33. doi:10.1136/medhum-2011-010026

Dewees, G. (2005, July 21). Disability film festival works to erase stigma. *New York Daily News.* Retrieved from http:// www.nydailynews.com/archives/boroughs/disability-film-festival-works-erase-stigma-article-1.584964

Doyle, D., & LaMourie, E. (Producer & Director). (2008). *OTs walk with NAMI* [video]. Retrieved from http://www.youtube.com/watch?v=DO76_980hKw

Ellison, B. (n.d.). Retrieved from http://www.brookeellison.com

Ellison, B., & Ellison, J. (2002). *Miracles happen: One mother, one daughter, one journey.* New York, NY: Hyperion Books.

Frank, A. W. (1995). *The wounded storyteller: Body, illness and ethics.* Chicago, IL: University of Chicago Press.

Frank, A. W. (2004a). Asking the right questions about pain: Narrative and phonesis. *Literature and Medicine, 23,* 209-225.

Frank, A. W. (2004b). *The renewal of generosity: Illness, medicine and how to live.* Chicago, IL: University of Chicago Press.

Frank, A. W. (2013). *The wounded storyteller: Body, illness and ethics* (2nd ed.). Chicago, IL: University of Chicago Press.

Gandolfini, J. (Producer), & Alpert, J., & Kent Goosenberg, E. (Directors). (2004). *Alive day memories: Home from Iraq* [Motion picture]. United States: HBO.

Garcia Sánchez, J. E., & Garcia Sánchez, E. (2006). Two years of the *Journal of Medicine and the Movies*: An overview and the future. *Journal of Medicine and the Movies, 2,* 123-124.

Garden, R. (2010). Disability and narrative: New directions for medicine and the medical humanities. *Medical Humanities, 36,* 70-74. doi:10.1136/jmh.2010.004143.

Gigliotti, D., Cohen, B., & Gordon, J. (Producers), & Russell, D. O. (Director). (2012). *Silver Linings Playbook* [Motion picture]. United States: The Weinstein Company.

Giles, A. K., Carson, N. E., Breland, H. L., Coker-Bolt, P., & Bowman, P. J. (2014). Use of simulated patients and reflective video analysis to assess occupational therapy students' preparedness for fieldwork. *American Journal of Occupational Therapy, 68*(Suppl. 2), S57-S66. doi:10.5014/ajot.2014.685S03

Gilkey, A. (Producer), & Neudel, E. (Director). (2011). *Lives worth living* [Motion picture]. United States: Storyline Motion Pictures and PBS: ITVS. Retrieved from http://www.pbs.org/independentlives/lives-worth-living

Goldstein, K., Kielhofner, G., & Ward, A. (2004). Occupational narratives and the therapeutic process. *Australian Occupational Therapy Journal, 51,* 119-124. doi:10.1111/j.1440-1630.2004.00443.x

Gorenstein, E. (2005, July, 23) Superwoman. *The Brooklyn Paper.* Retrieved from http://www.brooklynpaper.com /stories/28/29/28_29brookeellison.html

Haller, B. (2012). Documentaries, TV, & films about people with disabilities and disability issues for use in university courses. *Media and Disability Resources.* Retrieved from http://media-and-disability.blogspot.com/2012/03/documentaries-tv-film-about-people-with.html

Halpern, J. (1993). Empathy: Using resonance emotions in the service of curiosity. In M. Spiro, C. C. McCrea, E. Peschel, & D. St. James (Eds.), *Empathy and the practice of medicine: Beyond pills and the scalpel* (pp. 160-173). New Haven, CT: Yale University Press.

Hiadki, J. (2008). Social justice, artistic practices and new technologies: Gender and disability and identities in film and digital video. *Atlantis: A Women's Studies Journal/Revue d'etudes sur les femmes, 32*(2), 45-56.

Hull, A. J. (2013). Fictional father? Oliver Sacks and the revalidation of pathography. *Medical Humanities, 2,* 105-114. doi:10.1136/medhum-2012-010301

Jiménez Serranía, M. I. (2007). *Awakenings* (1990): The epidemic of children who fell asleep. *Journal of Medicine and Movies, 3,* 102-112. Retrieved from http://campus.usal.es/~revistamedicinacine/Vol_3/3.3/ing.3.3.htlm/despert _ing.htm

Jung, C. (1965). *Memories, dreams, reflections.* New York, NY: Random House.

Kassirer, J. P. (2010). Teaching clinical reasoning: Case-based and coached. *Academic Medicine, 85,* 1118-1124.

Kilty, S. (2000). Telling the illness story. *The Patient's Network Magazine, 5*(3), 17-18. Retrieved from http://www.aissg .org/articles/TELLING.HTM-TellingtheIllnessStory

Kramer, U. M., Mohammadi, B., Donamayor, N., Samii, A., & Munte, T. F. (2010). Emotional and cognitive aspects of empathy and their relation to social cognition: An *f*MRI study. *Brain Research, 1311,* 110-120. doi:10.1016/j.brainres.2009.11.043

Lennon, J. (1971). Imagine. On *Imagine.* (Medium of recording: Record). London, UK: Apple Records.

Lethborg, C., Aranda, S., & Kissane, D. (2008). Meaning and adjustment to cancer: A model of care. *Palliative and Supportive Care, 6,* 61-70. doi:10.1017/S1478951508000096

Literature, Arts and Medicine Database NYU. (1993-2014). *About the Literature, Arts, and Medicine Database.* Retrieved from http://medhum.med.nyu.edu/about

Mattingly, C. (1991). The narrative nature of clinical reasoning. *American Journal of Occupational Therapy, 45,* 998-1005.

Mattingly, C. (1998). *Healing dramas and clinical plots: The narrative structure of experience.* Cambridge, England: Cambridge University Press.

Mattingly, C. (2010). *The paradox of hope: Journey through a cultural borderland.* Berkeley, CA: University of California Press.

Mattingly, C., & Fleming, M. H. (1994). *Clinical reasoning: Forms of inquiry in a therapeutic practice.* Philadelphia, PA: F. A. Davis.

Mattingly, C., & Garro, L. (2000). *Narrative and the cultural construction of illness and healing.* Berkeley, CA: University of California Press.

McColl, M. A. (2011a). Conclusion. In M. A. McColl (Ed.), *Spirituality and occupational therapy* (2nd ed., pp. 269-279). Ottawa, Canada: CAOT Publications ACE.

McColl, M. A. (2011b). Defining spirituality. In M. A. McColl (Ed.), *Spirituality and occupational therapy* (2nd ed., pp. 53-62). Ottawa, Canada: CAOT Publications ACE.

McColl, M. A. (2011c). Models of spirituality, occupation and health. In M. A. McColl (Ed.), *Spirituality and occupational therapy* (2nd ed., pp. 91-101). Ottawa, Canada: CAOT Publications ACE.

McColl, M. A. (2011d). Other important words and concepts. In M. A. McColl (Ed.), *Spirituality and occupational therapy* (2nd ed., p. 64-69). Ottawa, Canada: CAOT Publications ACE.

McColl, M. A. (2011e). Spirituality among occupational therapists. In M. A. McColl (Ed.), *Spirituality and occupational therapy* (2nd ed., pp. 41-50). Ottawa, Canada: CAOT Publications ACE.

McColl, M. A. (2011f). Spirituality and disability. In M. A. McColl (Ed.), *Spirituality and occupational therapy* (2nd ed., pp. 31-40). Ottawa, Canada: CAOT Publications ACE.

McColl, M. A. (2011g). *Spirituality and occupational therapy* (2nd ed.). Ottawa, Canada: CAOT Publications ACE.

Mosey, A. C. (1981). Introduction: The art of practice. In B. Abreu (Ed.), *Physical disabilities manual* (pp. 1-3). New York, NY: Raven Press.

National Center on Health and Physical Activity and Disability. (2014). *Building healthy and inclusive communities.* Retrieved from http://www.nchpad.org

Osgood, R. J., & Hinshaw, J. (2009). *Visual storytelling, videography, and postproduction in the digital age.* Boston, MA: Wadsworth/Cengage Learning.

OTs Walk With NAMI. (2008). Website. Retrieved from http://www.downstate.edu/CHRP/ot/nami.html

Parkes, W. F., & Lasker, L. (Producers), & Marshall, P. (Director). (1990). *Awakenings* [Motion picture]. United States: Columbia Pictures.

Peloquin, S. (1995). The fullness of empathy: Reflections and illustrations. *American Journal of Occupational Therapy, 49,* 24-31.

Peloquin, S. (1996a). Art: An occupation with a promise for developing empathy. *American Journal of Occupational Therapy, 50,* 655-661.

Peloquin, S. (1996b). Using the arts to enhance confluent learning. *American Journal of Occupational Therapy, 50,* 148-151.

Pérez, J. (2013). The *Journal of Medicine and Movies,* a method for learning for students in health sciences. *Journal of Medicine and Movies, 9,* 149-150.

Polkinghorne, D. E. (1996). Transformative narratives: From victim to agentic life plots. *American Journal of Occupational Therapy, 50*(4), 299-305.

Puchalski, C., Ferrell, B., Virani, R., Otis-Green, S., Baird, P., Bull, J., et al. (2009). Improving the quality of spiritual care as a dimension of palliative care: The report of the consensus conference. *Journal of Palliative Medicine, 12,* 885-904. doi:10.1089/jpm.2009.0142

Quick, M. (2008). *Silver linings playbook.* New York, NY: Farrar, Straus and Giroux.

Rao, A. K. (2014). Occupational therapy in chronic progressive disorders: Enhancing function and modifying disease. *American Journal of Occupational Therapy, 68,* 251-253. Retrieved from http://ajot.aota.org/article.aspx?articleid=1867343

Reason, D. (2013). *A clinical reasoning framework for community occupational therapists: A formative evaluation study.* Dunedin, NZ: Otago Polytechnic School of Occupational Therapy.

Rilke, R. M. (1902, Nov. 6). *The panther.* Translated by M. Mitchell. Retrieved from http://www.poemhunter.com/poem/the-panther/

Rogers, J. (1983). Clinical reasoning: The ethics, science and art. *American Journal of Occupational Therapy, 37,* 601-616. doi:10.5012/ajot.37.9.601

Rogers, J., & Kielhofner, G. (1985). Treatment planning. In G. Kielhofner (Ed.), *A model of human occupation* (pp. 136-155). Baltimore, MD: Williams & Wilkins.

Rousseau, P. (2000). Spirituality and the dying patient. *Journal of Clinical Oncology, 18,* 2000-2002. Retrieved from http://www.http://jco.ascopubs.org/content/18/9/2000.full

Sacks, O. (1963). *Awakenings.* New York, NY: Vintage Paperbacks.

Sacks, O. (1987). *The man who mistook his wife for a hat.* New York, NY: Harper Perennial.

Salem, Y., Scott, A., Karpatkin, H., Concert, G., Haller, L., Kaminsky, E., et al. (2011). Community-based group aquatic program for individuals with multiple sclerosis: A pilot study. *Disability and Rehabilitation, 33,* 720-728.

Scaffa, M. E., Reitz, M., & Pizzi, M. (2010). *Occupational therapy in the promotion of health and wellness.* Philadelphia, PA: F. A. Davis.

Scott, A. (1999). Wellness works: Community service health promotion groups led by occupational therapy students. *American Journal of Occupational Therapy, 53,* 566-574.

Smith, B., & Sparkes, A. C. (2011). Exploring multiple responses to chaos narratives. *Health, 15,* 38-53. doi:10.1177/1363459309360782

Snyder, S., & Mitchell, D. (2008). How do we get all these disabilities in here? Disability film festivals and the politics of atypicality. *Canadian Journal of Film Studies, 17*(1), 11-29.

Soundy, A., Smith, B., Cressy, F., & Webb, L. (2010). The experience of spinal cord injury: Using Frank's narrative types to enhance physiotherapy undergraduates understanding. *Physiotherapy, 96*, 52-58.

Taylor, R. R., & van Puymbroeck, L. (2013). Therapeutic use of self: Applying the intentional relationship model in group therapy. In J. C. O'Brien & J. W. Solomon (Eds.), *Occupational analysis and group process* (pp. 36-52). St. Louis, MO: Elsevier.

Thibodaux, L. R. (1998). *Acknowledging the spiritual dimension of occupational therapy.* Paper presented at the 12th International Congress of World Federation of Occupational Therapists, Montreal, Quebec, Canada.

Unruh, A. M., Versnel, J., & Kerr, N. (2002). Spirituality unplugged: A review of commonalities and contentions, and a resolution. *Canadian Journal of Occupational Therapy, 69*, 5-19.

Weingarten, K. (2001). *Making sense of illness narratives: Braiding theory, practice and the embodied life.* Retrieved from http://dulwichcentre.com.au/articles-about-narrative-therapy/illness-narratives/

Wonder, S. (1969). My cherie amour. On *My Cherie Amour* (Medium of recording: Record), Detroit, MI: Motown.

RESOURCES

Advocacy and Arts by Disabled People. Retrieved from http://www.bioethicsanddisability.org/disartsadv.html

Christopher & Dana Reeve Foundation. (2014). *Quality of life grants.* Retrieved from http://www.christopherreeve.org/site/c.ddJFKRNoFiG/b.4425935/k.6491/Quality_of_Life_Grants.htm

Haller, B. (2013). Disability and mass media [course syllabus]. Retrieved from http://bethhaller.wordpress.com/syllabi/disability-mass-media

International Center for Bioethics, Culture and Disability. Retrieved from http://www.bioethicsanddisability.org

Museum of disABILITY History. Retrieved from http://www.museumofdisability.org

Reelabilities. Annual disability film festival; 14 US locations. Retrieved from http://www.reeabilities.org

The Cinematherapy Newsletter. Retrieved from www.cinematherapy.com

Social Reasoning in Occupational Therapy
Integrating Social Theories

Marilyn B. Cole, MS, OTR/L, FAOTA

I am waiting at the hospital for my husband to get out of surgery. In the meantime, I am getting his prescription filled, and soon I will meet with his doctor in recovery and get instructions for his aftercare. Then I will drive him home, help him up the stairs to the bedroom, change his dressings for a few weeks, and generally help him function for the 6 weeks it will take until he is healed. Are these occupations, or parts of my social role? I am a wife and, at least temporarily, a caregiver. I do these tasks because I care about my husband; without this significant relationship, the occupations themselves are meaningless. In this example, my occupations and my social roles cannot be separated. Similarly, I contend that nearly all occupations are embedded within social roles and relationships that provide both incentive and meaning for the individual. Without understanding our clients' social roles and relationships, how can occupational therapists truly comprehend their occupations?

This chapter explores the social dimensions of occupation and proposes that occupational therapists learn to think about occupations from a social perspective, a practice I refer to here as *social reasoning*. Adding a social dimension across occupational therapy practice areas is consistent with current professional trajectories. It affirms the complex nature of occupation that is embedded in individual and community life. In 2008, the American Occupational Therapy Association (AOTA) added *social participation* to its *Occupational Therapy Practice Framework* (2nd ed.), the document that defines the profession's domain of concern and process of service delivery in the United States. The AOTA affirmed social participation as a primary occupation in its *Occupational Therapy Practice Framework* (3rd ed.) update (2014). Primary occupations are "central to a person's identity and sense of competence and have particular meaning to that [person]" (AOTA, 2014, p. S5) The *Practice Framework* (3rd ed.) also inserts the concept of "co-occupation," referring to occupations that are shared and done with others (AOTA, 2014, p. S6). The World Health Organization (WHO) has recognized, for more than a decade, the importance of social determinants of health as well as the central role of occupations for "participation in life" (WHO, 2001, p. 123). Occupations

Cole, M. B., & Creek, J. (Eds.).
Global Perspectives in Professional Reasoning (pp. 145-164).
© 2016 Taylor & Francis Group.

have been defined as "including things people need to, want to, and are expected to do" (World Federation of Occupational Therapists, 2012), implying the element of social expectation as well as internal motivation. However, the relationship of social participation and/or context to occupations remains unclear, and its impact on occupational therapy practice is not well understood.

Exploring social dimensions of occupation takes us on a journey through the research of other disciplines including medicine, neuroscience, sociology, and social psychology. Our journey includes theories of social identity, social cognition, complexity, socioemotional selectivity, and social support. These theories from other disciplines can inform occupational therapists' understanding of the complex transactions between social and occupational realms.

To better define the concepts within social reasoning, I propose the following hypotheses:

1. Social roles and occupations are inseparable.
2. Social connections promote occupational and lifestyle choices.
3. Strong social identities motivate occupational engagement.
4. Social cognition determines the success of occupational endeavors.
5. Intentional self-management of social relationships and environments heightens occupational performance and meaning.

Within these broad topics, relevant social theories and evidence will be summarized, along with implications for application in occupational therapy practice.

1. Social Roles and Occupations Are Inseparable

In a recent qualitative study of productive aging, my colleague and I asked 40 older adult participants to describe their productive occupations (Cole & Macdonald, 2015). Almost without exception, they needed further explanation. They understood working to be a productive occupation, but most of our participants were retired. By way of explanation, we gave them some examples: home manager, lifelong learner, caregiver, or volunteer. They thought of these as social roles and, yes, now that we explained it, also occupations. But not one of them saw occupations and social roles as separate: the tasks of a caregiver for a grandchild or an aging relative, the division of chores for family members maintaining a home, the activities performed as part of a work team, whether paid or voluntary, are part of the social contexts and relationships within which they occur. And their meaning comes as much from the social interactions and internalized social expectations as from the occupation itself.

Social Expectations in Everyday Activities

Don't we perform some occupations alone? We may sleep alone, eat breakfast alone, shower, and dress for the day without the company of others. How are these social roles? One of my colleagues sustained a head injury as a result of an automobile accident. After some rehabilitation, she returned home to her apartment, without knowing when or if she might be able to return to her former roles and routines. For a few weeks, she wore the same sweat suit day and night, ate out of cans and jars when hungry, forgot to bathe, forgot to turn off the TV, and only occasionally remembered to keep follow-up appointments. Toward the end of her medical leave from work, she spoke to her former supervisor on the phone, and they agreed to her returning to work part time. With the help of some friends, she prepared herself by setting an alarm clock, following a checklist for bathing and grooming, stocking up on groceries, preparing and eating breakfast, doing her laundry, and dressing appropriately for work. Although she did perform some of these activities alone, they were socially motivated. Without a social purpose, none of these self-care occupations had meaning.

Creative Expression: Solitary or Social?

What about creative expression? A musician sits at the piano alone to compose a piece of music. An artist uses internal vision to create a painting. But where does artists' inspiration really come from? Is it not from his or her experiences in the social world? Love gained or lost? Anger or joy at the human condition or the state of society? And then, there is the philosophical question: What is the meaning of an artistic work if no one ever sees or hears it?

I've always wanted to write a novel. A few years ago, I tried writing about some of the experiences I had as an occupational therapist working in mental health. I focused on one specific patient, a beautiful young woman with a diagnosis of schizophrenia who often got involved with the wrong kind of man, with predictably disastrous consequences. Soon it became clear, however, that as a novice writer I needed some expert criticism. Therefore, seeing an ad in the local paper, I joined a writer's critique group. The other writers, some published, some novices like myself, thoughtfully critiqued one another's chapters at our bimonthly meetings. In these discussions, I had to articulate my motivation for writing: I wanted to change society's attitudes about both persons with serious mental illness and the role of occupational therapists in working with them. The inspiration for the novel came from a social experience, and my motivation for writing about it was also social. The critique group offered me a mirror for how well my message was coming across and how I might communicate it more effectively. The other members encouraged me to keep going, writing a new chapter every 2 weeks. Eventually I learned to critique myself, hearing their voices inside my head, and I became a much better writer because of this group experience.

Creation of Meaning in Occupations and Life

According to Hasselkus (2011), meaning has both shared dimensions and personal dimensions. "Perceptions are molded by social conventions, beliefs, and attitudes" (p. 3). People create meaning by trying to make sense of out of their experiences, a dynamic process of "constructing and reconstructing understandings and explanations of everyday living" (Hasselkus, 2011, p. 3). From a philosophical viewpoint, Frankl wrote that the search for meaning is a "primary motivational force in man" (1963, p. 20). To understand the meaning of an occupation, Mattingly (1998) found that occupational therapists first needed to use narrative reasoning to learn the life stories of their clients. In narrative theory, when people describe the events of their lives, they also convey their interpretations and beliefs about their experiences, giving important clues to their subjective meaning.

Think about what you might want to do on a Saturday. What in your mind might be worth doing? Taking a run through the park, doing your laundry, housecleaning, grocery shopping, going out for dinner with friends, or just relaxing with a good book—all of these occupations say something about what is important to you, what occupations hold meaning. Your choice of activity could involve other people, but maybe not. But its meaning cannot be fully understood without also understanding the context, what part this specific activity plays in your ongoing life story. And that life story is embedded within a host of relationships and social groups. For example, a woman may want to run through the park to keep her body fit but also because she wants to look attractive in her jeans or bathing suit; for her, running is for social as well as for health reasons. Even reading a book, or watching a movie, offers myriad vicarious social experiences, as we will see later in the section on social cognition. Clients also have their reasons for engaging in occupations, based on their evolving life stories.

2. SOCIAL CONNECTIONS PROMOTE OCCUPATIONAL AND LIFESTYLE CHOICES

As a health care profession, occupational therapy's primary concern is health and wellness. The health care literature has focused more prominently on social issues within the past decade than ever before. Although we already know the detrimental effects of social isolation for health and well-being, only recently have we come to realize the positive effects of social connections. Through years of study, some reasons for the importance of social connectedness are emerging, in particular, the way that other people influence our occupations and lifestyles.

Health Evidence

Health and well-being are highly dependent on the quantity and quality of social relationships. Evidence abounds across the health care disciplines that social connections and relationships can protect individuals of all ages from both mental and physical health conditions. In a meta-analytic review (148 studies), Holt-Lunstad, Smith, and Layton (2010) drew the astonishing conclusion that persons with stronger social relationships have a 50% higher likelihood of survival, regardless of age, gender, initial health status, or follow-up period. This makes social connections more influential in predicting health and mortality than smoking, diet, physical activity, or any other previously identified risk factor.

Two possible ways for social relationships to influence health are identified: a stress buffering model and a main effects model. Social resources and support may buffer the stress brought on by acute or chronic illness. Or, alternatively, the social relationships themselves could incidentally protect people from the stresses that might otherwise lead to illness, providing cognitive, emotional, behavioral, and biological influences that encourage healthy behaviors within social norms of the relationships. Just being a part of a social network also provides members with meaningful roles, self-esteem, and purpose in life (Cohen, 2004). Holt-Lunstad and colleagues (2010) recommended efforts within the medical community to promote enhanced social connections as an "opportunity to enhance not only quality of life but also survival" (p. 15). From this we understand that social connections can prevent illness, reduce disability, and prevent premature death, whereas social isolation has the opposite effect. Never has there been a stronger incentive for occupational therapists to make social participation a priority for both recovery and prevention. But it does not shed light on the relationship of social participation with occupation. We must look outside of medical research to better understand this relationship.

The Complex Science of Social Connections

Theories of social connectivity or networking, in the human rather than Internet sense, are proposed by Christakis and Fowler (2009), professors at Harvard and the University of California. They studied social networks by using computers to track multiple aspects of social relationships within networks and to identify patterns within the real social connections that people have with one another. Their research shows how these networks both drive and shape every aspect of our lives. These authors defined a social network as an organized set of people and their connections to one another that evolve through their natural tendency to seek out relationships. Initially, they defined some basic rules of "life in the network" (p. 17).

- **We shape our network.** When put into a random group, such as a college dormitory or a corporation, people seek out and connect with others who are similar to themselves. They choose the size of network they are comfortable with and the position they will hold within it. Those closer to the center of a social network have a greater number of connections and yield more influence than those toward the perimeter. Social relationships vary within networks in a variety of ways: (a) Closeness—the average American identified four close associations within the network. (b) Transitivity, or the degree to which people within a person's network also know one another—some people have several friends who don't know one another, whereas others have friends who are also friends with one another. (c) Homophily—the tendency to associate with others like ourselves. Some people relate mostly to others with similar background, appearance, or beliefs; others have more diverse friendships. The feature that allows scientists to track the trends and influences of social networks is that each member of one person's network has a whole different network of connections through which these trends and influences can flow, theoretically spiraling outward endlessly.

- *Our network shapes us.* People's life experience depends on their place within the social network. For example, first-, second-, or third-born children have different experiences within a family and follow different sets of rules when their parents are married and living together, compared with divorced parents. People on the margins of a network have less influence and are less influenced by the people toward the center. This might be detrimental if the person needs the help of others in finding a better job or gaining membership to an organization, but it is also fortunate when escaping the spread of germs, for example. Through computer-based research, Christakis and Fowler demonstrate how a central location within the network affects "everything from how much money you make to whether you will be happy" (2009, p. 21).

- *Our friends affect us.* What flows from one person to another generally influences both sender and recipient. People have a natural tendency to imitate one another and to seek one another's advice on a variety of issues. Some examples: Diners sitting next to heavy eaters tend to eat more, students with studious roommates tend to study more, voters who discuss their views with each other tend to vote the same way.

- *Our friends' friends' friends affect us.* The influences spreading outward from a single individual are called *hyperdyadic spread*, similar to the way childhood diseases get passed around at a playground. An example is Milgram's 1968 sidewalk experiment in New York City (Milgram, Bickman, & Berkowitz, 1969): When one research assistant on a crowded street looked up, 42% copied the behavior; when groups of 15 research assistants looked up, 86% of passersby looked up. However, a group of five assistants looking up elicited the same response as the group of 15. Milgram illustrated the limitations of this type of influence, leveling off at about five. Similarly, social norms, expectations, and sanctions pass through social networks in complex patterns not traceable without the assistance of computers.

- *The network has a life of its own.* Characteristics not immediately traceable to individuals within a network can only be studied by observing the entire network as a whole. The example given is *la ola*, or "the human wave," which can be observed within crowded sports stadiums, a phenomenon not unlike the spread of fire through a forest, having nothing to do with the properties of each individual within the group. Such characteristics of entire networks are called *emergent properties*, the whole adding up to more than the sum of the parts.

Six Degrees of Separation, Three Degrees of Influence

This familiar phrase, both a play by John Guare (1996) and the title of a book about Kevin Bacon (Foss, Ginelli, & Turtle, 1996), refers back to Milgram's original theory of the limitations of social influence based on his classic *small world experiment* (Milgram et al., 1969). In a more recent academic study, Dodds and Muhamad (2003) used email to recruit more than 90,000 subjects to help search for one of 18 targets located worldwide. They used Milgram's original methodology, asking each person to help to locate the target by contacting someone they knew personally who might know his or her location. On a global scale, these researchers found that it took an average of six steps (or contacts) to reach the targeted individuals.

Despite this limit of six, Christakis and Fowler (2009) found that influence over others was limited to three degrees (with our friend being one degree, our friend's friend being two degrees, and so forth). According to their own study, these researchers found that influence peters out after three jumps, in the case of word of mouth, because the integrity of the message itself becomes compromised. Another reason is that after three degrees, the connections become unstable. Friendships end, people die, people change jobs, get married, get divorced, or simply lose touch. Social connections are never permanent, especially when they are not really our own, but those of our friends' friends, and out of our control. But even with a limit of three degrees of influence, our own impact can be significant. Christakis gives the example of a person with 20 social connections (5 friends, 5 coworkers, and 10 family members). Your influence extends to $20 \times 20 \times 20$, or 8,000 individuals within 3 degrees of separation. And those 8,000 people also have an impact on you.

For practice, try drawing your own social network, using just six people, with each of them having connections to six other people, demonstrating two degrees of separation (follow the directions in Learning Activity 1 at the end of the chapter). If you told one of these people to forward a photograph to some of their contacts, how many people might see it? If you received a shocking piece of news from one contact, with whom would you discuss it, and how many people in the network might hear about it? What else can you learn about your influence and that of others from Learning Activity 1?

In relation to health promotion, people imitate one another's substance use habits, whether drinking, smoking tobacco, using marijuana, or sniffing cocaine. Data from the Framingham Heart Study showed that smoking cigarettes decreased in adults over the past four decades from 45% to 21%, a ripple effect starting with the news that just a few people had quit smoking. The wave of quitting spread through interconnected groups, often living miles away from each other. Obesity has spread in the opposite direction, not only because people imitate one another's overeating or poor diet, but because of changes in the social norms of what body sizes are acceptable. Contributing factors include subtle changes in culture, such as spending more time on computers and smart phones and less time participating in active work tasks or sports, or grabbing high calorie fast foods with larger portion sizes to eat at one's desk while working longer hours. Christakis and Fowler pointed out that obesity remains epidemic even though Hollywood icons are thinner than ever, because people are less influenced by the media than by "the actions and the appearance of the very real people to whom they are actually connected" (2009, p. 115).

Six degrees of separation demonstrates what a small world we live in and how connected we all are. Three degrees of influence demonstrates how "contagious" we are. Connection and contagion are "the structure and function of social networks" (Christakis & Fowler, 2009, p. 30).

3. Strong Social Identities Motivate Occupational Engagement

Social psychology research portrays social identity as a key motivator for occupational engagement. Social identity is defined as "the sense of self that people derive from their membership in social groups (e.g., family, work, community)" (Jetten, Haslam, & Haslam, 2012, p. 4). Most people have multiple social identities, some connected with small groups such as families, classmates, or coworkers, and others defined within larger society. But to what extent do these roles define who we are as people? For example, a teacher who has achieved tenure and status in the eyes of peers, and acclamation of value and affection by students, will likely have derived a strong positive social identity from this occupation and/or work role. Likewise, a woman who has taken the time and effort to nurture her children develops a strong social identity as a mother. Each of these positive social identities (both social roles and occupations) contribute to a person's sense of well-being. Furthermore, people seek out friendships and social relationships that support "valued aspects of the self that are related to identification with social groups, categories, and roles" (Weitz & Wood, 2005, p. 416). According to these researchers, the social identity support given or exchanged between friends predicted the closest and most lasting friendships over a 4-year period.

Social Identity, Health, and Well-Being

There is strong evidence to show that "membership in social groups . . . has the capacity to affect mood, life quality, cognitive decline, even life span. . . . This evidence, gathered across a broad range of experimental and laboratory research . . . was inspired by a social identity approach to health and well-being" (Haslam, Jetten, & Haslam, 2012, p. 319). According to Sani (2012), the quality of social relationships within groups determines the extent to which the social identity benefits health and well-being. Social identities are usually positive, subconsciously chosen by individuals as the way they would like others to view them—a good mother, a competent worker, a devout Catholic. But what about the child with autism who is bullied at school or treated as a failure by teachers and parents? A child might conclude from his home or school experience that he is stupid, clumsy, and an outcast undeserving of a more positive judgment. Social identity can be negative and can result in social isolation that may be other or self-imposed.

Group Identities and Sense of Belonging

Another important aspect of social identity occurs when people categorize themselves with larger segments of the population: Catholic, Jewish, African American, Hispanic, Southerner, middle class, blue-collar worker, wealthy, poor, gay or lesbian. The concept of social identity was first introduced by Tajfel (1981) as a "group-based" identity that explains how groups tend to stereotype one another. It was useful in helping to understand societal problems such as racial bias or gang violence and to guide public policies that discourage discrimination in the workplace, housing and neighborhoods, and schools. The concept of social identity in relation to health and well-being was largely unexplored until recently.

We might assume that self-categorization in specific religious or racial groups should be avoided because it can cause members to face discrimination or exclusion. However, a social identity derived from being a member of a minority or marginalized group has the surprising effect of increasing members' sense of belonging (common enemy?), and buffering against environmental threats (disadvantage, poverty). Research shows that such groups provide support for members to combat or cope with group-based discrimination (Haslam & Reiker, 2006). St. Claire and Clucas (2012) highlight the importance of self-categorization in identifying with groups based on a specific illness or disability. For example, persons with multiple sclerosis, once they have accepted this chronic illness identity, become more willing to join a support group where they can benefit from emotional support and group problem solving and, subsequently, more likely to engage in health-promoting behaviors.

Social Identity and Occupation

A few recent studies involving social identity have focused directly on specific occupations. For example, Jetten and Pachana (2012) found that older adults who had to give up driving faced an identity change that crossed the line between a vibrant, mature, fully functional self, and one that confirmed the undeniable reality of growing old. Researchers found that participants anticipated a gloomier outcome than actually occurred after driving cessation. They concluded that older adults with stronger social identities and larger social networks had an easier time adjusting to driving cessation than their less connected counterparts. Another study, of clients with dementia in a nursing home, focused on the occupation of reminiscence, both individually and in groups. These researchers found that even residents with moderate to severe dementia benefited from the group format, where members, contributing their long-term memories of earlier times and events, were able together to reconstruct shared social identities. The group concurrently provided a sense of belonging and buffered the effects of cognitive decline and social isolation for residents in long-term care (Haslam, Jetten, Haslam, & Knight, 2012).

Thus far we have looked at the relationship between social identity and meaning in life, and the effect of social identity on health and well-being. But how does this information help occupational therapists to think about the social dimensions of occupation?

Occupation as Identity

The concept of occupation as identity, proposed by Christiansen in 1999, reverses the way occupational therapists usually think about their role in restoring and maintaining health. We do not only use occupations to make people healthy; we enable healing to restore the occupations that define the lives of our clients. In doing so, our efforts provide support for our clients' social identities. Christiansen proposed a new idea, that "the ultimate goal of occupational therapy services is well-being, not health" (p. 547). He suggested that

> occupations come together within the contexts of our relationships with others to provide us with a sense of purpose and structure in our day-to-day activities, as well as over time. When we build our identities through occupations, we provide ourselves with the contexts necessary for creating meaningful lives, and life meaning helps us to be well. (Christiansen, 1999, p. 547)

From this perspective, meaningful occupations, embedded in social contexts, become essential for health and well-being because they are central to a person's social identity. "Occupations are more than movements strung together, more than simply doing something. They are opportunities to express the self and to create an identity" (Christiansen, 1999, p. 552).

Articulating One's Social Identity

If someone asks you to describe your social identity, how would you answer? What questions might you pose to find out what really gives someone's life meaning? Please see Table 9-1 for some ideas.

For practice, I asked myself this question: What is my social identity? My social roles are wife, mother and grandmother, college professor, occupational therapy educator and researcher, writer, home maintainer, friend, sometime caregiver, always lifelong learner. But this list seemed too superficial and lacking in the meaning I sought. To go deeper, I imagined myself lying in a hospital bed, injured or ill. Aside from coping with the medical issues, what would be most important for me to get back to doing? First, I would want to confirm my important social relationships—to communicate with my family and friends through email, telephone, or face-to-face visits. I'd ask someone to bring me my laptop computer and give me a Wi-Fi connection. Next, I'd want to read, play computer games to challenge my mind, and I would definitely want to write. It surprises me that I'd also want to shop and cook for myself, not just because I don't like hospital food but because I want to control what I eat. Of course, I'd want to go home as soon as possible, and get back to my normal routines. I'd want to stay fit, take walks with my husband, ride my bike, and go to my yoga class. I'd wonder: What is on my calendar? What obligations have I missed? When is my next writing deadline? I'd want to go out with my friends for lunch. Plan our next vacation or trip to visit my daughter in Texas. I'd ask the doctors to heal me so that I could get back to being the person whom I have become over my lifetime. How would an occupational therapist help me to restore my social identities?

Applying the concepts of social identity within the professional reasoning process can guide occupational therapists to create interventions that strengthen social identity, establish and develop social roles, and facilitate the protective benefits of group membership. This viewpoint acknowledges the advantages of occupational therapy group interventions that facilitate positive interactions among members as they engage in occupations within the process of recovery and self-management of health conditions.

TABLE 9-1

TEN QUESTIONS THAT ENCOURAGE CLIENTS TO DISCLOSE THEIR SOCIAL IDENTITIES

1. How would you introduce yourself to someone you just met
   a. at work with a new coworker?
   b. at a neighbor's open house?
   c. at a community event or fundraiser?
2. What are your most important relationships with others?
3. What social groups do you belong to, and what is your role in each?
4. Which accomplishments are you most proud of? (Least proud of?)
5. What do you most look forward to doing today, this week, and this year? Why? (What do you most dread, or like the least?)
6. If you had to leave your home within 5 minutes because of an emergency (fire, flood, bomb), carrying only a duffel bag, what would you put in it?
7. What are your life roles? List five.
8. What are your gifts or talents? List five things you are good at.
9. What is your life's work?
10. Name five things that give your life meaning (people, objects, and activities).

---

4. SOCIAL COGNITION DETERMINES THE SUCCESS OF OCCUPATIONAL ENDEAVORS

How do people develop a social identity? Bandura (1971) helps to explain this by describing ways in which people learn from observing and interacting with each other, a process he called *social learning*. Unlike earlier learning theories, social learning acknowledges the thinking process that occurs when people watch the behaviors of others. They do not just imitate mindlessly. They do not only remember images and verbal sequences. They also think about various aspects of the situations they observe, the emotions involved, and the consequences or outcomes. A child in a classroom watches and listens when classmates answer the teacher's questions. Is raising a hand required, or can students just speak out? How does the teacher respond? What kind of answers gain approval? What happens when the answer is wrong? The child weighs the pros and cons before venturing into the class discussion, then evaluates the response of the teacher and the other students to his or her own new behavior. On the basis of such experiences, the child concludes, "I am smart" or "I am good at reading but not so good in mathematics" or "even when I am wrong, I can still make people laugh." People, as they develop within social systems, learn to interact and take on social roles, continually trying out new behaviors. Through social interactions, in combination with the performance of occupations, they come to appreciate what they are able to accomplish by watching and listening to the responses of others to their own initiatives. These reflections about their own abilities, and the way other people think and feel about them, influence the characteristics of a social identity. (See Learning Activity 2 at the end of the chapter).

As health and psychological paradigms have shifted, Bandura's social learning theory has evolved to embrace the essential nature of human agency, defined as the conscious capacity to exercise control over the nature and quality of one's life. Some of the processes integral to social cognitive theory are functional consciousness, vicarious learning, self-regulation, taking advantage of opportunities, and self-direction and reflection "about one's capabilities, quality of functioning, and the meaning and purpose of one's life pursuits" (Bandura, 2001, p. 10). Self-efficacy and intentionality are more fully described in the next section.

Functional Consciousness

With a nod to Freud's "ego," the conscious mind constructs both a personal and social identity, together known as a "sense of self." This conscious mind selects, constructs, regulates, and evaluates thoughts and courses of action. It is responsible for making accurate judgments about one's own capabilities, anticipating consequences, sizing up social opportunities and constraints, and accordingly regulating behaviors. In performing occupations, people consider many social aspects, both internal and external to themselves, not the least of which is the potential meaning of the occupation. Occupational therapists need to evaluate their clients' social perspective to truly understand their motivations for engaging or refraining from engaging in occupations.

Vicarious Learning and the Mirror-Neuron System

People do not necessarily have to imitate actions themselves to learn from the behaviors of others. Biological evidence of this phenomenon has emerged in the form of "mirror neurons," which activate specific areas of the brain in response to watching other people engaging in activities. Adolphs (2009) reviewed studies of the neuroscientific basis of social and vicarious learning, many using brain imaging techniques. The insula is that portion of the brain that tends to mirror the experiences of others, a largely automatic or unconscious process based on the perception of social signals such as pain or strong emotion. This mirror-neuron system enables people to empathize with others and to predict their intentions on the basis of emotional cues, as seen through neural pathways from the insula to the anterior cingulate, prefrontal, and temporoparietal brain areas where social processing and reflection occur (Frith & Frith, 2007). Adolphs further explored the role of the mirror-neuron system in modulation of social cognition, based on both knowledge of the individual being observed, and the specific situation or circumstance. Three areas of social cognition were substantiated by this review:

1. The human ability to shift conscious experience into the future (plan ahead, set goals, anticipate consequences) and to understand the viewpoints of others

2. The strong emotional motivation of certain aspects of social behavior, the ability to distinguish between self and others, and the processes involved in judgment and emotion regulation

3. Mental flexibility in using social cognitive abilities across contexts and time intervals and the ability to retrieve and use episodic memories in keeping track of a large number of individuals with whom people maintain social connections

This biological evidence helps to explain some other areas of social experience, such as self-efficacy, intentionality, self-direction, and reflection, which strongly affect people's occupational choices. These aspects of "human agency" might also be described as self-management, a role that includes selecting, structuring, and prioritizing one's occupations and lifestyle within the context of social roles and relationships.

Self-Direction and Reflection

In social cognitive theory, people work on their intended action plans by giving them shape and direction over time. This self-direction includes both engagement and motivation in goal setting and an ongoing reevaluation and refinement. People set goals that are rooted in their personal identity and value system, thereby investing the subsequent activities with meaning and purpose (Bandura, 2001). Within this process, the nature of the goals becomes important. More distant goals are less motivating in the short run. More challenging goals provide the best incentives when they are broken down into more achievable subgoals to guide present actions. These actions also provide a sense of pride and self-worth. Yet self-direction also guides people to refrain from behaving in ways that bring them dissatisfaction or shame. According to Bandura (2001), moral agency forms an important part of self-directedness. For example, when competing with others for a desired goal, to what extent does morality influence or constrain efforts. A runner might strongly desire to win a race but will not purposely injure fellow competitors to do so. For most adults, standards of right and wrong remain stable during life pursuits, and this personal standard of morality guides the regulation of goal-directed behaviors.

How can a person apply social reasoning with respect to self-direction and goal setting? How do goals motivate people to engage in occupations?

Self-Regulation

Individuals set goals for themselves based partly on their belief in their own capability to achieve them. Self-awareness of one's strengths and limitations determines the types of goals people choose to undertake. Furthermore, people regulate the extent of their motivation and expectations of themselves based on the extent to which they believe they possess the prerequisite abilities and can control their own functioning. People who believe they are not smart may not attempt to learn something new or, if they do try, may give up after their first setback. In many life situations, belief in oneself needs also to be conveyed to others. For example, in applying for a job, it is necessary for the applicants to sell themselves and to articulate their own skills and assets to be offered the opportunity to perform an occupation. Their belief in their own effectiveness also extends to the control they can exert over other people and over other aspects of their environment.

The desire to act humanely toward others does not develop in isolation; there is a strong culturally based dimension of social expectation that shapes one's personal moral standards. Self-regulation often involves a kind of moral monitoring during the pursuit of life goals that prevents people from crossing self-imposed lines of acceptable conduct. For example, in constructing a profile for an online dating service, people might put the best spin on their social history but draw the line at outright lying.

Taking Advantage of Opportunities

The final process of Bandura's social cognitive theory deals with the handling of fortuitous or chance events. He gives the example of meeting potential marital partners while waiting for a delayed flight in an airport. If their flight had not been delayed, if they had not decided to sit in that particular café, they may not have met at all. Many married couples can tell a similar story of how they met by chance, or as a result of a series of unforeseen events beyond their control. Of course, the outcome of such meetings depends on whether they see it as an opportunity at all and what they do to continue the relationship afterward.

With many aspects of life, it is not always possible to control the internal or external phenomena that impact our lives. But if people wish to increase their chances of succeeding in their goals or intentions, there are almost always things they can do. People who go places and do things increase their opportunities for chance encounters. Then, what they do next depends on their self-efficacy and their ability to direct and regulate their behaviors to make the most of the opportunities afforded them. Social connections often form fortuitously, but once formed they evolve into friendships, intimate relationships, employment offers, career changes, or other opportunities for pursuing new learning or novel and enjoyable experiences. People who wish to enrich their lives need to be open to such opportunities without taking risks or becoming involved in scams or unsafe situations. Self-regulation helps people to make good judgments about such opportunities by guarding against participating in chance encounters that go against their internal moral standards.

5. Intentional Self-Management of Social Relationships and Environments Heightens Occupational Performance and Meaning

For occupational therapists, this hypothesis holds the most relevance for practice. If social relationships come under the control of clients themselves, and these have the potential to motivate, enhance, and give meaning to their occupational engagement, why would occupational therapists not want to understand and use this valuable tool? Some concepts from social cognitive theory help to explain the concepts of intentionality, self-efficacy, and self-determination. People may identify the intentional shaping of their own social connections and occupational goals setting as important aspects of self-management. In clinical and community settings, occupational therapists are well trained in designing and leading group interventions that facilitate member interaction, empathy, and support for one another. Groups offer the advantage of promoting various aspects of occupational performance with a supportive social context, thereby demonstrating the benefits of social group membership and modeling the skills necessary for developing and maintaining social relationships outside of therapy.

Self-Efficacy

Benight and Bandura (2004) consider self-efficacy the "foundation of human agency" (p. 1131). This belief in one's own abilities is necessary to manage one's own functioning and to control environmental events and circumstance that have an impact on one's life. Collected evidence confirms the importance of efficacy beliefs to the "quality of human functioning" (Benight & Bandura, 2004, p. 1131). This aspect of self and social identity influences the strength of motivation, the expression of emotion, and the direction and nature of goals and aspirations people have for themselves. In other words, people are more likely to engage in occupations when they believe they have a chance of achieving a successful outcome. In the face of threats to one's identity, such as the onset of a health condition, self-efficacy plays a key role in controlling stress responses, coping with problems, and persistence in attempting to manage or control both internal and external aversive events. For example, people who have experienced traumatic events are better able to control posttraumatic stress when they have a high sense of coping efficacy (Benight & Bandura, 2004).

A parallel to this became obvious in the productive aging study discussed earlier (Cole & Macdonald, 2015), when older adult participants described the prominence of their role as self-managers. This allowed them to take responsibility for their own aging processes and to make the necessary adaptations to continue to engage in the productive occupations that gave their lives meaning.

Intentionality

Intentions are future-directed plans of action. They emerge from a complex conscious cognitive process that considers not only desired outcomes but anticipated facilitators and barriers, as well as judgments of the likelihood that the plan will succeed. Intentions are vague at the outset; people refine the details in response to new information and may even reconsider their intentions when faced with obstacles along the way. Although an intention is self-motivated, it usually involves other "participating agents": people, groups, or organizations who share the intention and collaborate in working on a shared goal. For example, when a person intends to get promoted at work, he or she might take evening classes to obtain additional qualifications or make extra efforts to exceed the employers' expectations. This personal intention requires the cooperation of others: coworkers and supervisors, teachers and classmates, even family members who may make emotional and economic sacrifices to enable the "breadwinner" to work toward his or her intended outcome.

In the example of paid work, intentions require self-guidance, with tasks, activities, or occupations motivated and chosen according to a complex configuration of social expectations. For example, after 10 years of teaching at a university, I intended to achieve both promotion and tenure. To do so required that I have a significant publication or acquire an advanced degree. I chose to write and publish a book, as well as other research and scholarly efforts. Tenure, at that time, was awarded sparingly; it required an endorsement by a departmental evaluation committee composed of my peers, my director, and three other tenured faculty members from other departments. This committee also considered my student evaluations, my participation on university committees outside the department, and my voluntary contributions to both professional and neighboring communities. To achieve my "intention," I had to meet many social expectations, to enlist the cooperation of many other people, and also to write a book that was worthy of publication and that could be reviewed favorably by other members of my profession. Although writing a book might be considered an individual occupation, its publication and its relationship with my intended goal were also deeply embedded in institutional and social systems. My success in eventually achieving promotion and tenure depended heavily on the cooperation of many others. In the context of intention, the occupations of writing, teaching, and volunteering could not be separated from the social milieu within which they occurred. The questions in Learning Activity 3 at the end of the chapter will help the reader to explore his or her own intentions, goals, and future plans, with consideration for social influences, both positive and negative.

Intentionality requires a certain amount of forethought. People cognitively construct outcome expectations, and these serve as motivators for continuing in a set direction. In future planning, people consider the likely consequences of different plans of action, based on their own past experiences and those of others. They also anticipate possible barriers or detrimental outcomes, and think about how these might be circumvented or avoided. They may have multiple or conflicting goals and need to balance their current activities so that achieving one goal does not interfere with progress toward another, equally meaningful one.

People also plan ahead in the short term, both their daily activities and their structure for the next week or month. Actions in the short term could move them closer to long-term goals, or they could distract from or delay them. People who keep their intentions in mind are more likely to stay focused and to structure their lives around the achievement of distant or larger goals. For example, the intention of maintaining health requires short term steps or actions, such as planning healthy meals, going on daily walks, and taking medications as prescribed or carrying out treatment protocols for acute or chronic health conditions.

The term *intention* came up repeatedly in the productive aging study. Participants intentionally reached out to former coworkers after they had retired, recognizing the importance of maintaining these social connections. They intentionally built physical fitness activities into their daily schedules. Intentions helped these older adults to maintain their positive attitudes. They surrounded themselves with others who would keep them involved in their communities; they made activity or travel plans with family and friends so that they always had something to look forward to (Cole & Macdonald, 2015).

Socioemotional Selectivity in Friendship and Community Relationships

People naturally shape their own social networks, and socioemotional selectivity gives us some general guidelines as to how and why. The theory of socioemotional selectivity articulated by Carstensen (1998) explains social choices as a function of age or developmental life stage. Younger people choose friends for different reasons than older people do and receive different benefits from their social relationships. According to one recent study, younger cohorts tend to be future oriented, forming expanded and diverse social networks that offer novel experiences, whereas older cohorts prefer smaller social networks comprising familiar, emotionally close, and meaningful friendships (Lockenhoff & Carstensen, 2004). Researchers looked at three styles of friendship as a function of age: (1) discerning—enduring friendships with specific people, (2) independent—friends are closely linked with specific activities or life contexts, or (3) acquisitive—keep a core group of close friends but are open to new friends within specific contexts. As a function of age, younger adults tend toward acquisitive, middle adults toward independent, and older adults toward discerning. The discerning friendship style offers the highest degree of social and emotional support (Wright & Patterson, 2006). These trends can give occupational therapists some insights to how social support might be intentionally sought out by clients at different stages of life, depending on their goals and occupational priorities.

Social Support to Enable Occupational Performance and Well-Being

Social support theory contributes knowledge of the process and effects of various types of helping and caregiving. Evidence shows that partners and caregivers have a strong impact on occupational functioning for persons with disabilities, both positive and negative. Provision of social and emotional support can, in fact, have benefits for both the provider and the recipient (Reblin & Uchino, 2008). Concepts from this area help occupational therapists to collaborate with clients in evaluating their social contexts, including caregiver skills and attitudes, and the expectations of family members, friends, neighbors, and social and cultural norms in classroom, work, and community environments. Social support is clearly necessary for people recovering from illness or adapting to a disability to engage in meaningful occupations within their chosen environments. The success or failure of occupational therapy interventions often depends on the client's social supports or lack thereof.

Some studies suggest that social supports and interactions can serve as motivators to engage in occupations, both in wellness and while recovering from illness or injury. In a qualitative study of the potential of occupation for seniors, seven themes were identified: (1) Participation—"doing, not just watching"; (2) contributor to well-being; (3) means to express and manage identity; (4) connector to people; (5) organizer of time: (6) connector to past, present, and future; and (7) control essential for activity to fulfill its potential (Rudman, Cook, & Polatajko, 1997). This study supports the idea that the meaning of occupations is deeply embedded within social and temporal contexts. Looking at occupational engagement in women with spinal cord injury aged 25 to 61, researchers concluded that social support gives motivation in occupation through four mechanisms: (1) emotional support through confidence and togetherness, (2) practical support for basic self-care, (3) participation in reciprocal give-and-take relationships, and (4) cooperation and mutual problem solving with others in their social network (Isaksson, Lexell, & Skar, 2007). Here we learn that supportive social relationships can effectively facilitate occupational engagement during the healing process.

EVIDENCE FOR
OCCUPATIONAL THERAPY GROUP INTERVENTIONS

The best evidence for occupational therapy promotion of social participation comes from the well elderly studies over the past decade. Although not the original focus, small group meetings within the 9 months of the study enabled social connections, friendships, and mutual support among the older adult participants. Within the initial study, at a low-income, multicultural, high-rise apartment for seniors in Los Angeles, "the participants learned to balance their activities, enact healthy decisions in their lives, and face fears that create stagnation by challenging themselves within the group setting under the care of an occupational therapist" (Mandel, Jackson, Zemke, Nelson, & Clark, 1999, p. 17). In evaluating outcomes, researchers observed "we tested groups that had fairly consistent membership over nine months. There was a tremendous bond between group members and leader as well as between the group members themselves. Telephone numbers were exchanged to facilitate interaction between participants outside the group" (p. 55). The study reported highly successful outcomes with regard to life satisfaction, functional status, and health. In retrospect, it would have been interesting to also know to what extent these successes resulted from, or were enhanced by, the benefits of positive group interactions.

The second well elderly study, published in 2011, describes many examples of the benefit of group membership in providing support for making positive lifestyle changes and breaking down barriers to occupational participation. For community-dwelling seniors, that often meant exploring mobility issues, using group problem solving and support to overcome barriers, resulting in "improved health and greater participation in their communities" (Clark et al., 2011). The US studies were replicated in the United Kingdom with similar results (Mountain & Craig, 2011). Through occupational therapy–facilitated groups, participants were provided with the "space, time, and opportunity to share their experiences. Issues can be raised and conflicts re-enacted. Active experimentation can also take place here (within the therapeutic group)" (Craig & Mountain, 2007, p. 29).

Appreciating the wealth of evidence in support of the central role of social connectedness with health and well-being, occupational therapists need to draw on their training in group facilitation to reap its social benefits for clients. Groups have been shown to strengthen the effectiveness of occupational therapy interventions by providing the carefully orchestrated social environment that encourages members to support one another. As occupational therapists, we are in a rare position of being able to address both occupational and social dimensions within a group format. Through groups, occupational therapists can model the expression of empathy, emotional support, and giving and receiving constructive feedback; they can also encourage and enable the self-manager role for group members. Therapeutic use of self, applied through group leadership in occupational therapy, may be the ultimate application of social reasoning in our profession.

LEARNING ACTIVITY 1:
DRAW YOUR SOCIAL NETWORK

Put your own name in the center circle. Identify 6 people to whom you are close in the circles surrounding you. Then ask each of these people to identify 6 people to whom they are close and interact with often. Enter their names in the surrounding circles and draw lines connecting them as appropriate, including interconnections when friends or associates also connect with one another.

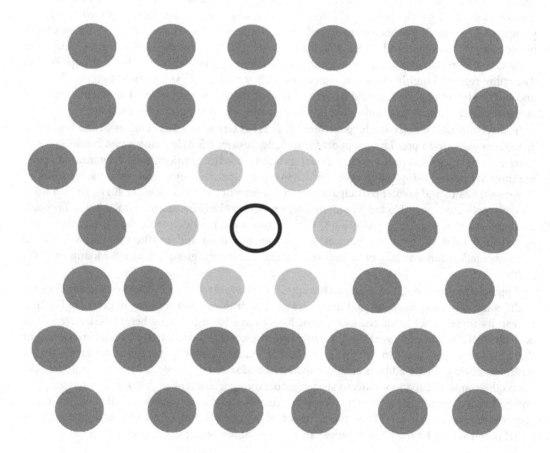

LEARNING ACTIVITY 2:
SOCIAL IDENTITY:
<u>SOME QUESTIONS TO THINK ABOUT</u>

a. How does a person acquire a social identity?

b. How do social groups support or reinforce members' social identity?

c. What causes social identity to change? Give an example.

d. Can social identity exist without performing occupations?

e. How does the performance of occupations strengthen one's social identity?

f. What is the role of memory in stabilizing social identity over time?

g. Looking at your own social identities, give an example of one positive identity and one negative identity you have held during your lifetime.

h. What are some occupations that serve to validate the meaning of your own life? List and describe at least five.

LEARNING ACTIVITY 3:
<u>INTENTIONS AND SOCIAL FACILITATORS</u>

a. What kinds of occupations do you consider worth doing?

b. What goals do you set for yourself?

c. Name one goal you are likely to achieve, and one goal that you may not achieve. Discuss your reasons for each.

d. What are the contexts within which you will engage in the occupations that will promote goal achievement?

e. With which other persons, groups, or organizations would you interact in the process of achieving your intentions?

f. How might your intentions be diverted, by yourself or others?

g. What events or circumstances might cause you to change your intentions or goals?

h. What has been an unintended consequence for one of your achievements or efforts?

i. In pursuing a goal, what might be some self-regulations that constrain people based on personal moral standards?

j. From the concepts of social cognitive theory, what can occupational therapists learn about client motivation to engage in occupations?

k. How can occupation be evaluated within the context of groups, organizations, and communities?

CONCLUSION

Because people generally do not view their occupations as separate from social roles, we might assume that they automatically consider their social relationships when making occupational and lifestyle choices. Current social science research provides considerable evidence for the influences inherent within social networks that shape such choices, with or without our awareness. Social reasoning encompasses not only how other people influence us, but also how we influence others through our words and actions. Occupations do not have meaning without considering their social contexts.

From a social cognitive perspective, people do have conscious intentions. Through a process of social learning, as described by Bandura (1971, 2001), they develop a sense of self-efficacy through trying out new social behaviors and observing and reflecting upon the responses of others. Neuroscientific evidence confirms the phenomenon of social learning through a mirror-neuron system in the brain, in which people watch or read about the experiences of others, both internalizing and empathizing with them. It is through social interaction that people develop a social identity, an internal vision of how others view them along with the constellation of occupations and social roles for which they feel capable, whether or not these are regularly performed. Throughout their lives, people set short- and long-term goals for themselves, often shaping the structure of their daily occupations to progress toward these goals. How, then, can we understand their occupations without also hearing the rest of their life stories? Social identity is a key concept because it reveals the motivation behind the occupations people choose. And evidence abounds that strong social identities often account for people's resilience, protecting them from the negative effects of stress and promoting health, well-being, and longevity.

Social reasoning compels occupational therapists to take a holistic view of clients, looking at their life stories with careful attention to their social identities, roles, relationships, and networks. As clients are becoming more empowered and self-determined, they need occupational therapists to support their role as self-managers, with a focus on intentionally building more supportive social environments within which to engage in the occupations that are meaningful within those contexts, and often because of them. Some recommendations for occupational therapists in each of the hypotheses for social reasoning are summarized in Table 9-2.

REFERENCES

Adolphs, R. (2009). The social brain: Neural basis of social knowledge. *Annual Review of Psychology, 60*, 693-716.

American Occupational Therapy Association. (2008). The occupational therapy practice framework: Domain and process (2nd ed.). *American Journal of Occupational Therapy, 62*, 625-683.

American Occupational Therapy Association. (2014). The occupational therapy practice framework: Domain and process (3rd ed.). *American Journal of Occupational Therapy, 68*, S1-S48.

Bandura, A. (1971). *Social learning theory.* New York, NY: General Learning Press.

Bandura, A. (2001). Social cognitive theory: An agentic perspective. *Annual Review of Psychology, 52*, 1-26.

Benight, C. C., & Bandura, A. (2004). Social cognitive theory of posttraumatic recovery: The role of perceived self-efficacy. *Behavior Research and Therapy, 42*, 1129-1148.

Carstensen, L. L. (1998). A life-span approach to social motivation. In J. Heckhousen & C. S. Dweck (Eds.), *Motivation and self-regulation across the life-span* (pp. 341-364). New York, NY: Cambridge University Press.

Christakis, N., & Fowler, J. (2009). *Connected: The surprising power of our social networks and how they shape our lives.* New York, NY: Little, Brown, & Co.

Christiansen, C. (1999). *Defining lives: Occupation as identity: An essay on competence, coherence, and the creation of meaning.* Retrieved from https://www.aota.org/-/media/Corporate/Files/Publications/AJOT/Slagle/1999.pdf

Clark, F., Jackson, J., Carlson, M., Chou, C., Cherry, B.J., Jordan-Marsh, M., et al. (2011). Effectiveness of a lifestyle intervention in promoting the well-being of independently living older people: Results of the well elderly 2 randomized controlled trial. *Journal of Epidemiology and Community Health.* Retrieved from http://jech.bmj.com/content/early/2011/06/01/jech2009.099754.full

Cohen, S. (2004). Social relationships and health. *American Psychologist, 59*, 676-684.

TABLE 9-2

SOCIAL REASONING RECOMMENDATIONS FOR OCCUPATIONAL THERAPY PRACTITIONERS

- Social roles and occupations are inseparable: Ask clients how their occupations and social roles and relationships are intertwined. Look for the meaning of and motivation for occupational goals within these social relationships.

- Social connections influence occupational and lifestyle choices: Define client social networks and evaluate the expectations and influences of social relationships for client occupational participation.

- Social cognition determines the success of occupational endeavors: Evaluate clients' social cognitive abilities with regard to setting realistic occupational goals, judging and regulating social behaviors, advocating for oneself, and ability to take advantage of opportunities and to enlist the help of others for occupational pursuits.

- Strong social identities motivate occupational engagement: Understand clients' occupational history with respect to social identity, encourage clients to remain engaged in groups and relationships that support that identity, and design occupational interventions that confirm it.

- Intentional self-management of social relationships and environments heightens occupational performance and meaning: Support client self-management and his or her ability to intentionally build and maintain supportive social networks and reciprocally beneficial social relationships. Use group interventions to model supportive social environments and build social skills that contribute to the development of reciprocal relationships.

Cole, M., & Macdonald, K. (2015). *Productive aging: An occupational perspective.* Thorofare, NJ: SLACK Incorporated.

Craig, C., & Mountain, G. (2007). *Lifestyle matters: An occupational approach to healthy ageing.* Milton Keynes, UK: Speechmark.

Dodds, P., & Muhamad, R. (2003). An experimental study of search in global social networks. *Science, 301,* 827-829.

Foss, C., Ginelli, M., & Turtle, B. (1996). *Six degrees of Kevin Bacon.* New York, NY: Penguin, Putnam, Inc.

Frankl, V. (1963). *Man's search for meaning.* New York, NY: Washington Square Press.

Frith, C. D., & Frith, U. (2007). Social cognition in humans. *Current Biology, 17,* R724-R732.

Guare, J. (1996). Six degrees of separation. Dramatists Play Service, Inc. Retrieved from http://www.dramatists.com/cgi-bin/db/single.asp?key-959

Haslam, C., Jetten, J., & Haslam, A. (2012). Advancing the social cure. In J. Jetten, C. Haslam, & A. Haslam (Eds.), *The social cure: Identity, health, & well-being* (pp. 319-343). New York, NY: Psychology Press.

Haslam, C., Jetten, J., Haslam, A., & Knight, C. (2012). The importance of remembering and deciding together: Enhancing the health and well-being of older adults in care. In J. Jetten, C. Haslam, & A. Haslam (Eds.), *The social cure: Identity, health, & well-being* (pp. 297-315). New York, NY: Psychology Press.

Haslam, C., & Reiker, S. D. (2006). Stressing the group: Social identity and the unfolding dynamics of responses to stress. *Journal of Applied Psychology, 91,* 1037-1052.

Hasselkus, B. (2011). *The meaning of everyday occupation* (2nd ed.). Thorofare, NJ: SLACK Incorporated.

Holt-Lunstad, J., Smith, T., & Layton, J. B. (2010). Social relationships and mortality risk: A meta-analytic review. *PLoS Medicine, 7,* 1-20. Retrieved from http://www.plosmedicine.org.e1000316

Isaksson, G., Lexell, J., & Skar, L. (2007). Social support provides motivation and ability to participate in occupation. *Occupational Therapy Journal of Research, 27,* 23-30.

Jetten, J. Haslam, C., & Haslam, A. (Eds.). (2012). *The social cure: Identity, health, & well-being.* New York, NY: Psychology Press.

Jetten, J., & Pachana, N. (2012). Not wanting to grow old: A social identity model of identity change (SIMIC) analysis of driving cessation among older adults. In J. Jetten, C. Haslam, & A. Haslam (Eds.), *The social cure: Identity, health, & well-being* (pp. 97-113). New York, NY: Psychology Press.

Lockenhoff, C. E., & Carstensen, L. L. (2004). Socioemotional selectivity theory, aging, and health: The increasingly delicate balance between regulating emotions and making tough choices. *Journal of Personality, 72*, 1395-1424.

Mandel, D., Jackson, J., Zemke, R., Nelson, L., & Clark, F. (1999). *Lifestyle Redesign: Implementing the well elderly program.* Bethesda, MD: AOTA Press.

Mattingly, C. (1998). *Healing dramas and clinical plots: The narrative structure of experience.* Cambridge, England: Cambridge University Press.

Milgram, S., Bickman, L., & Berkowitz, L. (1969). Note on the drawing power of crowds of different size. *Journal of Personality and Social Psychology, 13*, 79-82.

Mountain, G., & Craig, C. (2011). The lived experience of redesigning lifestyle post retirement in the U. K. *Occupational Therapy International, 18*, 48-58.

Reblin, M., & Uchino, B. (2008). Social and emotional support and its implication for health. *Current Opinions in Psychiatry, 2*, 201-205.

Rudman, D. L., Cook, J. V., & Polatajko, H. (1997). Understanding the potential of occupation: A qualitative exploration of seniors' perspectives on activity. *American Journal of Occupational Therapy, 51*, 640-650.

Sani, F. (2012). Group identification, social relationships, and health. In J. Jetten, C. Haslam, & A. Haslam (Eds.), *The social cure: Identity, health, & well-being* (pp. 21-38). New York, NY: Psychology Press.

St. Claire, L., & Clucas, C. (2012). In sickness and in health: Influences of social categorization on health-related outcomes. In J. Jetten, C. Haslam, & A. Haslam (Eds.), *The social cure: Identity, health, & well-being* (pp. 75-96). New York, NY: Psychology Press.

Tajfel, H. (1981). *Human groups and social categories.* Cambridge, England: Cambridge University Press.

Weitz, C., & Wood, L. (2005). Social identity support and friendship outcomes: A longitudinal study predicting who with be friends and best friends 4 years later. *Journal of Social and Personal Relationships, 22*, 416-432.

World Federation of Occupational Therapists. (2012). Definition of occupation. Retrieved from http://www.wfot.org/aboutus/aboutoccupationaltherapy/definitionofoccupationaltherapy.aspx

World Health Organization. (2001). *International classification of function, disability and health (ICF).* Geneva, Switzerland: Author.

Wright, K. & Patterson, B. (2006). Socioemotional selectivity theory and the macro dynamics of friendship: The role of friendship style and communication in friendship across the lifespan. *Communication Research Reports, 23*, 3, 13-170.

10

Creative Reasoning in Occupational Therapy

Estelle B. Breines, PhD, OTR, FAOTA

We have inherited a complex of traits which have been enabled by human creativity.

(Breines, 2005)

Although creativity is of compelling interest to various groups of people and is defined in many ways, its role in professional reasoning has not been fully explored to date as evidenced by the dearth of literature on this topic. Still, one finds creativity widely cited, often tucked in among language about learning, innovation, design, experimentation, and novel experiences (Iovine & Young, 2013). There are many approaches to creativity. May (1994) sees creativity as foundational to human development. Robinson (2013) advances ideas about how schools kill creativity, suggesting that popular notions held about learning are not certain. One young autistic savant, Jake Barnett, discusses what drives his own creative efforts (Safer, 2012).

Creativity in many of its forms is a fundamental issue for occupational therapy as well as many other disciplines (Runco & Pritzker, 1999). A variety of perspectives not ordinarily addressed may further an understanding of the topic. A selection of such elements are addressed in this chapter, as follows:

- The history of creativity in human development and its role in cultural evolution, ontogenetically and phylogenetically
- The interaction between automatic and deliberate behaviors in creative development through the integration of mind and body in performance
- The countervailing influences of environment and creativity
- Relationships among creativity, efficacy, and mastery as sources of professional reasoning
- Creative reasoning: efficacy and mastery for occupational therapists
- Developing creative professional reasoning through guided instruction

Creek and Cole (personal communication, 2013) noted that "Professional reasoning is understood to cover a broad spectrum of thinking, including clinical reasoning, ethical reasoning, creative thinking, problem-solving, collaborative working and understanding power relationships." It is the aspect of creative thinking, discussed here as creativity, that this chapter elaborates on.

Cole, M. B., & Creek, J. (Eds.).
Global Perspectives in Professional Reasoning (pp. 165-181).
© 2016 Taylor & Francis Group.

HISTORY OF CREATIVITY IN HUMAN DEVELOPMENT

Many features contribute to our understanding of creativity. In 1999, Runco and Pritzker composed a comprehensive encyclopedia dealing with the growing literature of creativity. It appears from their work that the largest portion of that literature is devoted to cognition and its influence on creativity, ignoring the influence of body on this process with one exception, the brain.

The literature on creativity tends to focus on the role of the mind in the creative process, without considering the unity of mind and body in task performance. This literature is largely grounded in cognitive psychology, within a Cartesian perspective of the world. From this perspective, the study of creativity appears to be grounded in reductionism, an odd configuration given the topic.

CREATIVITY IN EVERYDAY LIFE

This literature also exhibits an interest in the nature of genius on the creative process. To unlock the mystery of human creativity, Gruber (1981; Gruber & Voneche, 1986) examined the works of such geniuses as Darwin and Piaget. Yet study of the creativity of ordinary people is limited (McCrae, 1999). The mundane, those actions engaged in by all people in their usual tasks of living, is largely of secondary interest or of no interest at all. The requisite integration of mind and body in creative performance in work, play, leisure, and self-care receives limited attention. Yet creativity is of abiding interest to occupational therapists and others who recognize its importance in ordinary human events and advance its use as a therapeutic tool. Examining creativity from the perspective of the mundane tasks of living in which all people engage is an alternative way of exploring creativity.

This alternative way to think about creativity was promoted by John Dewey (1929), the renowned American pragmatist philosopher and educator, who describes this driving force as human beings' quest for certainty, a process of creating understanding through active occupation. There appears to be an inherent underlying drive for people to engage in new and stimulating experiences. According to Dewey (1916), these efforts are made in the hope of serving both self and society.

Performance alone is not sufficient, however. Intermittent success experiences are needed, sufficient to encourage repeated efforts. Hence, we speak of the just right challenge, often used to test oneself against difficult tasks or situations and so extend one's repertoire of skills. Creativity is a feature of individual effort, reinforced by success and positive social feedback. Creativity requires that one engage in risk-taking behaviors in anticipation that risk will foster future success. Without success, further effort is unlikely. Healthy humans are continually seeking the just right challenge in their efforts to achieve, contributing to their personal well-being and the welfare of their community in their pursuits.

Humans are endowed with a creative force, which they have used over the millennia to solve increasingly more complex and specialized problems. This evolving creative force has been described as a process of occupational genesis (Breines, 2005) in which creativity enables humans to engage in a series of evolving occupations, throughout individual lifetimes and throughout the millennia.

OCCUPATIONAL GENESIS

Occupational genesis, the evolution of human activity, is built on a uniquely human ability: creativity. With a long history of applying their creative abilities to their personal and social survival, human beings are reputedly the only creatures on earth endowed with this ability. While other

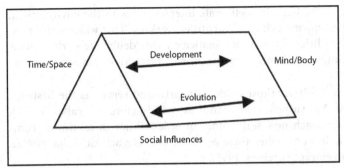

Figure 10-1. Occupational genesis: Interaction among mind/body, time/space, and society continue through the lifespan and evolve throughout the millennia. (Copyright © Estelle B. Breines.)

beings are able to use tools in limited ways, human beings have honed this skill to continually foster new, creative, and meaningful problem solving in a perpetual process. Through this process, civilization in all its forms has evolved and continues to evolve in a process that begins with understanding the lifelong development of the individual.

Human beings develop and change throughout their lifetimes from birth to the end of life. Initially their physical and mental capacities follow a largely prescribed path. Their genetic makeup inherited from their ancestors structures much of this path at the outset. However, as time passes, the minds and bodies of individuals diversify in capacity according to the individual directions that people's interests, skills, and talents take.

Throughout this developmental process, their sociocultural environment has as much influence as do their inherited abilities on the directions people take in developing their capacities. Ontogeny recapitulates a phylogenetic path set down in our DNA and is influenced by our experience in the various tangible and social worlds in which we live and in which we have lived throughout our history.

In a complex set of circumstances, human development takes an interactive path. The egocentric (mind–body), exocentric (time–space), and consensual (sociocultural) aspects of individuals' lives interact, each aspect influencing the others (Figure 10-1). Phylogenetic development is a long and adaptive evolutionary process that extends from its beginnings in the prehistoric past through ancient and modern history toward an unpredictable future, for the individual as well as society. Since our earliest past, human beings' lives have changed, as has their world, stimulated by the creativity of human beings, the characteristics of their tangible world, and the influences of others.

An important and universal relational paradigm is inherent in understanding creativity. This dialectical phenomenon underlies and influences one's ability to grow in skill and capacity. This phenomenon can be explained through the interaction of automatic and deliberate behaviors (Breines, 1986). Skill in performance emerges from the interaction of these two phenomena, one that is grounded in the past and one that reaches into the future.

AUTOMATIC BEHAVIORS IN HUMAN DEVELOPMENT

All creatures are endowed with certain automatic abilities, some of which are evident at birth, and some of which are acquired later. These reflexes or traits are inherited from ancient ancestors who preceded humankind. These automatic traits are developed according to preprogrammed and inherited schedules. For example, reaction to a touch on the cheek is spontaneous and universal among well infants. When touched, an infant turns his or her head to a mother's breast to prepare to suck and swallow, thus contributing to his or her own survival. Primitive automatic responses, identified as reflexes, serve as the foundation for acquiring interaction with the environment. Piaget (Ginsburg & Opper, 1979) described this process as assimilation, accommodation, and equilibration.

These enabling behaviors serve as the basis for deliberate interactions with the environment, enabling the acquisition of further automatic behaviors identified as skills. That which nature has given us is converted to acquired abilities. That is, automaticity yields deliberate performance, which in turn yields further automaticity, hence a transactional interaction continues among automatic and acquired abilities.

A series of developmental reflexes follows those evident at birth and serves as the basis for behaviors acquired soon afterward. We sit before we stand; we stand before we walk; we walk before we run. In early development, each new skill comes in order, although its timing commonly varies from person to person. It is only when these reflexes have been activated that human uniqueness and the creative process emerge (Breines, 1995).

Beyond those inherited predictable abilities that establish our fundamental performances and our survival, we spend our lives acquiring new, often individualized skills that we ultimately can perform with some level of automaticity, akin to those inherited traits. Learned performances serve the same functional purpose as those automated traits with which nature initially endowed us. Once acquired, they can be disregarded, enabling automaticity in their performance, and once automated, they serve as grounding for creativity and new learning.

How Skill Building Incorporates Automatic Aspects

True skill in the performance of any task requires that a portion of the task be performed automatically. If one were perpetually required to think consciously about all aspects of a task, one would be unable to proceed further in learning. As Huss (1981) reminds us, a youngster who cannot sit ably has difficulty learning to read and write, or even to feed him- or herself. Just walking across the room would occupy all of our effort if we needed to focus on the placement of each foot as we traveled. But that is not what nature had in mind. We are gifted adaptively with the ability to ignore, so that we may learn to function on higher and higher levels of performance, enabling further ongoing creativity. Essentially, this is the foundation of occupational therapy's belief in goal-directed activity as a therapeutic tool. The acquisition of automaticity enables one to develop creativity and grow in skill building.

Skill development is grounded in automatic behaviors, some of which are inherited, and some of which are acquired. This is true for society as a whole as well as for the individual. As Whitehead stated, civilization advances according to the things we can do without paying attention to them, not the reverse (Medawar, 1957). According to this belief, telling someone to "pay attention" to further his or her proficiency may be contrary to best practice.

Examples of human occupation that rely on automatic performance are endless. In fact, they are universal. Every activity in which we engage throughout the life span consists of aspects that are automatically performed. With a foundation of automatic performances on which one can rely, one is able to concentrate deliberately and creatively on solving new problems and acquiring new knowledge and skill. And simultaneously, this diversion strengthens reliable automatic performances on subordinate levels.

Learning New Skills: Some Everyday Examples

Recall how one learns a skill and makes it one's own. When learning to use a keyboard, for example, all one can think of at the outset is the fingering and the location of the keys. One focuses at first on individual letters, building sets of automatic mini-skills as fingering is established, until the keyboard is mastered. These motor and spatial learning skills take much time and effort to acquire and to use purposefully. In the beginning, much of the effort is cognitive; little is automatic. However, in time, as one learns to keyboard with speed and efficiency, automaticity is exhibited. This automaticity enables one to create words and sentences, until ideas pour forth, without a single letter being noted as the work proceeds.

The same process occurs when one is beginning to learn to drive a new vehicle. Consider how it feels to drive a new car. Driving a new car requires careful attention. The stick shift may be in a different location and have a different feel; the mirrors can be located higher or lower than one is accustomed to; the pedals respond to different forces; and the width and length of car may be different. All of these changes from the familiar initially require careful focusing to drive safely and are apt to generate anxiety in the driver. With experience, the familiar can be ignored, and indeed must be if further skill is to be developed. What has become automatic can now be ignored. Mastering the controls requires close attention, but truly proficient driving only takes place when one is able to ignore the details and can sally forth to a destination and accomplish a role.

This process of new learning begins with precision and focus, extending to skilled performance, and is the same process for each skill one masters. What our brains initially deal with on a cognitive or deliberate level converts to a process described here as automaticity, which Ayres (1973) identified as subcorticalization. Only when one can perform certain skills automatically can that skill be applied to new learning. Paying close attention, while enabling at first, is limiting rather than expanding, despite the oft-cited motto to the contrary. It is the ability to perform without conscious attention to details that engenders creativity.

Whether one is learning to operate a toy or sew a hem, the details are initially attended to by the learner, eventually converting to a set of automatic behaviors that enable one's creativity to emerge, unfettered by the details that initiated the process. Throughout, mind and body perform together, automaticity leading to deliberation, and deliberation leading to further automaticity, in a dialectical phenomenon that was described earlier.

THE COUNTERVAILING INFLUENCES OF ENVIRONMENT AND CREATIVITY

As human beings developed various occupations from earliest prehistory to the modern era, they engaged in a process that integrated environmental constituents in their performance. Applying these skills in a range of tasks "from clay to computers" (Breines, 1995), creativity enabled humans to invent a series of evolving occupations, in a process of occupational genesis, to meet the demands of a perpetually changing world. Each creative invention led to the development of further implements and techniques, enhancing engagement in life tasks. Drawing on the ideas of Dewey, occupational therapists adopted this knowledge to create a model of therapy based on this acquisition of occupations (Breines, 1986).

CREATIVITY IN EVOLVING SOCIETIES

The objects that early human beings had available to them to aid in their survival were very precious and hard won. For example, harvesting honey from a nest high up in a tree requires tremendous effort and skill and considerable risk to life and limb. Yet despite these hazards, the problems inherent in accomplishing these tasks were solved. Certainly society would not support the risk such efforts would cause to the community unless there was some benefit to be obtained. Limited resources are of great concern to a society that is striving to survive and in which each individual is a precious commodity. Survival is not a solitary effort; it is a goal of a social group and the result of collaborative effort. Everyone must contribute to the benefit of all, or the group will not survive.

Auel's respected series of novels, collectively entitled *Earth Children* (1980–2011), presented information that largely was built from archaeological research and a knowledge of indigenous peoples. These books metaphorically describe how the earliest people gained knowledge and applied it to life's tasks. Ayla, Auel's protagonist, gained experience through trial and error, acquiring skills in the many environments in which she traveled over time, as a representation of how human knowledge builds on previous knowledge, influenced by the varying nature of the environments in which people live.

This evolutionary process serves as a foundation for understanding the development of all human endeavors, illustrating the creativity of the makers in using the materials available within their environment in the process. In time, human beings coursed through the Stone Age, the Bronze Age, the Iron Age, to an era of industrialization, through to the technological era in which we find ourselves today.

Invention is structured by the elements available in a given environment. For example, while baskets are a common early artifact created by people all over the world, many are markedly different in material as well as style. Each climate produces different sorts of vegetable materials. These materials stimulate ideas. In different times and climes, vines, reeds, wood—all have been modified to produce tools and artifacts that are used by their creators to meet their life needs. Recognizing how people and their world evolved reveals the role of creativity in this process.

CREATIVITY AS AN ADAPTIVE TRAIT

Essentially, those who are well adapted to the environment are likely to live longer than those who are not well adapted; the latter therefore are less likely to live to procreate. Consequently, the traits of those who are maladapted will be lost to the gene pool, which may not be an advantage to the individual but is a great advantage to the species as a whole (Dawkins, 1996).

Not only did natural selection aid in inherited survival, the ability to solve problems creatively contributed to adaptive health and survival. Thus, a body of curious, erect people descended from their ancestors, later known as humans (Petit, 1999). They spread out in different directions, meeting ever-new environments and their inherent problems. From a life in the trees to one where one stands tall in the grass to peer beyond to find food and observe danger required learning new skills. Standing and ambulating became an asset. Their lower limbs supported them and enabled locomotion, while freeing their upper limbs for manipulation and hand specialization. Their opposable thumb and hand dominance enabled them to do remarkable things with the objects they found in their world (Bower, 2003).

Performing purposeful tasks while they moved about on two legs enabled their adaptive survival in their new world. Erect posture, bipedalism, and opposing thumbs led to the development of skills in cognition and communication that furthered their competence. Or, as Washburn (1960) suggests, perhaps it was the reverse. Regardless, people who could manipulate their hands and minds could devise tools and artifacts from the natural things that surrounded them. With communication they could share their ideas and skills, informing their offspring and their community, thereby influencing the survival of their kind thereafter.

THE ROLE OF COMMUNICATION IN SURVIVAL

With their new ability to communicate, ancient peoples shared an understanding of the hazards that surrounded them and created potential solutions. They shared their knowledge of the environment, identifying where nut and fruit trees and berry bushes grew, and the seasons of their ripeness. Communication enabled them to plan their hunts along the annual paths of animals in their migration so they could hunt communally to feed themselves and their offspring, thus thriving on this knowledge (Ziker, 2003).

Communication enabled them to provide information from past to current and later generations through a shared oral tradition. Storytelling, music, song, and dance served as a library of information to be remembered and transmitted from parents to offspring, from elders to youth, and from community to community.

The progeny of these early people brought these memories and ideas with them as they dispersed widely throughout the world, ultimately covering all of the habitable continents and their various climates and terrains. They moved into the mountains, and they lived along the shores learning about the earth and the seas. In each new place, they were confronted with new and arduous conditions. In response, they devised new means of dealing with the hardships they encountered by creating objects and methods from the world around them. They conquered each season and each change in climate in their various geographies by creating adaptations of what they found in nature to meet their needs in the various environments they called home.

CULTURE AND CREATIVE ARTS

As expertise grew, people ornamented their artifacts and their bodies to reflect the worlds they saw about them. Weaving methods were devised to take advantage of the qualities of the materials at hand. People created designs by interweaving natural colors and textures. They dyed their materials using vegetable matter, insects, and other things. Their weaving imbedded objects such as beads and feathers. A visit to any museum containing cultural artifacts will illustrate the many different kinds of baskets and clothing made throughout the world, demonstrating their regional uniqueness. Objects housed in museum collections from Asia, Africa, North America, South America, and other regions differ in their characteristics (e.g., American Museum of Natural History and Brooklyn Museum in New York City; Khouri-Dagher, 1998) and are readily identified as to their origins by experts.

Objects were decorated according to their environmental experiences. The blue of ice influenced the creative artistry of peoples in the north; the red and gold of the sun are found in products from warmer regions. Symbols from nature are found in the pictographs they used for decoration and writing. Mountains, water, animals, birds, and fish—the items of life's sustenance—were inscribed in their work. Clay from the mud of streambeds became pots of beauty and endurance as they learned to master heat (Rossotti, 1993). Clay from different regions produced pots with different characteristics using different techniques. Some are quite distinctive, such as the beautiful black pottery made by the Santa Maria tribe (Native Web, 2003).

Fire provided them with food, warmth, and tools, as they applied it to objects in the world around them (Goudsbloom, 1994). In learning to control fire, people created metal from rocks, forming tools of ever-greater strength and complexity. Their knowledge of the smelting of copper, bronze, and brass was applied to the working of iron, later adapted to the manufacture of steel and more complex metals (Breines, 1995; Cramb, 2003). The objects they created were both purposeful and means of expression and were used for sharing with others and for gaining recognition from others.

CREATING OCCUPATIONS IN THE EVOLUTION OF MODERN CULTURES

The means people needed to survive were invented in all the places they roamed, influencing their cultures. They harvested the tangible and worshipped the intangible. And as they traveled, their languages became increasingly differentiated, and the standards for behavior of their families and neighbors evolved in each place, along with their skills.

Hunters and gatherers who harvested what naturally grew around them ultimately became farmers, planting rice in paddies and wheat, corn, and barley on the plains. And as they settled, they developed a commitment to the land on which they grew their crops. They became expert in growing what they understood, raising potatoes in one locale and tomatoes in another. The harsh climate in Russia and other northern countries produced root vegetables and vodka, whereas tomatoes, zucchini, and wine thrived in the Mediterranean. Recipes grounded in wheat, rice, and maize emerged that characterized their diverse peoples.

These varying products introduced commodity trading, with some people devoted to travel as their means of survival. Nomads became experts in animal husbandry, moving their flocks and families about to meet the needs of people and animals. Camels, sheep, reindeer, and yaks served the same survival needs, yielding different products and contributing to different cultural identities. Each provided meat and clothing to feed and clothe the community.

Many processing techniques were developed. Milk was turned into cheese so it would last longer before spoiling. Other means of preserving food were developed as well, as each season was not equal in providing for people's welfare. They learned to dry meat and fruit, pickle vegetables, make jams and jellies, all to preserve food from a bountiful season in anticipation of the barren winter of deep cold. They devised explanations for the seasons, praying for the return of bounty. They developed festivals to celebrate the harvests and their annual return, learning calculation and calendation in the process.

RELATIVE PERMANENCE OF HUMAN CREATIVE EFFORTS OVER TIME

Some human activities changed over time, but many of them remained the same, although often not for the same purposes for which they were originally developed. Ancient activities originally designed for survival in one community often became leisure activities in another. For example, fishing rods that enabled survival in one generation became a source of leisure and relaxation at a later time. These activities provided satisfaction and competence to the masters of these skills, regardless of their origins and purposes (Breines, 1981, 1995). The ancient activities of clay, leatherwork, and yarn crafts remained meaningful when incorporated into culturally relevant activities, so did later activities such as carpentry, metal craft, and printing and the more recent ones of website construction and videography (Breines, 1995). Each activity filled the need humans have for creative engagement, reinforced by social commentary and influence. Whether of ancient or modern origin, these activities filled people's lives and provided personal satisfaction and feedback from others.

This process of human and cultural development has been described as a genesis of occupations (Breines, 1990). It is an unending process of evolution and development in which human beings are perpetually engaged. Occupational genesis is dependent on a mixture of human abilities of both mental and physical construction. These are incorporated with the contributions of the environment in which people live, along with a social network through which communication allows the sharing of knowledge from person to person from the past to the future.

We have inherited a complex of traits that have been enabled by human creativity. These traits survived millennia in which we encountered untold numbers of problems, solving some and disposing of others, leading us to enhanced health and longevity. When provided with the filtering of time and experience, our ancestors were assured the healthful development of the community from generation to generation (Breines, 1981, 1986, 1990, 1995, 2005).

CREATIVE REASONING: EFFICACY AND MASTERY FOR OCCUPATIONAL THERAPISTS

Creativity, efficacy and mastery are the keys to successful human endeavour. Creativity is built on feelings of self-identity and self-confidence that emerge from experiences of success, for without these qualities, one is less likely to stretch one's imagination in pursuit of further accomplishment. Efficacy refers to proficiency, whereas mastery describes a higher order of accomplishment. Together, they speak to the accomplishments of all human endeavor.

TAKING A HISTORICAL PERSPECTIVE

The history of creativity in human development described in the previous sections leads us to appreciate the fact that all of the objects that surround us, and the ways that we use them in our daily lives, have evolved from creative solutions to past problems encountered by our ancestors. For example, in developed countries, hunting and gathering are no longer necessary for our survival because our predecessors have, over time, created vast systems of agriculture, fishing, farming, and ranching, leading to today's convenience of purchasing our food at a local grocery store. Likewise, if we are lucky enough to live in a developed country with sufficient resources, the objects and equipment in a modern kitchen make meal preparation quick and easy, even automatic. We don't need to cut wood and build a fire to cook. We have a stove, an oven, and a microwave. And it is precisely because many aspects of feeding ourselves and our families have become automatic that we can, at times when we choose to, be creative in trying out new recipes, adding herbs, mixing flavors, and experimenting with new preparation strategies. Thus our creative cooking efforts are built on the automatic aspects provided by the creative problem solvers of previous generations.

Likewise, occupational therapists have learned their trade from the knowledge and skills of others who have gone before. Some of our education involves reading and understanding scientific bodies of knowledge, other parts require physical and practical skills. Yet the unique part of being an occupational therapist is not the knowledge and skills we have acquired but, rather, how we think, reason, and approach clients and situations. To create the best interventions and solutions for the recipients of our services, we must stand on the shoulders of those master clinicians who have paved the way with theories, models of practice, and successful strategies and outcomes. Creative reasoning includes the choices we make in selecting from the repertoire of our own past experiences and those of others who have gone before. It also includes how we evaluate outcomes and how we choose to learn from our mistakes as well as our successes.

SELF-EFFICACY'S ROLE IN MASTERY

People experience self-satisfaction when they are successful at occupations in which they engage (White, 1959). This trait tends to engender feelings of wellness that accrue to people who achieve satisfaction through their personal efforts. This belief is at the core of occupational therapists' commitment to therapeutic activity as a means of promoting health. On the other hand, dissatisfaction and anxiety are apt to contribute to ill health. For example, the work schedules in which people in various cultures engage to earn their living may be making demands on them that are detrimental to their health and welfare (Association of Professional Executives of the Public Service of Canada, 1997; Schiltz, 1999).

Every skill in which one seeks mastery is practiced until automaticity is achieved. Mastery enables further creativity and its inherent risk taking. Mastery on one level leads one to establish goals for achievement on ever increasing levels of performance. For example, playing chess requires that one first know which way each of the pieces can move before the game can begin. Practice with other skilled players can eventually lead to winning a game of chess. Creative activities are made possible by developing skills on lower levels of performance, performing them automatically, and committing those subskills to the refinement of goal-directed performance. This foundation in subskills underlies the development of new performances and invention. Invention, the essential result of creativity, may only occur when one has mastery of the necessary underlying skills upon which one can rely. Mastery has been achieved when one does not need to pay attention. Skill building means building performance skills on subordinate levels of automatic performance by diverting attention to new and compelling learning.

Students of occupational therapy must master skills in therapeutic use of self. Although it helps to have a natural tendency to socialize with others, professional students also need to appreciate the difference between conversing with friends and the art of establishing a therapeutic relationship. This often means starting over and building the skills of therapeutic interactions, for example, learning to ask open questions, express empathy, and strategically use self-disclosure to develop trust and connection. When these skills become automatic, students can then practice using them in establishing client-centered partnerships, a more nuanced application in which they convey respect for persons' values and preferences, collaborate with them in setting realistic goals, and guide them in finding their own creative solutions to the problems they encounter in their everyday occupations and lives. For occupational therapy professionals, creative reasoning often means refraining from solving problems for our clients, and instead finding ways to encourage and facilitate the client's own creativity.

Just as with all skills, one acquires skill in professional reasoning. Recognizing the relationships among creativity, efficacy, and mastery can contribute to this process. Although initially professional reasoning is addressed consciously and deliberately, it is truly evidenced when it is exhibited automatically. A master clinician can be identified by his or her proficiency in reaching for the right tools, setting up the environment so it is most effective, or touching the patient in exactly the right way to elicit a favorable response. In fact, research in clinical reasoning has shown that automatic performance is evident in mastery, that to understand the process, it is necessary to bring to conscious attention that which has been demonstrated automatically. This compels clinicians as subjects of study to examine their actions consciously in retrospect.

CREATIVE PROBLEM SOLVING: BUILDING CREATIVE ADAPTATIONS

Automaticity is evidence of mastery, both for the individual and for society as a whole. Engaging in satisfying activity can provide the automaticity that enables creative problem solving toward a healthy society, enabling humans to survive as a species. In all life roles, we depend on certain necessities being accomplished automatically to more fully attend to new problems and to creatively address new personal and professional goals. For example, a busy mother who works full time might do all the cooking for the week over the weekend, so that she and her family members can heat up prepared meals whenever their busy weekday schedules permit. As occupational therapists, we might see this strategy as a creative adaptation to a hectic lifestyle. Occupational therapy students and professionals often save time by consciously building adaptive habits and routines, such as showering and laying out clothing in the evening and organizing a backpack or briefcase the night before a busy workday. Building the habit may take some time but, once it is mastered, doing these preparatory tasks becomes automatic.

When confronted with a new problem, all people need to reason creatively: a child gets sick, and mother cannot go to work; a car breaks down, preventing a retired elder from doing his grocery shopping. Such problems, although temporary, require creative solutions. Think about a homeless person, evicted from his apartment for nonpayment of rent since he lost his job. When he falls through the cracks in public assistance, is it not creative to keep his belongings in a shopping cart or sleep in an abandoned car? When people encounter unexpected health issues, such as broken hip, heart attack, or stroke, they often feel overwhelmed and may need the help of an occupational therapist just to get their basic needs met before they can begin to think about creative problem solving with regard to their disrupted occupations. Helping clients to creatively solve the problems brought on by health conditions and to reorganize and build creative adaptations that enable them to continue engaging in meaningful occupations is one of the most rewarding aspects of being an occupational therapist.

Creativity is enabled by the physical and mental abilities that humans bring to problem solving. It is reinforced by the confidence, or feelings of efficacy, one acquires as one performs successfully (Fidler, 1981; White, 1959). Satisfaction with self is both personally and socially experienced. Feelings of efficacy derive from mastery of skills, illustrated by performance that provides people with feelings of control and satisfaction. It is also reinforced by feedback from others.

In practice, occupational therapists benefit from feedback from their peers or supervisors when their creative efforts produce positive outcomes. This principle also applies when working with clients: We should take every opportunity to guide, support, and validate their efforts to use creativity in adapting to changes and solving life's problems. In this way, both professionals and clients will gain the confidence to take further risks in finding creative solutions.

RESOURCEFULNESS

A resource is a "stock or reserve that can be drawn upon as needed" (*Shorter Oxford English Dictionary*, 2002). To be resourceful is to be "capable, full of practical ingenuity" (Creek, 2014, p. 1). For occupational therapists, being resourceful is necessary to find and acquire the things they need and to identify and engage the people they need to accomplish their goals. In traditional settings, resources are provided by health care organizations or with public funding. However, professionals who seek out underserved populations in communities or in nontraditional settings often need to be exceedingly resourceful in obtaining equipment, materials, spaces, and personnel for which funding has not been automatically provided. For example, an occupational therapist is asked to establish a community program to assist people who are unemployed and living in a homeless shelter to learn the skills they need to find new jobs. How will creative reasoning help him or her with this task? What information will be needed, and where might it be found? What materials and equipment will be needed, and where might they be acquired? Who might be available to administer such a program, and where should it take place? Please see Learning Activity 5 to practice your own creative reasoning skills with the homeless shelter employment project. Examples of occupational therapists who have established programs in nontraditional settings may be found in Chapters 5, 6, 7, and 12.

ENVISIONING THE FUTURE

Just as our ancestors sought to better their living conditions for themselves and their children, we also strive to make the world a better place for our own as well as upcoming generations. Nothing requires more creativity than forming a dream for the future because our imaginations are free to wander unconstrained by today's realities. However, an accurate assessment of those realities will be necessary for the dream to have any chance of coming true. Here is a good place to apply the principles of occupational genesis, considering egocentric, exocentric, and consensual dimensions.

- Egocentric (mind–body)—What practical and creative abilities do you have to pursue your dream? What personal resources could you call on? What life experiences would help you achieve your vision?
- Exocentric (time–space)—Where are you in life's course, relative to how much time it might take to reach your goal? Where you living and with whom? What are the physical surroundings or structures like? What financial resources are available to you?
- Consensual (social/cultural)—What political system surrounds you, and how much control or input can you have to public policy? How does your cultural background affect your ability to move forward with your goal? To what social networks do you belong and what is your position within them?

Because human development is an interactive journey, each of these dimensions of occupational genesis continually affects the others through time, from past to present and future. The questions posted represent only the beginnings of the creative reasoning involved in envisioning a future that is different from the present. For yourself, in your early adulthood, you might set a goal to become a doctor. In midlife, you may decide to run for public office in an attempt to right the wrongs of a broken political system. In retirement, you may wish to learn a new skill, such as gardening, drawing, playing a musical instrument, or learning how to play golf. More enterprising retirees may wish to find new ways to stay engaged with communities, such as starting their own business or advocating for a social cause. Visions for ourselves are highly dependent on the answers to the questions just posed, and many others. Envisioning a future for groups, populations, or whole societies becomes more dependent on the extent of our influence on and collaboration with others or working as part of a team. Some such projects are described in Chapters 3, 4, 5, 6, and 12. The evolution and unfolding of goals and intentions are more fully described in Chapter 9 as a part of social cognitive theory.

For occupational therapists, envisioning the future with clients requires a more interactive type of creative reasoning. The unique set of abilities and circumstances that contributed to their own personal goals or intentions may have been compromised by illness or disability, causing the entire trajectory to become disrupted. In this situation, only the occupational therapist may be able to imagine what is possible for clients based on evidence and experience with other similar clients, while the clients themselves remain immersed in the discouraging and challenging struggles of the rehabilitation process. A wounded soldier with a newly amputated leg, for example, may not be able to envision being able to walk again, let alone ski, ride a bicycle, or climb a mountain. Yet for some, these things are possible and have been accomplished, thanks to medical and technological advances available today.

The occupations we choose for the future are often generated by the problems we see all around us in the present. How many young people choose health care careers based on their interactions with a parent, sibling, or close friend whose ongoing health problems they were unable to solve as children? The parent of a child who died needlessly because of bullying, gun violence, or drunk driving often becomes the champion of a cause to prevent these things from happening to anyone else. What inequities do you see around you? How could you use your own knowledge and abilities to change things or to make a difference?

DEVELOPING CREATIVE REASONING THROUGH GUIDED INSTRUCTION

A distinguishing feature of human beings in the course of this evolutionary and developmental process is their ability to manipulate the environment in creative and skillful ways, to meet their physical, mental, emotional, and interactive needs as thoughtful and adventurous social beings. Teaching students this process so they internalize it is vital if they plan to use active occupation as a therapeutic tool. Yet identifying effective methods for teaching is often a dilemma. I recommend reviewing the concept of occupational genesis at the outset. This can be done in multiple ways. First, the conceptual framework should be identified. Here is where the relationships among ego-centric, exocentric, and consensual elements, both ontogenetically and phylogenetically, are made clear to the students. Using a simple model such as Figure 10-1 to frame the ideas can be helpful in clarifying these relationships (Breines, 1995). Use the concept of occupational genesis to demonstrate that activities we now recognize as recreational were initially active occupations in which people engaged for their survival benefits. Furthermore, many of these same activities still have a role in modern work, play, leisure, and self-care and, ultimately, a role in therapy.

LEARNING ACTIVITY 1:
OCCUPATIONAL GENESIS

Imagine that you are an uninjured survivor of a plane crash, stranded on a deserted tropical island with no rescue in the near future. This could be either an individual or a small group activity.

a. In your life raft there are five basic tools. What should they be?

b. List your five top priorities for survival on the island until you are rescued.

c. Imagine what the island might look like. How would you use the natural resources on the island to meet your basic needs? Explain in detail how you might use your skills, tools, and resources to accomplish your top five priorities.

d. Think about how ancient peoples also used the natural resources that surrounded them to ensure their survival. What creative arts and crafts could have developed from their attempts to solve the practical problems they faced on the same island you have imagined in this exercise? List and describe at least five.

LEARNING ACTIVITY 2:
ARTS AND CRAFTS IN HUMAN EVOLUTION

Organize the laboratory instruction of activities "from clay to computers" so that students can obtain skills in a variety of tasks that can be used therapeutically, while recognizing that these activities are not frivolous but were life skills in the eras in which they were initially developed. Examples are clay sculpting, woodworking, simple hand-loom weaving, crocheting, leather working, and basket weaving. Communication through the ages might be demonstrated through use of drawing or painting to convey ideas or teach skills or through the use of gestures in dance or mime to convey emotions or intentions. This helps to develop respect for activity as a valuable tool, negating the impression that crafts are unimportant uses of time and effort.

LEARNING ACTIVITY 3:
ACTIVITIES OF THE INDUSTRIAL WORLD

Another useful learning task for students, embedded in a lab reflecting activities of the industrial world, requires going to a building supply store containing myriad objects such as pipes, screws, and other things that have been designed for a particular purpose (found or discarded objects may also be used). From this array of items, the students choose an item and reconfigure it in such a way that it now can serve another purpose, thus stimulating their creative instincts along with their manipulative skills. This exercise results in an unlimited supply of ideas, as illustrated in different classes from year to year. Each student demonstrates his or her product to the class, helping everyone to expand his or her notions of creativity.

The most memorable results of this lesson for me as the teacher are the variability and uniqueness of each project and the effect that each project has had on the other students in the class. Each student expects to be capable of performing this simple task; however, students are always much more impressed with their classmates' productions than their own, often being astonished by the creativity of their colleagues.

LEARNING ACTIVITY 4:
DEVELOPING A NEW SKILL

This assignment is a lengthy one. At the beginning of the semester, students select an activity that they want to learn. The choices are completely up to the students and range from simple to the most complex tasks. The level of mastery they achieve is completely up to them, but should be declared at the outset. The goal of the assignment is for the students to self-observe and report the process they have gone through in obtaining this new skill. At the end of the semester, each student presents his or her project to the class. Among those activities I recall are the following:

a. A 30-year-old who never rode a bicycle before achieved this skill with his classmates' help so that he could take a group bicycle trip through Europe like his elderly aunt did with her friends.

b. A young woman who wanted to learn to paint initially produced work that appeared to be done by a kindergarten child. She became increasingly skilled as the semester proceeded, and after showing a collection of works she had produced, concluded by announcing to the class, "I am an artist!" Her work had improved remarkably, and her pride in herself was evident.

c. A young man learned fly-tying so that he could develop a more complete relationship with his grandfather, a fly fisherman.

d. A number of students learned to dance, engaging their classmates at the end of the semester, while various other students learned to play musical instruments: piano, drums, marimba, and guitar.

e. One student learned Indian beadwork from people in her father's tribe, bringing her closer to a parent from whom she had been distanced all the years she was growing up.

In any class, the meaningfulness of each activity is demonstrated in different ways, to self and to classmates. The breadth of activities and each one's unique importance is made clear, making it possible to generalize about active occupation. A sense of pride evolves for each student, regardless of the choice of activity he or she made. A new appreciation for the potential of activity as a therapeutic tool develops, serving as a foundation for the development of mastery in professional reasoning.

LEARNING ACTIVITY 5:
HOMELESS SHELTER EMPLOYMENT PROJECT

Refer to the previous section on Resourcefulness for an introduction to this activity. Assume there are about 20 adult men and women with varying skill levels who are housed in a homeless shelter in a major city. (In the United States, choose from New York City, Chicago, Atlanta, Houston, or Los Angeles.) As an occupational therapist, you have a small grant ($10,000 USD), and your goal is to assist as many as possible to find some type of employment within 1 year. You have 4 hours per week to devote to this project. To make this a meaningful learning experience, it is necessary to choose one specific location and explore the current conditions and resources within that space and culture.

a. Make a list of steps you would take in planning your program.

b. What limitations will set the boundaries for your role?

c. What other nearby organizations or entities have similar interests or goals? With whom might you partner or obtain additional resources?

d. How could you find a suitable space within which to run the program?

e. Choose five resources you would find essential to the project.

f. How would you assess the skills and problems of each participant?

g. With limited funding, how might you find other people to assist you in planning and administering the program?

h. Where could you find reliable information about employment opportunities in the area you have chosen?

i. On what might you spend your grant funds to get the most for your money?

j. How could you acquire donated materials, and how would you use them?

This activity addresses an occupational deprivation issue that exists for people in homeless shelters within the United States. However, it may adapted for any developed, underdeveloped, or undeveloped country using the parameters of homelessness and employment opportunities in that location and calculating the US dollar equivalency.

Conclusion

We currently live in a world undergoing great and rapid change. Because of this, we can have little perspective on what events or circumstances will have long-term benefits to our survival. The early years of our evolution led to the natural selection of survivors that took eons to develop. Now the changes we are experiencing do not have the benefit of the same extended periods of time to determine what will result in enduring health and welfare.

Human beings are engaged in an unending process of solution seeking. Engagement in activity that incorporates mind and body with the influences of the tangible and social environments has led to human survival over vast millennia. This inherited problem-solving ability now must focus on questions that face us today, so that we can continue to survive as a species. The problems of nuclear fuel and weapons, environmental contamination, the impact of drugs on disease mutation, potential hazards of genetic manipulation of our food sources, and other hazards must now be faced.

These seem to be formidable questions but in fact may be no greater than the questions that our ancestors faced in each of their generations. Human beings in the past proved themselves to be intelligent creative beings capable of finding solutions to problems of all sorts. Now we must prove it for the future to ensure the survival of our species. Intuitively it seems that creative active occupation is effective as a survival tool and is the method we will use to solve our dilemmas. Our well-being and survival depend on it. One hopes that creative reasoning will enable us to master new skills so we can move beyond potential disaster, thriving into yet another level of human development.

References

Association of Professional Executives of the Public Service of Canada. (1997). *Work habits: Working conditions and the health of the executive cadre in the public service of Canada.* Retrieved from http://www.apex.gc.ca/interest /synopsis_e.html

Auel, J. (1980-2011). *Earth children series.* New York, NY: Crown.

Ayres, J. (1973). *Sensory integration and learning disorders.* Los Angeles, CA: Western Psychological Services.

Bower, B. (2003, April 12). The stone masters. *Science News, 163,* 243-236.

Breines, E. B. (1981). *Perception: Its development and recapitulation.* Lebanon, NJ: Geri-Rehab.

Breines, E. B. (1986). *Origins and adaptations: A philosophy of practice.* Lebanon, NJ: Geri-Rehab.

Breines, E. B. (1990). Genesis of occupation: A philosophical model for therapy and theory. *Australian Occupational Therapy Journal, 37*, 45-49.

Breines, E. B. (1995). *Occupational therapy activities from clay to computers: Theory and practice.* Philadelphia, PA: F. A. Davis.

Breines, E. B. (2005). Occupational genesis, creativity and health. In T. Schmidt (Ed.), *Promoting health through creativity: For professionals in health, arts and education.* London, England: Whurr.

Cramb, A. W. (2003). Department of Materials Science and Engineering, Carnegie Mellon University.

Creek, J. (2014.) *Occupational therapy and mental health.* Amsterdam, The Netherlands: Elsevier.

Dawkins, R. (1996). *The blind watchmaker: Why the evidence of evolution reveals a universe without design.* London, England: Norton.

Dewey, J. (1916). *Democracy and education: An introduction to the philosophy of education.* Toronto, Canada: Collier-Macmillan.

Dewey, J. (1929). *The quest for certainty: A study of the relation of knowledge and action.* New York, NY: Minton Bauch.

Fidler, G. (1981). From crafts to competence. *American Journal of Occupational Therapy, 38*, 567-573.

Ginsburg, H., & Opper, S. (1979). *Piaget's theory of intellectual development.* New York, NY: Prentice Hall.

Goudsbloom, J. (1994). *Fire and civilization.* London, England: Penguin.

Gruber, H. (1981). *Darwin on man: A psychological study of scientific creativity* (2nd ed.). Chicago, IL: University of Chicago Press.

Gruber, H. E., & Voneche, J. J. (1986). *The essential Piaget.* New York, NY: Basic Books.

Huss, A. J. (1981). From kinesiology to adaptation. *American Journal of Occupational Therapy, 35*, 574.

Iovine, J., & Young, A. (2013). University of Southern California. *New York Times,* May 21, A11.

Khouri-Dagher, N. (1998). Botswana: The zebra on wheels. *UNESCO Sources, 105*, 7-9.

May, R. (1994). *The courage to create.* New York, NY: W. W. Norton.

McCrae, R. R. (1999). Consistency of creativity across the life span. In M. A. Runco & S. R. Pritzker (Eds.), *Encyclopedia of creativity* (pp. 361-366). San Diego, CA: Academic Press.

Medawar, P. B. (1957). *The uniqueness of the individual.* London, England: Methuen.

Native Web. (2003). *Caveman to chemist projects: Fire.* Retrieved from http://nativeweb.org

Petit, C. W. (1999). *U.S. News and World Report, 126*(17).

Robinson, J. (2013, June 10). 10 questions. *Time,* p. 68.

Rossotti, H. (1993). *Fire.* Oxford, England: Oxford University Press.

Runco, M. A., & Pritzker, S. R. (Eds.). (1999). *Encyclopedia of creativity.* San Diego, CA: Academic Press.

Safer, M. (2012, January 15). *Jake: Math prodigy proud of his autism. 60 Minutes* [Television broadcast]. New York, NY: CBS.

Schiltz, C. P. (1999, Autumn). Those unhappy, unhealthy lawyers. *Notre Dame Magazine.*

Shorter Oxford English Dictionary. (2002). Oxford, England: Oxford University Press.

Washburn, S. L. (1960). Tools and human evolution. *Scientific American, 203*, 3-15.

White, R. (1959). Motivation reconsidered: The concept of competence. *Psychological Review, 66*, 297-332.

Ziker, J. P. (2003). Assigned territories: Family, clan, communal holdings and common pool resources in the Tarimyr autonomous region, northern Russia. *Human Ecology: An Interdisciplinary Journal, 31*, 331-368.

11

Nonlinear Reasoning in Cognition
Restoring the Essence of the Occupational Therapy Process

Ivelisse Lazzarini, OTD, OTR/L

Understanding the mind and its cognitive processes is the human odyssey. For a few decades, *cognitive sciences* embedded in culturally shaped notions has been able to manifest crystallized generalizations and ideological legacies that not always correlate with our intuitive view of the fluidity of human action. The reason is the plethora of cognitive approaches that continue to be sustained by theoretically reductionist, atemporal, disembodied, static, rationalist, emotionless, and culture-free views of human action. It is time to move to a fundamentally richer understanding of cognition enveloping the *intentionality, meanings, and perceptions* of living bodies *acting on* their daily occupations. An examination of cognition is important to the field of occupational therapy because understanding cognition is quintessentially stating how changes in cognitive capacity are driven by everyday occupations.

MAJOR APPROACHES TO UNDERSTANDING COGNITION

In the field of occupational therapy, the major theories of the 20th century have provided metaphors as a means to understanding cognition and guiding practice. For instance, from the early 1900s to the 1950s, under the influence of behaviorism, cognition was viewed as behavioral conditioning. In the 1960s, the guiding theory shifted to information processing, and cognition became information computation. Another shift in the 1980s brought the constructivist metaphor of cognition as knowledge construction, integrating the views of Piaget (1930), Vygotsky (1986), and information processing (Haltiwanger, Lazzarini, & Nazeran, 2007; Mayer, 1992). All of these theories have contributed to our knowledge of cognition as a whole and have been applied to the study and practice of occupational therapy. However, cognition and the therapeutic processes have traditionally been studied and taught in segmented ways and the complexities of the *cognitive-therapeutic* process have been overlooked. Nonlinear dynamics (NLD) system theory offers a unifying approach to explain both cognition and therapeutic approaches that has not been explicitly discussed. Before elaborating on this idea, a discussion of major cognitive approaches as well as the guiding theoretical principles of NLD is discussed.

Cole, M. B., & Creek, J. (Eds.).
Global Perspectives in Professional Reasoning (pp. 183-202).
© 2016 Taylor & Francis Group.

Cognition as Behavior Conditioning

Behaviorism or behavioral learning theory was the dominant platform in educational research and academia for the first 50 years of the 20th century. The primary assumptions sustaining its tenets articulated the learner as a passive player and tabula rasa in the learning process, learning resulted in permanent changes in behavior, complex behavior could be reduced into simpler parts, and behavioral change occur by interaction with the environment (Gage & Berliner, 1998; Woolfolk, 1998). Teaching approaches and curricular development were based on stimulus–response views with the learner considered to be a "passive recipient of knowledge or an object to be manipulated" (Shuell, 1996, p. 735).

In the 1960s, the concepts of behaviorism collapsed for a number of reasons (Miller, 1993). First, research on verbal learning had not satisfactorily accounted for memory or learning. Second, new evidence indicated that biology limited the laws of learning (Thelen & Smith, 1994). Third, Noam Chomsky (1959, 1965) began attacking Skinner's ideas on language development. Finally, information processing evolved by the fast development of computers and the interest in complex tasks, which began offering alternative views of learning (Gagne, 1985). Hence, a shift occurred to viewing cognition and its processes as information computation (Freeman, 1995).

Cognition as Information Processing

Information computation developed into a field called *cognitivism*. It was meant to be an interdisciplinary field receiving contributions from psychology, neuroscience, analytic philosophy, linguistics, and computer science (Freeman, 1999). However, in the end, computer sciences play the dominant role (Varela, 1989). The cognitivist-oriented study of the mind emerged as a concrete proposal for overcoming many of the analytic problems left unsolved by the approaches of the preceding era, such as introspection, psychoanalysis, and behaviorism. The goal was to operationalize and emulate the workings of the mind and its behavior in precise, pervasive, and uniform ways that were objective, transparent, and controllable. Thus, the mind as a rational calculating device served as a framework, and computers provided the key tool for making the enterprise flourish.

The computer metaphor was built on substance dualism, which postulates an essential division between mind and body, and on functionalism, which defines mind as set of mechanisms that can perform functions independently of the physical platform on which it is implanted (Block, 1980). The digital computer was the perfect platform on which these doctrines could be realized by positing "a level of analysis completely separated from the biological or neurological, on the one hand, and the sociological or cultural, on the other" (Gardner, 1985, p. 6). This approach reduced the level of analysis to focus on the individual mind as a passive input–output device that processed information and that characterized reasoning as the logical manipulation of arbitrary symbols. Hence, technology gave rise to the most powerful and alluring metaphor, a legacy that still deeply influences us today: the metaphor of mind as a computer.

As a result, all aspects of the mind were seen as software that happened in humans to be implemented in wetware having unreliable neurons and that could be vastly improved if implemented in hardware with reliable transistors. Thus, computers served as the most sustainable model of how the human mind functions (Gardner, 1985). As a consequence, the entire domain of the cognitive science became narrowly defined as "the study of intelligence and intelligent systems, with particular reference to intelligent behavior as computation" (Simon & Kaplan, 1989, p. 1). This reductionist approach became synonymous with cognitive science. Cognitivism not only defined cognitive science but also neatly prescribed how to conceive and carry out a feasible research agenda.

The cognitive revolution was launched with great optimism, predicting the development of devices for general problem solving, speech recognition, language translation, reading cursive script and photographs, and making free-roving household robots (Dreyfus, 1979). There were many failures throughout the development and sustainability of the prescribed cognitive notions;

however, it did not stop the already enamored scientific community (Dreyfus, 1979; Winograd & Flores, 1986). This seductive approach engendered new journals, university departments, and academic societies to exploit the new concepts and their related technology. As a result, the mind as computer metaphor provided not only a redefinition of fundamental concepts such as reasoning, thought, perception, knowledge, and learning, but it also later became an entire conceptual apparatus for how to understand individuals, communities, brains, neurons, languages, and academic experiences. The computer-oriented vision has enslaved in various ways the minds of two generations of scientists.

New approaches following the cognitive revolution were parallel distributed processing, artificial neural networks, hybrid systems, and more recently, neurocomputation, although cognitivism in the form of artificial intelligence is not as widely endorsed as it was previously (Searle, 1992). The legacy of cognitivism is pervasive. Cognitive scientists failed to identify and explain some inherent aspects of the mind, such as the human brain as an organ of social actions, intentions, meanings, emotions, bodily grounded experiences, and the transcendent essence of memory that underscores the development of habits and rituals defining human nature.

Cognition as Knowledge Construction

Constructivism evolved from the notion that learners construct their own knowledge from their lived experiences. It involves the active creation and adaptation of ideas, thoughts, and critical reflection that originate as the result of experiences that occur within a sociocultural context. The assumptions of constructivism embrace two major ideas:

1. Knowledge is not passively accumulated, but rather is the result of active cognizing by the individual.

2. Cognition is an adaptive process that organizes and makes sense of our daily experiences, albeit not rending an accurate representation of ontological reality (von Glasersfeld, 1984, 1995).

The constructivist approach has a great degree of theoretical variability. There is exogenous, endogenous, and dialectical/social constructivism. Exogenous constructivism emphasizes the external nature of knowledge. In this view, cognition, and thus knowledge, is perceived as the internalization and reconstruction of the external reality. Exogenous constructivism is most associated with information processing and its levels of description, including schemata, declarative and procedural memory, and propositional networks (Gagne, Yekovich, & Yekovich, 1993).

Endogenous or radical constructivism emphasizes the internal nature of knowledge. The main theoretical construct and discourse is based on discovery-oriented approaches. Cognition is constructed not from external experiences, but from earlier mental structures. Cognition is acquisition, reconstruction, and reorganization of old knowledge in light of new experiences and is most associated with the work of Jean Piaget (1930, 1952, 1972, 1983) and his stage theory of cognitive development. His work has been influential in occupational therapy cognitive approaches.

Finally, dialectical/social constructivism underscores the interactional nature of cognition. Cognition is the result of the interaction between the learner (internal) and the environment (external). Dialectical constructivism is most associated with the work of Lev Vygotsky (1986) and his sociocultural perspective. Vygotsky's views challenged Piaget's assumptions that development unavoidably precedes learning. Every function in the child's cultural development appears twice: first on the social level, and later on the individual level; first, between people (interpsychological) and then inside the child (intrapsychological) (Vygotsky, 1986). This approach has been most significant in academia; however, it has also deeply influenced the social/cultural aspects of occupational therapy practice. Please refer to Table 11-1 for a quick comparison between Piaget and Vygotsky views.

TABLE 11-1		
PIAGET AND VYGOTSKY COGNITIVE VIEWS		
COGNITION PROGRESSES FROM:	VYGOTSKY	PIAGET
	Outward to inward	Inward to outward
	Social	Developmental
	Social to individual	Individual to social
DEVELOPMENTAL STAGES	Based on social interaction	Based on age
INTERACTION	Interpersonal	Intrapersonal
THERAPIST ROLE	Significant	Limited
THERAPEUTIC MILIEU	Socially interactive	Discovery oriented
Copyright © Ivelisse Lazzarini.		

The previous three views of constructivism provide a continuum from which to view learning and cognition. However, the limitation of the constructivist view is that it does not account for biological changes that may occur as a result of learning.

Biological Approaches to Cognition

The overall trend away from behaviorism and advances in our understanding of biological contributions to behavior has helped shift attention from environmental factors to the biological processes of cognition. However, the biological view of cognition brings a fair amount of baggage. Case in point, many educators equate the term *biology* with genes and view genetic heritage as a determinant of cognitive abilities. Context or environment is perceived as less significant. In a study conducted by Plomin (1989), it was reported that family environments had a slight ($r = .25$) long-term impact during childhood and near zero during adolescence for cognitive abilities in adoptive siblings. Studies such as this seem to portray biology as a form of predestination acting as a single predictor of human cognition. Biology and genetics are clearly important for a complete theory of cognition, but their role must be appropriately articulated and outlined.

Genes operate within context. In a study performed by Bronfenbrenner (1975), research data from twin studies were reanalyzed and found that correlations of IQ differed as a function of the environment in which they developed. The correlation between twins growing up in the same kind of environment ($r = .86$) differed markedly from those in dissimilar communities ($r = .26$). By 1986, at least one study had replicated the same findings (Bronfenbrenner, 1986). Clearly, genes are not the sole determinants of cognitive ability.

In 1992, Gerald M. Edelman published the theory of neuronal group selection (TNGS). His work is anchored in three major assumptions:

1. Developmental choice leads to the formation of neuroanatomical characteristics of a given species. In human brains, neurons, synapses, and neural networks make possible for language, abstract thinking, and metacognition.

2. Through actions, synaptic connections or maps are strengthened or weakened.

3. Neuronal maps interact by a process called reentry or circular causality affording the "simultaneous coordination of responses across several sensory modalities" (Thelen & Smith, 1994, p. 149).

Edelman's theory (1992) proposes a biological explanation of what could be happening in the brain as cognitive processes develop. As a student learns to add and multiply, neural maps are stimulated. As he or she writes down mathematical calculations, reentry occurs so that the brain map for writing and the brain mapping for mathematical calculations are coordinated. Over time, neuronal connections are strengthened as the process is repeated. This integration of the role of biology in cognitive development is necessary to a complete theory of cognition. Of great importance is to mention that in 1972, Dr. Edelman received the Nobel prize for his work in medicine/physiology.

GUIDING PRINCIPLES OF NONLINEAR DYNAMICS AND COGNITION

In the past 25 years, there has been a tremendous increase in explorations of the mind and its by-product, cognition. Understanding the workings and connections of the brain–mind–body as a cognitive whole ranks high on the agendas of neuroscience and worldwide society. Cognitive science and neuroscience have developed into a new interdisciplinary field, conflating knowledge and skills from multiple scientific approaches to develop mathematical and nonmathematical explanations for the workings of the mind. The umbrella term in which this work occurs is called the *nonlinear approach to cognition*.

A system is a way of looking at the world, a theoretical construct that simplifies nature. An NLD system is one that changes over time (Freeman, 1995; Kelso, 1999; Ward, 2002). NLD systems are characterized by complexity, randomness, and nonlinearity (Kelso, 1999; Thelen & Smith, 1994). The underlying assumption is that biological organisms are complex, multidimensional, interdependent, cooperative systems that exhibit self-organization (Lazzarini, 2004; Wright & Liley, 1996).

NLD articulates human cognition as a self-organizing, intentional process in which pattern formation and neural organization develop through internal interactions (Freeman, 2000b, 2000d). Cognition, as a process, is an emergent pattern of multiple cooperating components, all of which count and none of which are privileged. It is the relationship of the multiple parts that gives the system order and pattern. This is what is meant by self-organizing. The mind simply does not exist as something decoupled from the body and the environment in which it resides (Freeman, 2000a, 2000e). The components of mind are not hierarchical linear elements as traditional input–output models depict but deeply embedded and continuously dynamically coupled (Haken & Tschacher, 2011). A coupled system refers to a system guided by influence as opposed to control. For example, the nervous system as a nonlinear system is embedded in and coupled to the body and together they are embedded in and coupled with the environment. What follows is a discourse of how principles of NLD can be applied to cognitive processes of clients, the therapeutic milieu, and the therapist–client dynamic relationship, potentially providing occupational therapists with a framework for research and practice.

Linear vs. Nonlinear and the Self-Organizing Processes

It is important to explain the differences between what is meant by *linear* and *nonlinear* approaches to cognition (Table 11-2). Linear approaches to cognition state that the behavior of a system is easily predictable from the behavior of individual neurons or brain structures. In a linear system, small changes produce small effects, and large changes produce large effects. In this view, intentional behaviors are representations that set into motion a causal chain. Representations, according to linear models, function as internal causes of behavior (Markman & Dietrich, 2000; Wegner & Wheatley, 1999). As a consequence, behavior, metaphorically speaking, is the end result of chains of billiard ball–type interactions among representations (Freeman, 1999; Kelso, 1999).

TABLE 11-2
COMPARISON BETWEEN LINEAR AND NONLINEAR VIEWS

LINEAR VIEWS	NONLINEAR VIEWS
Causality	Emergent properties
Linear	Nonlinear
Objective	Includes subjectivity
Isolate events	Emphasizes context
Matter	Process
Focuses on stability	Focus on sensitivity
Logic	Deeper pattern
Closed system	Open system
Reductive	Complex
Predictability	Chaotic/stochastic
Explicit/observable	Implicit/hidden
Time is uniform	Sensitive to critical periods
Cause and effect	Positive feedback loops of autocatalysis
Sequential	Experience dependent
Mechanistic	Self-regulating
Fixed relations	Network interconnections
Objects/parts	Fields/relationships with parts
Particulate	Parallel

Most cognitive models, particularly information-processing approaches, use Newtonian efficient cause as a metaphor that largely defines the content and boundaries of discussion, thus restricting discoveries and the study of human cognition to cause-and-effect relationships (Juarrero, 2002; Van Orden & Holden, 2002). Some of the limitations of the science delineating linear assumptions are prediction, reduction, and inferential design and analysis methods of the research of stable systems. However, human beings are not stable, closed linear systems; they are open, variable, and nonlinear systems that are far from a state of equilibrium (Prigogine, 1994, 1997). Humans are open in the sense that they can interact with their environment, exchanging information, energy, and matter, and they are far from equilibrium in the sense that without these sources, humans and other animals cannot maintain their structure or function (Freeman, 1995; Haken & Tschacher, 2011; Prigogine, 1994). As a result, NLD metaphors that are more inclusive are needed to understand purposeful or goal-directed behavior in occupation. Otherwise, intentional performance as an endogenous process remains forever unsubstantiated, vague, and inexplicable, even supernatural.

Perhaps the chambered nautilus with its highly ordered shell but nonlinear structure can serve as the new metaphor (Figure 11-1). The structure of the shell provides key functionality to the actual organism, which resides in the outer chamber of the shell. The chambers of the nautilus are of ever-increasing size and are ordered in a spiral array. Each chamber is connected to the

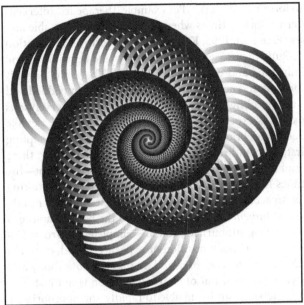

Figure 11-1. The chambered nautilus. (Copyright © Ivelisse Lazzarini.)

foregoing and after-coming segments by a siphuncle that transports gases, thus permitting the shell to act as a float, affording the organism the ability to traverse the vast ocean. This communication mechanism between earlier segments permits a dynamic response by the living organism to changes in the environment with which it directly interacts. This process resembles the nonlinearity of the ever-changing nonlinear cognitive process.

Like the nautilus and its ever-increasing size and self-organization, the common denominator of the nonlinear approach to cognition is a simple one—mind as a self-organizing and emergent process. That is viewing the human nervous system as a dynamic self-organizing process and the cognitive process as the emergent property of the assembly of the infrastructure, none of which contain a prescription or command center (Skarda & Freeman, 1987; Szentagothai, 1984). Instead of describing the purely abstract structures of the mind, the nonlinear approach seeks to understand the emergence of a dynamic and neural flexible coupling between direct real-time processes and cognitive process that are less tightly coupled to the receiving input (Haken & Tschacher, 2011; Thelen & Smith, 1994). It is precisely the continuity in time of the embedded and coupled systems that is essential for fluid, adapted behavior, which gives meaning to the notion of an embodied cognition.

Nonlinear Dynamics and Pattern Formation

A nonlinear system exists as patterns in time, such that the current state is a function of previous states (both immediate and more distant past) and in turn is the basis of future states (Freeman, 1995; Haken, 2002; Kelso, 1999; Thelen & Smith, 1994). There are two more critical features of such an embedded and coupled system that separate it from the traditional input–output causal metaphor and information-processing models. First, the system is self-organizing and multiply causal. This principle explains human behavior as an emergent pattern of multiple cooperating components, all of which are important and none of which are privileged. The mind and its cognitive processes do not exist decoupled from the body and the environment in which it inhabits.

The understanding of cognition dramatically changes when everything is considered as a process in time rather than as static structures. Second, as a time-based system it can vary in its relative stability (Kelso, 1999). The stability is determined by how tightly the components bind—in other words, how deeply ingrained are the habits formed. For change to occur, the system needs to lose stability so that the elements are free to form new patterns. For example, therapeutic interventions involve continuous shifts in the pattern stability: times when the system is quite stable and other times when a new combination arises (Freeman, 1995; Kelso, 1999). The critical implication of this nonlinear conceptualization is that cognitive processes are a product of the nervous system, body, and environment that are always embedded and dynamically coupled. They start out this way, and there is no point in the cognitive process and no context when they are not embedded and coupled. What can change is the nature of the coupling (Kelso, 1999). In therapeutic interventions where development or adaptation of new skills is expected, the coupling must be highly flexible and dynamically responsive to task. Some activities or occupations take some distinctive coupling characteristic useful to briefly explore. First, we could refer to *body–environment coupling*; there are times when the activity or occupation and the body are tightly linked to the environment—the case of learning to drive or play golf. At times like these, you cannot easily isolate your thinking from the immediate task at hand for fear of an accident or poor performance. Second, the mind–environment coupling, when the *mind to environment* coupling is tight and the body coupling is less, the case of a body part going numb or getting sunburned. You are completely engrossed in an occupation for its own sake and oblivious to your body position or exposure. Third, coupling speaks of times when *concentration or meditative states take over and we shut out both* (body and mind), the world and body, case in point, yoga practice. But of course, cognition is not just having these moments of more protected mental activity but being able to rapidly and appropriately change the coupling strengths. In lay terms, we call this notion *mental flexibility*.

Nonlinear Dynamics and Initial Conditions

NLD also articulates initial conditions or initial state (Freeman, 2000d; Haken, 2002; Kelso, 1999). Sensitivity to initial conditions means that the smallest differences in input can produce entirely different outcomes for the system, yielding various learning or outcome routes to a degree of complexity that exhibits characteristics of randomness. When relating this concept to therapeutic interventions, it means that the therapist can destabilize the present state of the client's habits and potentially initiate growth and changes that facilitate the adaptation of the individual as a whole, thus, in the end, potentially producing large modifications in the individual's occupation, improving quality of life.

Cognitive adaptation during critical therapeutic times means having the ability to categorize the world in order to flexibly and rapidly recruit useful categories of activities/occupations to make a mental plan based on prior experience before actually acting, when required, and also quickly responding without a lot of hesitation, when necessary. Hence, the emphasis on the connectedness of elements is central to the study of cognition.

In the initial state the components of the system are coupled in a particular obligatory way based on previous knowledge. Changes in cognitive processes consist of the progressive ability to modulate the coupling so as to meet different and changing situations. Cognition means acquiring not only enhanced offline processes (taking time to think, solve problems, and reflect), but also better online ones (making decision in real time) and, most important, the ability to seamlessly shift between them (Haken & Tschacher, 2011). The term *offline cognitive processes* proposed explanations for when cognitive operations are decoupled from real time and the world environment. It is a process of reflecting and problem solving the acquired knowledge during the online experiences. During offline cognitive processing, the individual is able to make careful considerations about recent decisions or actions. Online cognition refers to the notion of situated cognition (Varela, Thompson, & Rosch, 1991), where all cognitive operations occur in real time, are environmentally embedded, and demand immediate action. It requires a high degree of flexibility and fluidity to effectively interact and adapt to the environment.

THERAPEUTIC APPROACHES USING NONLINEAR DYNAMICS

Occupational therapy interventions are deeply rooted in the concept of online cognition, which is certainly a dynamic process that occurs across the lifespan. Therapists must gain a deeper understanding of how cognitive operations take place to better articulate change from an NLD perspective. For example, learning as a cognitive self-organized process is sensitive to initial conditions, and it is also fractal—fractal in the sense that once new learning occurs the whole system changes, hence, the occupational therapist's job is to teach new learning or relearning from a nonlinear, self-organized perspective. This perspective accounts for sensitivity to initial conditions, degree of the system's components coupled, which accounts for intrinsic tendencies or constraints, and the multiply causal relationships, which explains the emergent pattern of multiple cooperating components. The value of a deeper understanding of a nonlinear approach to cognition resides in the ability of therapist to scientifically substantiate and sustain rehabilitation interventions and also to articulate how change is facilitated in and through initial conditions, which in turn influences the state of the whole system.

Constraints and Patterns

Cognitive models based on NLD maintain that behavior arises from interactions between interdependent components that may also include feedback effects based on the constraints (variables that limit the degrees of freedom for interactions among the processes of the human brain–mind–body) of control parameters. Control parameters are variables that lead the system through the variety of possible patterns or states but do prescribe or contain the code for emerging patterns (Freeman, 1988a, 1988b; Kay, Lancaster, & Freeman, 1996; Kelso, 1999). This kind of behavior is not easily predictable from the individual interaction of the parts, and it can be quite rich (Van Orden, Holden, & Turvey, 2003). In a nonlinear system, the output is not proportional to the input and the system does not conform to the principle of additivity, that is, it may involve synergistic reactions in which the whole is not equal to the sum of its parts (Haken, 2000; Prigogine & Stengers, 1984). This is what most people recognize as the butterfly effect, inspired by the meteorological experiments of Edward Lorenz in 1961. The butterfly effect implies that two states differing by imperceptible amounts may eventually evolve into two considerably different states. If, then, there is any mistake in observing the present state—and in any real dynamic system, such error seems inescapable—then an acceptable prediction of the instantaneous state in the distant future may well be impossible. Thus, instead of making predictions about the future state of a system, NLD attempts a qualitative study of the system by concentrating on behavior that is unstable and aperiodic, meaning studying how the system changes over time and how the behavior does not repeat itself (just like one snowflake is not the same as the previous).

Hence, purposeful occupations and behaviors of living systems are viewed as self-organized and pattern forming and cannot be reduced to basic cause-and-effect assumptions. When researchers discuss patterns, they refer to the relations among things (Haken, 2002; Haken & Tschacher, 2011; Kelso, 1999; Ward, 2002). Pattern formation is the brain's basic means of storing information, and pattern recognition is the basic means of sharing it. At the genetic level, patterns contain the seed of who and what we are (Kelso, 1999; Ward, 2002). Repetition and variation of these patterns are the processes by which selections occur (Kelso, 1999). Patterns convey information about an individual's lifestyle, habits, rituals, and present situation; consequently, the interdependence of brain activity as a self-organizing whole demonstrates that pattern formation is at the heart of cognitive rehabilitation. See Table 11-3 for a quick reference of these terms.

NLD patterns of brain activity are constructed from a very large number of material components (Haken, 2002; Kelso, 1999). The brain has approximately 10^{10} neurons, each of which can have up to 10^4 connections with other neurons and 50-plus neurotransmitters (chemicals that are

TABLE 11-3 NONLINEAR DYNAMIC SYSTEM DEFINITIONS OF PATTERN FORMATION AND PATTERN RECOGNITION	
Pattern	Relations in time
Pattern formation	Brain basic means of storing information
Pattern recognition	Basic means of sharing the information
Copyright © Ivelisse Lazzarini.	

necessary for neurons to work; Freeman, 1995; Haken, 2002; Kelso, 1999). Hence, pattern formation (storing of information) is not about one specific pattern but many patterns (relations) produced to accommodate different circumstances. These patterns allude to the multifunctionality of human performance. Human beings are multifunctional in that they use the same anatomical components for different behavioral functions, such as eating and speaking, or different components to perform the same function (i.e., listening to a book instead of reading it, or using a keyboard or cell phone vs. pencil and paper). Therefore, self-organization of pattern formation in cognition is ubiquitous.

Open Systems

The nonlinearity of cognitive processes is deeply embedded in the concept of openness. The system is open in the sense that it exchanges matter and energy with its environment. It is the iterative feedback processes in which the product of the process is necessary for the process itself that typically characterizes NLD systems. This process is called circular causality, which is a form of self-cause or self-actualization (Freeman, 1999). When the parts interact to produce wholes, the resulting distributed wholes in turn affect the behavior of their parts and so inter-causality is at work. This process is also described as the global dynamics from microscopic–macroscopic (Freeman, 2000b, 2000c). Interactions among levels of neural correlates can create a system-level organization with new properties that are not the simple sum of the components that constitute the higher level (Freeman, 2000c; Haken & Tschacher, 2011). In turn, the overall global neural dynamics of the emergent distributed system not only determine which parts will be allowed into the system but also regulate and constrain the behavior of the lower level components. The causal mechanism at work between levels of organization can be best understood as the operations constraints. The interlevel constraints explaining the dynamics of cognitive change are (1) context-free constraints, which takes a system's component far from equiprobability; (2) context-sensitive constraints, which synchronize and correlate previously independent parts into a systemic whole; and (3) context-dependent constraints, which is when parts become correlated as an integral whole imposed by the newly organized system in which they are now embedded (Freeman, 1995; Kelso, 1999; Llinás & Ribary, 1993; Wright & Liley, 1996; Table 11-4). At this level and from a top-down perspective, the dynamics of the global level closes off to some behavioral choices that would be open to the components were they not habituated in the overall system. Thus, the context-dependent constraint level (history of knowledge/habits) is the previous organized state that simultaneously opens up to new possibilities (Freeman, 1988a; Kelso, 1999; Shibata & Kaneko, 1998; Skarda & Freeman, 1987). The more complex the system, the more states and properties it can manifest. Cognitively speaking, when human experience is self-organized into habits, other human occupations can continue to develop through the continuous growth of experiential cognitive processes.

		TABLE 11-4	
		INTERLEVEL CONSTRAINTS EXPLAINING COGNITIVE CHANGES	
CONSTRAINTS	**DESCRIPTION**	**BOTTOM UP**	**TOP DOWN**
Context-free constraints	The flexibility of the system and openness to change Open with high degrees of freedom Far from equiprobability		
Context-sensitive constraints	Synchronize and correlate previously independent parts into a systemic whole Meaningful exchanges anchored in existing perceptual repertoire	Self-organization of the global level Experience, habits, self-control of action and self-actualization	
Contextual constraints First- and second-order context-dependent constraints	Global dynamical systems in turn *close off* to some behavioral choices if not habituated When organized into a complex, integral whole, parts become correlated as a function of the newly organized system in which they are now embedded Previous organized whole		The global level dynamics closes off some of the behavioral alternatives that would be open to components were they not captured in the overall system Examples: Performance of activities of daily living that once habituated, changes are more difficult Order parameters
Copyright © Ivelisse Lazzarini.			

From the bottom up, the establishment of context-sensitive constraints is the phase change that self-organizes the global level (experience, habits, and self-control of action). Therefore, self-organization of the global level is the appearance of context-sensitive constrains on the system's components. From the top down, and serving as contextual constraints, global dynamics close off to some behavioral alternatives that would be open to the components if they were not already captured in the overall system (Haken & Tschacher, 2011). Hence, once behavioral patterns are habituated, we can find them extremely difficult to change. (See Figure 11-2 for the NoLCoM diagram.)

Constraints work by modifying either a system's landscape or the probability distribution of events and movement within that space (Lazzarini, 2004). Because actions are lower-motor-level implementations of higher-level-intentional causes, reconceptualizing mental causation in terms

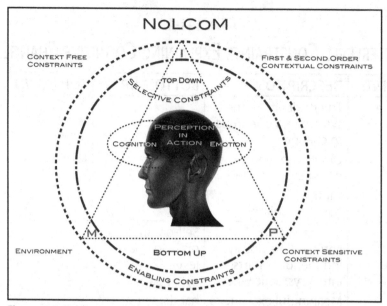

Figure 11-2. Nonlinear cognitive model. (Copyright © Ivelisse Lazzarini.)

of top-down, context-sensitive dynamics constraints can radically recast our thinking about cognitive processes. There is plenty of evidence to suggest that the human brain is a nonlinear, self-organized system that integrates stimuli with context-sensitive constraints. Each cortical pattern is a dissipative structure emergent from microscopic fluctuation suggesting a plausible hypothesis (Freeman, 1995; Kelso, 1999; Llinás & Ribary, 1993; Thelen & Smith, 1994; Tsuda, 1991, 1996; Wright & Liley, 1996).

Nonlinear Feedback

Not only does the brain have reentrant pathways that function as positive feedback channels (Edelman, 1987), it is also know to self-determine what counts as a meaningful stimulus and what constitutes meaningless noise. Research increasingly supports the hypothesis that nonlinear feedback and resonance and entrainment among neurons—as well as between the overall nervous system and the environment—are responsible for the self-organization of coherent behavior in neuronal populations (Freeman, 1995). As is true of all self-organized structure, the emergent dynamics of coherent neurological activity can be expected to show novel and surprising properties as a consequence of the neurological self-organization, resulting from context-sensitive constraints: experiences, habits, and self-control of action that give rise to intention, meaning making, and goal-directed actions. Thinking of individuals and their actions or occupations in this manner provides a previously unavailable way of conceptualizing the difference in the etiology and trajectory of habitual automatic actions and what we consider novel goal-directed (intentional) actions (Freeman, 2001). Furthermore, thinking about self-organized neurological systems as nonlinear landscapes makes the recalcitrant problem of meaning tractable. Therefore, meaningful intentions are embodied in self-organized neurological dynamics. The brain's self-organized dynamics originate, regulate, and constrain skeletomuscular processes such that the resulting behavior "satisfies the meaningful content" embodied in the complex dynamics from which it issued (Thelen & Smith, 1994).

Phase Changes

Formulating a prior intention to act is the counterpart of a neurological phase change. A phase change is the dynamical self-organization of a more complex level of coherent brain activity that integrates neuronal patterns embodying wants, desires, and meaning. Unlike Newtonian cause, however, these higher levels of neurological organization would not be simply triggering devices (Freeman, 1997, 2001). The global dynamics of self-organizing nonlinear adaptive processes constrain their contextual components top down (motor behavior). As contextual constraints, however, a system's dynamics are not occurring events like Newtonian forces. An intention's constraint would be embodied in the meta-stable dynamics that characterize the intention's neurophysiological organization, and as such would not immediately disengage. Serving as the brain's order parameter, those contextual constraints that embody an intention (acting top down) would provide the behavior with continuous, ongoing control and direction by modifying in real time the probability distribution of lower-level neurological processes and, as a consequence, the behavioral alternative available to and implemented by the individual. Far from representing messy, noisy complications that can be safely ignored, time and context are as central to the identity and behavior of these dynamical processes as they are to human beings (Freeman, 2000b, 2000e; Kelso, 1999).

Unlike the processes described by classical linear models, which in their relentless march toward equilibrium forget their past, nonlinear adaptive systems are essentially historical. They embody in their very structure the conditions under which they were created, including chance events around which each self-organized stage reorganizes. The unrepeatable, random fluctuation or perturbation around which each phase of a sequence of adaptations form an experience leaves its mark on the specific configuration that emerges (Lazzarini, 2004). Therefore, if human beings and their cognitive behavior are nonlinear adaptive phenomena, the precise pathway that their actions will take is simply unpredictable. Unpredictability and uncertainty are the hallmarks of their embeddedness in time and space. Consequently, goal-directed activities/occupations and meaning cannot be relegated or labeled as just a stimulus-response.

Embodied and Situated Cognition

Cognitive processes are embodied, and the body is embedded. The body serves as the principal tool of the brain for cognitive development. This view requires a shift from predicting how individuals' brains react to objects in the environment to understanding their actions in terms of self-organized probabilities or tendencies (Lazzarini, 2004)—that is, of a body–mind–brain immersed in the environment, experiencing the sensory consequences of goal-directed activities that affords them the possibility to change their and, therefore, the essence of the neural patterns of brain dynamics. Thus, cognition can be understood only as a manifestation of the interactions among the individual's past, present, and expectancy of future patterns of activity performance. Cognition is therefore not an isolated goal-directed action but rather an event that interconnects all other experiences in a particular way (Freeman, 2001, 2002; Guastello, 1995; Haken, 2003; Kelso, 1999). It grows from intentions, perceptions, and meanings and remains tied to it; the body, the world, and the mind are always united by these common dynamics. Hence, understanding the workings of the mind requires reconsideration of what one understands as *mind*. The NLD framework articulates mind as brain and body and as a dynamic web of interrelated events in space and time.

An embodied-oriented approach has an explicit commitment to all of cognition, not just to low-level aspects of cognition such as sensory-motor activity, which are lower levels of cognitive performance (Lakoff & Nuñez, 2000). NLD takes embodiment to be a living phenomenon in which the primacy of bodily grounded experience (e.g., intention, meaning, perception, emotion, and movement) is inherently part of the very subject matter of the study of the mind. Full embodiment has a robust commitment to all cognition, acknowledging from the most basic perceptive action to the most sophisticated form of abstract thinking (Johnson, 1987). Full embodiment explicitly develops a paradigm to explain the objects created by the intentionality of the human mind. In this realm, we find concepts, theories, ideas, and explanations in terms of the unrestricted bodily experiences sustained by the habits of brains and bodies (Lakoff & Nuñez, 2000).

An important feature of embodied cognition is that the very objects created by human conceptual structures and understanding are not seen as existing in an absolute transcendental realm but as being brought forth through specific human bodily grounded processes (Iverson & Thelen 1999; Varela et al., 1991). Conceptual systems and meaning are not considered a priori, but they become subject matters to be explained in real-time bodily-grounded terms. From this perspective, not only is meaning embodied and not out there in the world, but so is the concept of occupations.

Full embodiment is the complete and compelling argument enveloping conceptual structures as well as high-level cognition (Nuñez, 1997), clearly to understand the primacy of the inherent aspects of human occupations, which is at the core of the conceptual mapping of space and time events. The body serves as the principal tool of the brain for cognitive development (Varela et al., 1991). This view requires a shift from predicting how individuals' brains react to objects in the environment to understanding their actions in terms of self-organized probabilities or tendencies; that is, of a body–mind–brain immersed in the environment, experiencing the sensory consequences of goal-directed activities affords the individual the possibilities to change his or her history and, therefore, the essence of the neural patterns of brain dynamics (Lazzarini, 2004).

NONLINEAR COGNITION AND PROFESSIONAL REASONING

Understanding and applying NLD to the therapeutic process could assist occupational therapists in discovering how meaningful occupational patterns are formed in their clients. Moreover, occupation from the viewpoint of embodied, nonlinear cognition may serve as the vehicle of change to transport individuals through self-organizing intentional states, where the actualizing of habitual daily occupations may serve as the catalyst to construct new occupational patterns. When considering using occupation as the vehicle to elicit therapeutic changes, consideration should be given to the concepts of sensitivity to initial conditions, which mark the dynamical instabilities and the depth of mental and/or physical limitations.

Recognizing Instabilities as Therapeutic Opportunities

System instabilities, for example, create the precise opportunities for therapists to facilitate change through the increased degrees of freedom afforded to the system and from which a fresh therapeutic start can be made. The degrees of instabilities, therefore, could be referred to as states of neural flexibility. When a state of neural flexibility emerges in the depth of an occupational crisis due to illness, traumatic events, or other reasons, occupational therapists, using the process and states of NLD and occupation as the vehicle of change, can facilitate the creation of new experiences. These experiences, in turn, may lead to the development of new habits, beliefs, and value systems. Envisioning clients as a constantly shifting dynamical system and armed with the knowledge of how meaningful occupational patterns are formed, therapists could scientifically validate occupation not only as a therapeutic tool but also as a vehicle to elicit change. Quality of life often resides in the ability of those experiencing unexpected illnesses to be able to change their most significant private and public occupations. Although this is not a new fact, what becomes important is the way in which the process of NLD could facilitate individuals' ability to experience meaningful lives.

Understanding Intentional States

Consequently, the most critical piece of information for the success of therapeutic interventions is to determine the individual intentional state. Understanding intentional states means realizing that self-organized systems are not merely influenced by traditional generalized rehabilitation protocols. Individuals, regardless of their illnesses, are profoundly influenced by their past experiences, historical essence, and lifetime constructed meanings, which therapists ought to explore and discover to facilitate change.

Introducing Perturbations to Evaluate Openness to Change

One way of using intentional states paired with the ubiquitous power of occupation to elicit change is to explore the individual's degree of stability, instability, or resistance to change. Because individuals rely on past experiences, goals, and meanings, which ultimately are the habitual patterns of daily living, therapists could quickly determine the flexibility or rigidity of intentional states by perturbing the system. Perturbation is a way of providing the individual with an opportunity to demonstrate how fast he or she can recover from sudden or abrupt changes. An individual standing on a moving train and holding onto a railing is stable, but someone walking in the aisle is not. If the person walking in the aisle regains his or her chosen posture after each perturbation (state transition), that state is regarded as stable, and it is said to be governed by an attractor state. This is a metaphor to say that the individual is attracted to the state (particular action or behavior) through an interim state of transience. If the perturbation is so strong that it causes a broken hip and the person cannot stand up again, then the system has been placed outside the habitual pattern (attractor state/stable behavior), and a new state supervenes the previous attractor state. These perturbations become the occupational process that can actualize the individual's potential and create change. Ultimately, it is by the self-organizing process of intentionality that individuals "stretch forth" to experience the sensory consequences of their actions, assigning meaning to occupations. Thus, understanding dynamical instabilities may allow researchers and clinicians to accomplish the following:

- Distinguish among unhealthy occupational patterns—habits or routines—to facilitate change by using the cognitive NLD concepts
- Use occupation as it happens, in real time (online cognitive processes) and with the constraints found in daily clinical interventions
- Prepare clients to reflect, rehearse, and find the tendencies that they are most comfortable with and influence the nonlinear cognitive process as it evolves
- Use these concepts as the means to evaluate short-term predictions about the nonlinear collective dynamic variables of human beings

Consequently, the concepts of NLD as it pertains to cognition could help to open a path to new ways to model theoretically the collective dynamical variables relevant to our clients, clarifying present ambiguities in cognitive models and tools.

Recognizing Nonlinear Dynamics' Fundamental Change in Viewpoint

NLD represents a fundamental change in viewpoint. One of the most important features of this change is a shift away from theoretical models that, although they may express brain processes as active, continue to err by conflating cognitivism with NLD. This leads practitioners to the categorical error that meaning is an isolated process inherent in the environment and extracted by tuned resonances in brain circuits (Freeman, 1997). Hence, from an NLD viewpoint, it represents a shift from a linear and disembodied perspective to an embodied, intentional, and self-organized occupational process view.

Ultimately, the concepts of NLD may serve as a powerful tool to integrate a broader perspective within the interaction between occupational therapists and the ever-changing experiences of their clients. The application of NLD may assist in helping to organize and understand the complexities of heterarchical, intentional, and self-organized systems and their occupations, thus avoiding traditional linear and mechanistic approaches. NLD might also help to inspire occupational therapists to engage in the investigation and discourse of human experience from the multiple levels contained within human occupations (Lazzarini, 2004; McLaughlin, Kennedy, & Zemke, 1996; Royeen, 2002).

Currently in the field of occupational therapy, the majority of models, tools, and assessments hold a subtle linear causality perspective. Neurodynamics of brain activity are understood as input–output phenomena driven by external forces, as opposed to the view of self-organized nonlinear systems described here. The nonlinear perspective, however, discourages the hubris of presuming to be able to predict or control the details of an unfolding and self-organizing life. Consequently, models and tools enveloped in linear perspectives are limited in their ability to guide therapists to understand and carry out the practice of occupational therapy from the embodied and the NLD essence of human experience.

Creating Spaces for Self-Organization

All brains can know is the hypothesis that they construct and the results of experiencing it by acting into the environment and shaping past experiences by assimilation from the sensory consequences encountered through flexible states that are self-organizing and emerging (Lazzarini, 2004). As a result, the human brain–mind–body, through its dynamical instabilities in one state, drives the system into another state, leading to the actualization of routines, habits, and occupations. This is where clinical practitioners exploiting the power of occupation as a vehicle of change and through the NLD cognitive process can provide the means to actualize the potential of their clients. So rather than imposing an external organization on a client, the therapist needs to attend to the conditions under which the client's own self-organization can emerge. This is a fundamentally different way of reasoning about therapeutic change.

Ultimately, therapeutic interventions as socialized interactions require the neurochemical mechanisms of affiliation and bonding that evolved through early years. As such, when clients are in a *sensitive to initial conditions state* due to illness or disease, therapists, endowed with the knowledge of NLD, could invoke individuals' past experiences and elicit perturbations to facilitate change. Hence, recognizing and understanding that dynamical instabilities of cognitive states serve as therapeutic opportunities allows therapists to use these brief windows of opportunity to facilitate self-organization, change, and the creation of new experiences.

Habits and Routines

Habits, routines, and rituals are deeply meaningful and provide the foundation supporting the engagement in meaningful daily occupations. It is common for occupational therapists to explore the habits, routines, and rituals of their clients. However, it is important for occupational therapists to understand that occupational therapy evaluation and treatment interventions are often attempts to facilitate perturbation. These are used to explore the client's ability to flexibly transition between dynamic cognitive states and to facilitate change. Therapeutic exchanges may help to create or destabilize habitual patterns, depending on the co-created treatment goals of the client and therapist. Understanding the NLD process of the circular causality of habit formation helps occupational therapists understand the neurodynamics involved in habit formation, thus better enabling the ability to co-create therapeutic interventions leading to positive and meaningful treatment outcomes.

Implications and Applications of Nonlinear Dynamics

A substantial amount of scholarly work remains to be executed in the field of occupational therapy to fully embrace an NLD perspective. However, understanding the benefits, implications, and applications, could very well serve to inspire researchers, clinicians, and academicians to engage on the discovery and discourse of NLD.

1. Connectedness of elements is central to the study of cognition.

2. Cognitive processes are embodied and the body is embedded. The body serves as the principal tool of the brain for cognitive development.

3. The mind simply does not exist as something decoupled from the body and the environment in which it resides. A coupled system refers to a system guided by influence as opposed to control.

4. In therapeutic interventions where development or adaptation of new skills is expected, the coupling must be highly flexible and dynamically responsive to task.

5. NLD takes embodiment to be a living phenomenon in which the primacy of bodily grounded experience (e.g., intention, meaning, perception, emotion, and movement) is inherently part of the very subject matter of the study of cognition.

6. There is no controlling agent, input–output causality, or blank slate. Every individual enters a new situation with an existing degree of cognitive capacity and unique meanings.

7. The system is self-organizing and multiply causal. NLD articulates human cognition as a self-organizing, intentional process in which pattern formation and neural organization develop through internal interactions.

8. Cognition, as a process, is an emergent pattern of multiple cooperating components all of which count and none of which are privileged. It is the relationship of the multiple parts that gives the system order and pattern (self-organization).

9. Changes in cognitive processes consist of the progressive ability to modulate the coupling to meet different and changing situations.

10. To understand, measure, and propel therapeutic change, preexisting intentions, perceptions, and meanings need to be identified before the introduction of a novel task because they influence and determine successful perturbations and thus therapeutic change.

11. Cognitive adaptation during critical therapeutic times means having the ability to categorize the world to flexibly and rapidly recruit useful categories of activities/occupations to make a mental plan based on prior experience before actually acting, when required, and also quickly responding without a lot of hesitation when necessary.

12. All brains can know is the hypothesis that they construct and the results of experiencing it by acting into the environment and shaping past experiences by assimilation from the sensory consequences encountered through flexible states that are self-organizing and emerging.

13. Occupational therapy process fundamentally means the modification of preexisting cognitive stable states. It is not just reinforcing, repetition, or drilling.

14. When a human brain is learning or adapting a skill, activity in local neural populations and the coordination among distant neural areas is dramatically reorganized. Moreover, the individual brain, after it has integrated the skill, is functioning far more economically than one that has not.

15. Cognition is fractal in the sense that once new learning occurs the whole system changes.

16. Cognitive processes are a product of the nervous system, body, and environment that are always embedded and dynamically coupled.

17. New information either cooperates or competes with the individual's existing knowledge (coordination dynamics). Knowledge accounts for habits, rituals, and meaning. Cooperative or competitive states determine the assimilation rate of therapeutic exchanges: faster for the former and slow and laborious for the latter.

18. Cognition is not necessarily a gradual process. Rather, depending on the level of cooperation and cooperation of internal states, it may involve shifts in parameter space or highly nonlinear, abrupt transitions ("Aha!" moments).

19. Remembering refers to the stability of cognitive states, a process that can be and has been precisely quantified.

20. Rather than imposing an external organization on a client, the therapist needs to attend to the conditions under which the client's own self-organization can emerge. This is a fundamentally different way of reasoning about therapeutic change.

21. Because individuals rely on past experiences, goals, and meanings, which ultimately are the habitual patterns of daily living, therapists could quickly determine the flexibility or rigidity of intentional states by perturbing the system.

22. Recognize and understand that dynamical instabilities of cognitive states serve as therapeutic opportunities allowing therapists to use these brief windows of opportunity to facilitate self-organization, change, and the creation of new experiences.

23. The value of a deeper understanding of a nonlinear approach to cognition resides in the ability of therapist to scientifically substantiate and sustain rehabilitation interventions and also to articulate how change is facilitated in and through initial conditions, which in turn influences the state of the whole system.

This list, albeit brief and incomplete, is meant to encourage a reevaluation of therapeutic approaches and explanations presently used to validate occupational therapy practice. The focus on the individual previous intentions, meanings, and perceptions as constraints on the therapeutic process and the need to structure the learning environment in light of them have significant consequences for curricular undertakings and clinical practice, as well as implication for rehabilitation policy.

CONCLUSION

The theoretical cognitive approaches discussed in this chapter have unequivocally sustained occupational therapy for a number of decades. These views have served as the platforms from which occupational therapy developed its guiding frameworks and thus, clinical practice. Nonetheless, NLD, as a conceptual framework, provides a more encompassing perspective than any previous theories could support. It emphasizes the complexity and importance of cognitive processes and the client's historical essence. The historical essence of human beings drives intentional states, perceptions, and ultimately the meaningful choices they make.

NLD recognizes the importance of context in the process of change. It connects and reconciles the mental and the physical. It allows the therapeutic teaching–learning exchanges to be connected processes. NLD offers a unifying approach that affords scientists, academicians, and clinical practitioners to engage in a discourse of both cognition and therapeutic approaches that have not been previously available. Ultimately, NLD scientifically validates the role of occupational therapy in restoring the essence of occupational therapy practice and clearly articulating occupation as the agency for change propelling human action into new meanings.

REFERENCES

Block, N. (Ed.). (1980). What is functionalism? In *Readings in philosophy of psychology* (Vol. 1). Cambridge, MA: Harvard University Press.

Bronfenbrenner, U. (1975). Nature with nurture: A reinterpretation of the evidence. In A. Montague (Ed.), *Race and IQ* (pp. 114-144). New York, NY: Oxford University Press.

Bronfenbrenner, U. (1986). Ecology of the family as a context for human development: Research perspectives. *Developmental Psychology, 22*, 723-742.

Chomsky, N. (1959). A review of verbal behavior by B. F. Skinner. *Language, 35*, 26-35.

Chomsky, N. (1965). *Aspects of the theory of syntax.* Cambridge, MA: MIT Press.

Dreyfus, H. (1979). *What computers can't do: The limits of artificial intelligence.* New York, NY: Harper Colophon.

Edelman, G. M. (1987). *Neural Darwinism: The theory of neuronal group selection.* New York, NY: Basic Books, Inc.

Edelman, G. M. (1992). *Bright air, brilliant fire: On the matter of the mind.* New York, NY: Basic Books.

Freeman, W. J. (1988a). Nonlinear neural dynamics in olfaction as a model for cognition. In E. Basar (Ed.), *Dynamics of sensory and cognitive processing by the brain* (pp. 19-29). Berlin, Germany: Springer.

Freeman, W. J. (1988b). Strange attractors that govern mammalian brain dynamics as shown by trajectories of electroencephalographic (EEG) potential. *IEEE Transactions on Circuits and Systems, 35*, 781-783.

Freeman, W. J. (1995). *Societies of brains.* Mahwah, NJ: Erlbaum.

Freeman, W. J. (1997). Three centuries of category errors in studies of the neural basis of consciousness and intentionality. *Neural Networks, 10*, 1175-1183.

Freeman, W. J. (1999). Consciousness, intentionality and causality. *Journal of Consciousness Studies, 6*, 143-172.

Freeman, W. J. (2000a). A proposed name for aperiodic brain activity: Stochastic chaos. *Neural Networks, 13*, 11-13.

Freeman, W. J. (2000b). Brain dynamics: Brain chaos and intentionality. In E. Gordon (Ed.), *Integrative neuroscience: Bringing together biological, psychological and clinical models of the human brain* (pp. 163-171). Camberwell, Australia: Harwood Academic.

Freeman, W. J. (2000c). Brains create macroscopic order from microscopic disorder by neurodynamics in perception. In P. Arhem, C. Blomberg, & H. Liljenstrom (Eds.), *Disorder versus order in brain function* (pp. 205-219). Hackensack, NJ: World Scientific.

Freeman, W. J. (2000d). Mesoscopic neurodynamics from neuron to brain. *Journal of Physiology, 94*, 303-322.

Freeman, W. J. (2000e). *Neurodynamics: An exploration in mesoscopic brain dynamics.* New York, NY: Springer.

Freeman, W. J. (2001). Self-organizing brain dynamics by which the goals are constructed that control patterns of muscle actions. *IEEE American Control Conference, 1*, 240-245.

Freeman, W. J. (2002). Brains create macroscopic order from microscopic disorder by neurodynamics in perception. In P. Arhem, C. Blomberg, & H. Liljenstrom (Eds.), *Disorder versus order in brain function* (pp. 205-219). Singapore: World Scientific Publishing Co.

Gagne, R. (1985). *The conditions of learning* (4th ed.). New York, NY: Holt, Rinehart & Winston.

Gagne, E., Yekovich, C., & Yekovich, F. (1993). *The cognitive psychology of school learning* (2nd ed.). New York, NY: HarperCollins.

Gage, N., & Berliner, D. (1998). *Educational psychology* (6th ed.). Boston, MA: Houghton Mifflin.

Gardner, H. (1985). *The mind's new science.* New York, NY: Basic Books.

Guastello, S. (1995). *Chaos, catastrophe, and human affairs.* Mahwah, NJ: Erlbaum.

Haken, H. (2000). A physicist's view of brain functioning: Coherence, chaos, pattern formation, noise. In P. Arhem, C. Blomberg, & H. Liljenstrom (Eds.), *Disorder versus order in brain function* (pp. 135-184). Singapore: World Scientific.

Haken, H. (2002). *Brain dynamics: Synchronization and activity patterns in pulse-coupled neural nets with delays and noise.* New York, NY: Springer.

Haken, H. (2003). Intelligent behavior: A synergetic view. In W. Tschacher & J. S. Dauwaldere (Eds.), *The dynamical system approach to cognition* (pp. 3-16). Singapore: World Scientific.

Haken, H., & Tschacher, W. (2011). The transfer of principles of non-equilibrium physics to embodied cognition. In W. Tschacher & C. Bergomi (Eds.), *The implications of embodiment: Cognition and communication* (pp. 75-88). Exeter, England: Imprint Academic.

Haltiwanger, E., Lazzarini, I., & Nazeran, H. (2007). Application of complexity theory to neuro-occupation: A case study of alcoholism. *British Journal of Occupational Therapy, 70*, 349-357.

Iverson, J. M., & Thelen, E. (1999). Hand, mouth and brain: The dynamics emergence of speech and gesture. *Journal of Consciousness, 6*(11-12), 19-40.

Johnson, M. (1987). *The body in the mind: The bodily basis of meaning, imagination and reason.* Chicago, IL: University of Chicago Press.

Juarrero, A. (2002). *Dynamics in action: Intentional behavior as a complex system.* Cambridge, MA: MIT Press.

Kay, L. M., Lancaster, L., & Freeman, W. J. (1996). Reafference and attractors in the olfactory system during odor recognition. *International Journal of Neural Systems, 7*, 489-496.

Kelso, S. J. A. (1999). *Dynamic patterns: The self-organization of brain and behavior.* Cambridge, MA: MIT Press.

Lakoff, G., & Nuñez, R. (2000). *Where mathematics comes from: How the embodied mind creates mathematics*. New York, NY: Basic Books.

Lazzarini, I. (2004). Neuro-occupation: The nonlinear dynamics of intention, meaning and perception. *British Journal of Occupational Therapy, 67*, 1-11.

Llinás, R., & Ribary, U. (1993). Coherent 40-Hz oscillation characterizes dream state in humans. *Proceedings, National Academy of Sciences, 90*, 2078-2081.

Lorenz, E. (1972). *Does the flap of a butterfly's wings in Brazil set off a tornado in Texas?* Presented at the 139th Meeting of American Association for the Advancement of Science, Washington, DC.

Markman, A. B., & Dietrich, E. (2000). In defense of representation. *Cognitive Psychology, 40*, 138-171.

Mayer, R. E. (1992). Cognition and instruction: The historic meaning within educational psychology. *Journal of Educational Psychology, 84*, 405-412.

McLaughlin, J., Kennedy, B., & Zemke, R. (1996). Dynamic system theory: An overview. In R. Zemke & F. Clark (Eds.), *Occupational science: The evolving discipline* (pp. 297-308). Philadelphia, PA: F. A. Davis.

Miller, P. H. (1993). *Theories of development psychology* (3rd ed.). New York, NY: W. H. Freeman.

Nuñez, R. (1997). Eating soup with chopsticks: Dogmas, difficulties, and alternatives in the study of conscious experience. *Journal of Consciousness Studies, 4*, 143-166.

Piaget, J. (1930). *The child's conception of physical causality*. New York, NY: Harcourt Brace.

Piaget, J. (1952). *The origins of intelligence in children*. New York, NY: International University Press.

Piaget, J. (1972). Intellectual evolution from adolescence to adulthood. *Human Development, 15*, 1-12.

Piaget, J. (1983). Piaget's theory. In P. H. Mussen (Ed.), *Handbook of child psychology: Vol. 1. History, theory, and methods* (pp. 103-126). New York, NY: Wiley.

Plomin, R. (1989). Environment and genes. *American Psychologist, 44*, 105-111.

Prigogine, I. (1994). *Order out of chaos*. New York, NY: Bantam.

Prigogine, I. (1997). *The end of certainty: Time, chaos, and the new laws of nature*. New York, NY: Free Press.

Prigogine, I., & Stengers, I. (1984). *Order out of chaos: Man's dialogue with nature*. New York, NY: Bantam.

Royeen, C. (2002). Occupation reconsidered. *Occupational Therapy International, 9*, 112-121.

Searle, J. R. (1992). *The rediscovery of mind*. Cambridge, MA: MIT Press.

Shibata, T., & Kaneko, K. (1998). Collective chaos. *Physical Review Letters, 81*, 4116-4119.

Shuell, T. J. (1996). Teaching and learning in a classroom context. In D. C. Berliner & R. C. Calfee (Eds.), *Handbook of educational psychology* (pp. 726-764). New York, NY: Macmillan.

Simon, H., & Kaplan, C. (1989). Foundations of cognitive science. In M. Posner (Ed.), *Foundations of cognitive science* (pp. 1-45). Cambridge, MA: MIT Press.

Skarda, C., & Freeman, W. J. (1987). How brains make chaos in the order to make sense of the world. *Behavioral and Brain Sciences, 10*, 161-173.

Szentagothai, J. (1984). Downward causation? *Annual Review of Neuroscience, 1*, 1-11.

Thelen, E., & Smith, L. B. (1994). *A dynamic approach to the development of cognition and action*. Cambridge, MA: MIT Press.

Tsuda, I. (1991). Chaotic itinerancy as a dynamical basis of hermeneutics in brain and mind. *World Futures, 32*, 167-184.

Tsuda, I. (1996). A new type of self-organization associated with chaotic dynamics in neural networks. *International Journal of Neural Systems, 7*, 451-459.

Van Orden, G., & Holden, J. G. (2002). Intentional contents and self-control. *Ecological Psychology, 14*, 87-109.

Van Orden, G., Holden, G., & Turvey, I. (2003). Self-organization of cognitive performance. *Journal of Experimental Psychology, 132*, 331-350.

Varela, F. (1989). *Connaitre les sciences cognitives: Tendances et perspectives*. Paris, France: Seuil.

Varela, F., Thompson, E., & Rosch, E. (1991). *The embodied mind: Cognitive science and human experience*. Cambridge, MA: MIT Press.

von Glaserfeld, E. (1984). An introduction to radical constructivism. In P. Watzlawick (Ed.), *The invented reality* (pp. 17-40). New York, NY: Norton.

von Glaserfeld, E. (1995). A constructive approach to teaching. In L. P. Steffe & J. Gale (Eds.), *Constructivism in education* (pp. 3-16). Hillsdale, NJ: Erlbaum.

Vygotsky, L. (1986). *Thought and language*. Cambridge, MA: MIT Press.

Ward, L. (2002). *Dynamical cognitive science*. Cambridge, MA: MIT Press.

Wegner, D. M., & Wheatley, T. (1999). Sources of the experience of will. *American Psychologist, 54*, 480-492.

Winograd, T., & Flores, F. (1986). *Understanding computers and cognition: A new foundation design*. Norwood, NJ: Ablex.

Woolfolk, A. (1998). *Educational psychology* (7th ed.). Needham Heights, MA: Allyn and Bacon.

Wright, J. J., & Liley, D. T. J. (1996). Dynamics of the brain at global and microscopic scales: Neural networks and EEG. *Behavioral and Brain Sciences, 19*, 285-295.

12

Development Reasoning in Community Practice

E. Madeleine Duncan, BAOT, BA Hon (Psych), MScOT, DPhil (Psychology)

Development refers to the gradual unfolding or bringing out of latent potential in people, their environments, and social systems. It implies growth—maturation and advancement to a more organized and preferred state of being and may occur spontaneously or be facilitated. The fundamental goal of development as an approach is a world in which each individual has the inalienable right to live a life worthy of a human being. The achievement of this goal requires development approaches to target the material, structural, and social conditions through which people can live dignified and meaningful lives without compromising the natural environment. Development reasoning is the process of thinking about a facet of development in a logical way in order to form a conclusion, make a judgment, or guide an action toward the attainment of a particular development outcome.

Development studies is a multidisciplinary branch of social science that is concerned with social, structural, and economic change in developing countries (Kothari, 2005). A developing or less developed country is a "nation with a lower standard of living, industrial base, and Human Development Index (HDI) relative to other countries" (Sullivan & Sheffrin, 2003, p. 241). The 2013 Human Development Report indicates that the majority of developing countries are located in the global south (United Nations Development Programme, 2013). Development studies incorporate scholarly contributions from a range of social sciences, including anthropology, criminology, demography, ecology, economics, geography, history, international relations, philosophy, political science, public management, and sociology. Other interdisciplinary or emerging fields that have made their mark in theorizing development include area studies, cultural studies, epidemiology, ethnic studies, migration studies, pedagogy, postcolonialism, and women's studies.

Given the scope of scholarship involved, it is understandable that development is a contested concept that is understood differently depending on the people, disciplines, agencies, or stakeholders involved. For some, development is a vehicle for transformation that brings improvement and progress toward something better than the current reality of people's lives. For others, development has negative connotations as a masquerade to exploit people by taking their land and

Cole, M. B., & Creek, J. (Eds.).
Global Perspectives in Professional Reasoning (pp. 203-237).
© 2016 Taylor & Francis Group.

resources, with adverse impact on their indigenous social systems and local economies (Davids, Theron, & Maphunye, 2009; Mloka, 2004). Development reasoning must therefore proceed from the understanding that the discourse of development is historically, culturally, and locally contingent; that is, the ways people think and talk about and act to promote or resist development are determined by complex sociopolitical processes (Naz, 2006).

Development as discourse refers to the ways in which particular concepts, theories, and practices for social change are created and reproduced over time to convey knowledge and consolidate or exert power (Escobar, 1995; Naz, 2006). The institutionalization of development started after the Second World War when the rise of capitalism and modernity saw the birth of the development organization, the development expert, the national development plan, and university courses on development. Benchmarks for development were articulated by so-called first world countries (Western Europe, the United States, Canada, Australia, and Japan) and imposed on countries that were variously labeled as underdeveloped, developing, the third world, and the South. The idea of development became synonymous with economic, political, and social change brought about in the developing world (Africa, the Middle East including Muslim North Africa, Asia minus Japan and China, and Latin America) by development aid and knowledge colonization (imposition of ideology) from first world countries (Kothari, 2005). The hegemonic and extractive agendas of development aid and the consequences of colonization in Africa, South America, and the Orient have been extensively addressed (e.g., Freire, 2005; Gibson, 2011; Said, 1994). Although the history and politics of macrodevelopment may appear to be of limited relevance to occupational therapy, there is a growing body of professional literature that explores the implications of knowledge colonization for socially responsible, occupation-based community practice (Pollard, Sakellariou, & Kronenberg, 2008; Robertson, 2012; Whalley Hammell & Iwama, 2012).

Pertinent to the discussion, however, is the need to adopt a critical standpoint in development reasoning.

This chapter considers development and development reasoning in community practice in five sections. The first section presents a rationale for situating occupational therapy in development. The next section discusses some facets of development: individual, human, organizational, community, social, and rural. The third section describes macro and micro levels of development and identifies the modes of thinking appropriate to each of them. The fourth section describes three forms of reasoning that can be used to support microdevelopment practice: sociological imagination, public reasoning, and axiological reasoning. The final section is a case study of two participatory research projects in a remote rural area of South Africa that illustrate some of the points presented in the first four sections.

SITUATING OCCUPATIONAL THERAPY IN DEVELOPMENT

Occupational therapy is a health profession with an established philosophical, theoretical, and practical history of optimizing human potential and well-being. Occupational therapists believe that health is more than the absence of disease and ill-being. It is also a human right that is advanced through occupation—that is, through the ordinary (and extraordinary) things people do every day to give expression to their creativity, meet their needs, and achieve their aspirations (World Federation of Occupational Therapists [WFOT], 2006). The

> human right to occupation includes the right to fulfil basic human needs to act or otherwise engage in the world (doing), to discover one's true self as an individual or community member (being), to connect in relationships with other humans, and with animals and the inanimate environment (belonging), and to pursue human aspirations, visions and dreams for individuals, communities and populations (becoming). (WFOT, 2014, p. 7)

The goal of occupational therapy is to enable people to do well, individually and collectively.

Occupational therapists, combining knowledge and methods from the health, social, and human sciences, address the praxis between human doing (occupation), the doing human (individual, group, population), and the environments in which humans live, learn, work, play, and socialize. The core purpose of the profession is to enable human doing well. Environment refers to the external physical (material, structural), sociocultural, and temporal factors that demand and shape occupational performance (Creek, 2010). The optimal, health-promoting fit among person(s), occupation(s), and environment(s) may be disrupted by personal factors (e.g., impairments of body structure and function, behavioral dysfunction, developmental delay, or adverse life events) and/or contextual factors (e.g., marginalizing or oppressive historical, socioeconomic, cultural, and political circumstances). Context refers to the external influences or factors that surround a particular situation or event. Human doing is always transactional. It is "inseparable from the contextual foreground and background within which it occurs" (Cutchin, Aldrich, Baillard, & Coppola, 2008, p. 161). Development reasoning in occupational therapy therefore places particular emphasis on thinking about the prevailing contextual influences that shape human–occupation–environment praxis.

The identity of occupational therapy as a health profession emphasizes its remedial and rehabilitative role in addressing individual impairments that lead to occupational performance dysfunction and participation restrictions. Although recent occupational therapy literature reflects a trend toward development practice (e.g., Kronenberg, Pollard, & Sakellariou, 2011), the profession remains predominantly concerned with helping people who face health risks, ill health, and disability to perform their activities of daily living. This health-focused, individualistic, therapeutic, and occupational performance-centered concern sets the profession apart from other development-orientated professions and disciplines. Occupational therapists bring a much-needed perspective and skill set to the development agenda: a focus on humans as occupational beings and the ability to consider economies of scale when designing population-orientated, occupation-based, graded programs that address the social determinants of health (van Bruggen, 2009). Health practitioners, including occupational therapists, acknowledge that the biomedical and functional dimensions of health conditions are intimately entwined with the social determinants of health and human well-being. Writing about health justice, Venkatopuram (2011, p. 8) suggested that addressing the social determinants of health involves "protecting, promoting, sustaining, or restoring [people's] capability to be healthy to a level that is commensurate with equal human dignity in the modern world."

This is the core focus of development reasoning in social occupational therapy. By conceptualizing the political and strategic nature of development we are able "to maintain a focus on power and domination, while at the same time exploring the discourse's conditions of possibility as well as its effects" (Naz, 2006, p. 71). Reflexive thinking is necessary. Assumptions about development theory, method, and practice must be bracketed (by suspending taken for granted ways of seeing the world) so that potential nodes of hegemonic power and domination are identified. Occupational therapy thinking takes into consideration the prevailing discourse(s) in a particular development context, discerning the role that knowledge and power play in development orientated practice. Drawing on the work of Naz (2006) and Escobar (1995), three examples of development as discourse are suggested in Box 12-1. Questions are posed to facilitate occupational therapy vigilance in development reasoning.

Occupational Therapy: A Heart and Soul Profession

Contemporary development practitioners are referred to as change agents because they act as direct and indirect catalysts for releasing the creative energies of people (development beneficiaries) to achieve their self-determined future (Davids et al., 2009). Theron (2008, p. 3) distinguished between "nuts-and-bolts" development professions, such as economists, engineers, and city planners, and "heart-and-soul" development professions, such as social workers and community psychologists. Development theorists seldom consider occupational therapy as belonging in the

Box 12-1. Development as Discourse

1. **Development is presented as a humanitarian and moral concern, an ethical obligation on behalf of the rich, the developed, and/or informed (knowledgeable experts such as health professionals) to help and care for those less fortunate and to advance social justice.** Escobar (1995) argued that behind this aura of humanitarianism and justice rhetoric lurks a fear of poverty and the poor. The *underdeveloped* become a category of intervention, a place to be managed and reformed by self-acclaimed "developed" people (Naz, 2006). The discourse of development masks the ways in which underdeveloped people threaten the wealth and civilized way of life of developed people. Poor and marginalized people become observed, classified, and managed through various development techniques that ostensibly aim to combat social injustice. In short, development initiatives are conceived out of the self-directed charity of development agents and donors and not from the expressed concerns of those being aided (Chan, 2014). Occupational therapists are knowledgeable experts about humans as occupational beings. How should they position their thinking when entering contexts characterized by disadvantage and social injustice?

2. **Development is presented as the answer to lack, as a means of making "the other" like "us."** The discourse of *lack* implies that there are nothing but deficiencies before development. The developing world (also called third world) is defined primarily by what it is not rather than by what it is. A similar discourse is applied to marginalized people and to the places where they live, such as informal human settlements and urban ghettos. The central characteristics of a country, a group of people, or a location are defined by what is lacking, not by what is possessed (Naz, 2006). People become homogenized; they are all poor, illiterate, primitive, violent, and so forth. The structuring of discourse around a series of absences legitimizes development-orientated actions and interventions aimed at remediating and rectifying the presumed misery and suffering that are associated with underdevelopment (Chan, 2014). How may occupational therapists retain the profession's moral-philosophical commitment to eliciting human potential through occupation in underdeveloped contexts? What would hinder or facilitate thinking about what people can do, rather than cannot do, to become more than they are (if that is what they desire for themselves)?

3. **Western domination in the majority world is perpetuated under the guise of development.** The notion of development is couched in language that invokes images of change for the better, from stagnation to dynamism, from simplicity to complexity, from scarcity to abundance (Naz, 2006). This form of development discourse establishes a clear hierarchy, where the first or developed world is placed above the third or underdeveloped world (Escobar, 1995). A similar hierarchical mode of development reasoning in occupational therapy may place the profession's knowledge above indigenous knowledge and culturally informed, local ways of *doing life*. The beneficiaries of development are, however, not passive receivers, wholly oppressed by power; they are "active agents who may and frequently do contest, resist, divert, and manipulate the activities carried out in the name of development" (Naz, 2006, p. 80). How may occupational therapists, as change agents trained in Western modes of thinking originating in the developed world, recognize, facilitate, and work with people's agency and resistance to domination in less developed contexts?

TABLE 12-1 CLINICAL AND DEVELOPMENT REASONING		
FEATURE	**CLINICAL REASONING**	**DEVELOPMENT REASONING**
PURPOSE(S)	Remediation, restoration of function	Social change, unlocking human potential
ROLE	Therapist/clinician	Change agent/developer
FOCUS	Consequences of health conditions	Precipitants of health conditions
MODEL	Medical (biopsychosocial)	Sociopolitical

Adapted from Boyt Schell, B. A., & Schell, J. W. (2008). *Clinical and professional reasoning in occupational therapy.* Philadelphia, PA: Lippincott Williams & Wilkins and Theron, F. (2008). *The development change agent: A micro-level approach to development.* Pretoria, South Africa: van Schaik.

latter category, probably because they are unaware of what the profession has to offer, especially in health development. Health development refers to the active participation and empowerment of people in promoting and caring for their own health (Davids et al., 2009). It is time to change this omission. Both the clinical and social applications of occupational therapy affirm the profession's holistic understanding of humans as occupational beings in the context of their local life world—in particular, how social and environmental determinants affect people's health by either enabling or limiting their occupational opportunities, choices, and engagement. Table 12-1 depicts two forms of reasoning employed by occupational therapists, the combined use of which positions the profession as a development change agent that can straddle health and social science in seeking practical solutions to the precipitants and consequences of health conditions. The contextual relevance of these forms of professional reasoning must, however, be mediated with due consideration of local histories, indigenous knowledge systems, and sociocultural forms of reasoning. The transformation of the profession (i.e., the decolonization of dominant occupational therapy theories and practices) requires critical engagement with and privileging of subaltern social practices (Connell, 2007).

Occupational science, an evolving social science discipline in the service of occupational therapy and other professions, is concerned with theorizing human occupation. Recent theories conceptualize occupation as self-action and interaction, as the transactional and relational connection between the individual, the social, and the contextual (Cutchin et al., 2008; Cutchin & Dickie, 2013). Here, occupation is potentially the means through which "humans and context exist in an ongoing process of reproduction and occasional transformation, dependent on one another for their current states of existence" (Cutchin et al., 2008, p. 162). Occupation moves beyond being the means and focus of therapeutic intervention to become a construct for appreciating the agency, actions, and adaptive capacity of humans in and on their lived environments, and of the environment's effect on them. A challenge for occupational therapy is to scale up its population-level of impact (Galheigo, 2011; Watson, 2013). To this end, a growing number of texts are addressing socially orientated, occupation-based occupational therapy practice theories and frameworks (e.g., Kronenberg et al., 2011; van Bruggen, 2009; Whiteford & Hocking, 2012; Whiteford & Townsend, 2011). Occupation-based development focuses on human occupation to advance an occupational therapy vision of health, well-being, and social justice for individuals, groups, and communities. Occupation is used as a means to create the conditions necessary for individual, group, organizational, and community development through learning by doing. As an end in itself, occupation also works against discrimination, exclusion, and marginalization in several ways and on many levels (Leclair, 2010). For example, collective occupations—such as lobbying, fundraising, voting, or volunteering—provide a biographical, historical, and structural context through which people can share in the same activities and, in so doing, the same rights and privileges (Ramugondo

& Kronenberg, 2015). In summary, occupation-based practice provides occupational therapists with a theoretically substantiated means of working developmentally toward social change by addressing the socio-occupational determinants of health. It also provides the basis for a range of health development approaches such as primary health care, disability-inclusive development, and community-based rehabilitation (CBR).

Occupational Therapy and Primary Health Care

Primary health care, consisting of promotive, preventative, curative, rehabilitative, and palliative components, aims to provide accessible and appropriate health benefits to all people at a reasonable cost (Canadian Association of Occupational Therapists, 2006). Of relevance to this chapter is the contribution of occupational therapy in effecting the primary health care principle of participatory health development. Davids et al. (2009) argued that participation emphasizes the bottom-up approach to planning and implementing development programs, including health development, where people are seen as active participants, compared with the conventional top-down approach where people are viewed as passive recipients of programs designed for them by professionals and government officials. What may this perspective on participation mean for occupational therapy as a contributor to health development? If both clinical and social orientations to practice are held in creative tension, as suggested in Box 12-2, then occupational therapy will add value to the social compact of building a better world in partnership with the people being served. A particular focus may be to advance the health and disability literacy of communities from an occupational perspective (Levasseur & Carrier, 2012).

Occupational Therapy and Inclusive Development

Many people are excluded from development because of their gender, ethnicity, age, sexual orientation, disability, or poverty (United Nations Development Programme, 2014). Inclusive development ensures that marginalized and excluded groups are stakeholders in development processes by integrating the standards of human rights as these apply to their specific needs: participation, nondiscrimination, and accountability. The political activism of people with disabilities for their citizen rights has led to the calls for disability-inclusive development to ensure that all phases of the development cycle (design, implementation, monitoring, and evaluation) include a disability dimension and that persons with disabilities participate meaningfully and effectively in development processes and policies (Chervin & Geiser, 2012).

Disability-inclusive development is guided, among other policies, by the *United Nations Convention on the Rights of Persons with Disabilities* (CRPD; United Nations, 2006). A rights approach to disability affirms the democratic and developmental project at the societal level and, at the individual level, the right to develop personal skills, interests, and abilities. Occupational therapists are well versed in making the latter possible but less so with the former. Because most of the determinants of health, well-being, and occupational justice operate outside the person, it makes sense for occupational therapists to engage with the structural, social, and systemic environments that affect people's health, functioning, and social participation. Examples of disability-inclusive development in occupational therapy are presented by Lorenzo in this book.

Occupational Therapy and Community-Based Rehabilitation

CBR is a strategy for disability-inclusive development concerned with making health, education, social, livelihood, and empowerment services accessible, affordable, and appropriate for persons with disabilities (World Health Organization [WHO], 2010). CBR is not a service in itself but an approach that benefits everyone in a community because it emphasizes the inherent values of human development. CBR is first and foremost about promoting the social inclusion of people with physical, sensory, psychiatric, learning, and other disabilities by reducing structural,

BOX 12-2. CLINICAL AND SOCIAL OCCUPATIONAL THERAPY

Considering their theoretical and skills base, occupational therapists may offer one or a combination of the following:

- **Clinically oriented interventions for individuals, groups, or populations at tertiary, secondary, and primary levels of care.** The clinical focus is on the functional implications of health conditions. Programs that remediate and rehabilitate impairments, occupational performance dysfunction, and occupational participation restrictions in self-care, work, learning, play, and social domains are designed in collaboration with the person(s) concerned. Interventions at primary level may be offered directly by the therapist at a health clinic or in people's homes, and/or indirectly through supported task shifting by carers, midlevel health workers, and other role players, such as job coaches. School and occupational health may be included under the primary health care umbrella, in which case occupational therapists may work in the education, labor, or other public sectors.

- **Socially oriented interventions at the primary care level, in which occupational therapy adopts a development focus on the creation of opportunities for increased humanness in local meaning-giving contexts.** The social focus of occupational therapy is on health development as a process concerned with enhancing intrapersonal capabilities (individual), interpersonal relationships (group), and transpersonal social systems (societal). Health development unfolds in different pockets in a community, with different players addressing different needs associated with the social determinants of health, such as poverty, low literacy, environmental degradation, maternal and infant morbidity, violence, prolonged stress and psychosocial trauma, chronic diseases of lifestyle, and mental illness (World Health Organization, 2007). Projects may, for example, target income generation, food security, health literacy, physical fitness, psychological resilience, healthy lifestyles, and restoration of the environment. Occupation clearly anchors each of these examples, yet occupational therapy is seldom factored in by microdevelopment policy makers and planners as a profession equipped to enhance intrapersonal, interpersonal, and transpersonal social systems. Conversely, occupation-based practice requires occupational therapists to understand the complexities of the environments and local meaning-giving contexts within which health development takes place.

environmental, and attitudinal barriers to their full participation in society. Health development–orientated interventions position CBR as an integrative strategy for intersectoral collaboration in the democratic project of building an inclusive society. The CBR Guidelines (WHO, 2010) are an invaluable, practical resource to guide disability-inclusive practice, especially in resource-poor and underdeveloped contexts. Occupational therapy is positioned to work across and within the CBR domains by virtue of the profession's holistic appreciation of the interface between people, what they do, and the environments within which they engage with life and its various demands.

In summary, it can be argued that clinical and social occupational therapy intersect in development-orientated practice. The next section discusses some of the facets of development, all of which require development reasoning.

FACETS OF DEVELOPMENT

Our life chances and our very experiences of social life will differ dramatically according to what kind of society we are born into. Human lives do not unfold according to sheer chance, nor do people live isolated lives relying solely on what philosophers call "free will" in choosing every thought and action. On the contrary, although individuals make many important decisions every day, we do so within the larger arena called *society*—a friendship, a family, a university, a nation, an entire world. (Macionis & Plummer, 2008, p. 27)

Different development approaches focus on different facets of society, such as the life course progression of individuals, the quality of life of humans in general, or the well-being of organizations, communities, and society as a whole. The extent, direction, and duration of development is influenced by multiple, intersecting factors, such as critical life events, political unrest, economic downturns, famine or other natural disasters, and the historical passage of time. Although development approaches may differ depending on their focus, the process of gradual social change is essentially the same. Society changes outwardly because people change inwardly. Individuals develop with the active support of society and society develops through the contributions of individuals. For example, better educated women are more likely to keep their children in school, with the long-term benefit of a healthier and more productive nation. However, the access that women and girl children have to education depends on a country's sociopolitical ideology, legislative commitment to gender equality, and prevailing contextual circumstances.

Development, Time, and Occupation

From an occupational perspective, each facet of development reveals and requires different forms of occupation and patterns of occupational engagement. Knowledge, skills, and values associated with occupation across the spectrum of human endeavors are passed on between generations. Physical, sociocultural and structural environments change over time and, in so doing, may hinder or enable the occupational performance capabilities of individuals and shape the occupational engagement patterns of cultural groups. Table 12-2 summarizes some of the ways in which development, time, and occupation may intersect.

The various facets of development depicted in Table 12-2 are familiar practice territories for occupational therapists, ranging from the clinical application of life course development theory to occupational justice for marginalized people in contexts where structural poverty and social inequality intersect. Each of the facets or focus areas of development is briefly explained in the following six sections, highlighting aspects of interest for occupational therapists.

Individual Life Course Development

Humans develop ontogenetically over the course of their life span from conception through infancy, childhood, youth, adulthood, and old age to death. Each age and stage is characterized by biopsychosocial, behavioral, and other changes in human attributes and abilities that are considered normative in a particular society, culture, or historical period. Besides being shaped by personal biological and psychological processes, individual development and identity are also determined by intersectional features such as gender, class, race, ability, and sexual orientation and by other factors such as material circumstances, geographic location, and prevailing societal dynamics. There is no universally applicable age and stage understanding of individual development because people groups across the world interpret the human life cycle differently. For example, five rites associated with birth, adulthood, marriage, eldership, and ancestorship are performed in traditional African cultures. A rite is a fundamental act (or set of rituals) performed according to prescribed social rules and customs to mark critical life transitions and stages across the life span (Ampim, 2003).

TABLE 12-2
FACETS OF DEVELOPMENT, TIME, AND OCCUPATION

FACETS OF DEVELOPMENT	DEVELOPMENT OVER TIME				
	Seconds/ Minutes	Hours	Days/Weeks/ Months	Years/ Decades	Centuries
	OCCUPATIONAL PROFILE OVER TIME				
	Personal				
		Collective			
			Intergenerational		
INDIVIDUAL LIFE COURSE	Biopsychosocial processes and personal life experiences				
HUMAN		Group processes and dynamics			
ORGANIZATION		Formalized change processes through organized systems			
COMMUNITY		Social movements and processes; communal and kinship experiences			
SOCIETY			Constitution of institutions (e.g., political, religious, economic, educational, indigenous)		Historical-cultural processes and transitions

Adapted from Coetzee, J. K. (2001). A micro foundation for development thinking. In J. K. Coetzee & J. Graaf (Eds.), *Development theory, policy and practice* (pp. 118-139). Cape Town, South Africa: Oxford University Press and Macionis, J. J., & Plummer, K. (2008). *Sociology: A global introduction* (4th ed.). Harlow, England: Pearson Education Limited.

The earlier that people get help to overcome adversity the better their life course development trajectory is likely to be. An individual's developmental structure (biopsychosocial processes) directs and enables his or her performance of and engagement in occupations of necessity and choice. Evidence of individual development can be observed over time as the person is occupied from seconds to decades across the life span in a uniquely personal and ever-changing profile of occupations. The range and type of occupations performed varies in accordance with changes in the person's biopsychosocial developmental structure and emergent life experiences. Taking the social determinants of health into consideration, and with the aim of promoting individual development, the occupational therapist is able to discern, assess, and address, in profession specific ways, the impact of adverse life events such as illness, chronic disease, injury, psychological trauma, and social injustice on people's occupational performance and participation through occupation.

Human Development

Human development refers to the improvement of people's lives by expansion of their choices, freedoms, and dignity. The main goal of human development is to create enabling environments in which people can live long, healthy, and creative lives. The 2014 Human Development Report (United Nations Development Programme, 2014) argues that progress in human development hinges on reducing vulnerabilities and building resilience and that the timing of intervention in the life cycle matters. Timeous and appropriate human development interventions for a people, group, region, or country may be compromised by globalization, migration, urbanization, rural depopulation, environmental degradation, and sociopolitical and economic instability. Important catalysts for human development include, among others, a decent standard of living, education, political freedom, guaranteed human rights, opportunity freedom (choice), process freedom (development as participatory and dynamic), and personal self-respect. These and other criteria are reflected in the Sustainable Development Goals (SDGs), which will build on the Millennium Development Goals and converge with the post 2015 agenda to serve as international indicators for within and cross-country comparisons of human development (Sachs, 2012).

Although human development relies heavily on the economy and political stability of a country, its focus is much wider than the material conditions of people's lives. Amartya Sen, development theorist and Nobel Laureate in economics, suggests that human development, as an approach, is concerned with advancing the richness of human life rather than the richness of the economy in which human beings live (Fukuda-Parr, 2003). He sees development as the process of widening people's freedoms and choices through the formation of their capabilities, such as improved health or knowledge, and the enablement of their functioning, such as making it possible for people to use their acquired capabilities for work or leisure. The capabilities approach to human development has been extensively documented elsewhere and will not be reviewed further here (Nussbaum, 2011; Sen, 2011). It has also found traction in occupational therapy and occupational science scholarship (e.g., Townsend, 2012).

Suffice to note that Sen's capabilities approach recognizes the limitations of human freedoms (Wells, 2013). Sen acknowledges that development could well be expanded in ways that exacerbate inequality, are wasteful, or infringe on the human rights of one group to expand the freedoms of another (Wells, 2013). One example of inequality in human development is the income and resource disparities between rich and poor people (Narayan, 1999). The Gini coefficient is a human development index used to measure equality in human development in a country, using indices such as income and welfare distribution. It is a numerical approximation of equality on a number between 0 and 1, where 0 corresponds with perfect equality (everyone has the same income) and 1 corresponds with perfect inequality (one person has all the income and everyone else has zero income). South Africa is currently one of the world's most unequal societies, with an estimated pretax Gini coefficient of between 0.63 and 0.7 (World Bank, 2013). In simple terms, the human development index shows that approximately 20% of the world's population owns approximately 80% of the world's wealth. Mandela (2005), in a public address in London on the war on poverty, stated that "massive poverty and obscene inequality are such terrible scourges of our times—times in which the world boasts breathtaking advances in science, technology, industry and wealth accumulation—that they have to rank alongside slavery and apartheid as social evils." The reduction of poverty and inequality clearly warrants overt attention by all governments and professional organizations, including occupational therapy, irrespective of where they practice.

The task of closing the inequality gap is a function of the state and a co-responsibility of citizens. Working toward equality is almost always better for everyone, rich and poor alike (Wilkinson & Pickett, 2010). Promoting equality has two sides. One side is concerned with the equitable expansion of human capabilities that enable people to act. The other side is concerned with mediating how people act—responsibly or not—to advance their personal well-being and development while contributing to the development of society in general. A philosophical and theoretical foundation exists for occupational therapists to contribute to human development from an occupational perspective, by engaging in policy design and decision making with a broad group of governmental and nongovernmental actors, such as those involved with education, nutrition, agriculture, urban planning, disaster risk, and citizen rights. Occupational science scholarship has theorized constructs such as occupational apartheid (Pollard et al., 2008), occupational consciousness (Ramugondo, 2012), and occupational justice (Wilcock & Townsend, 2009) that make it possible to study and explain the occupational dimensions of human development and equality.

Organizational Development

Organization is the human capacity to harness available information, knowledge, resources, technology, infrastructure, and human skills to embrace new opportunities and deal with the challenges and hurdles that block progress (Davids et al., 2009; McLean, 2005). Development is advanced through improvements in the human capacity for organization. A primary, although not exclusive, goal of organizational development is to improve effectiveness in managing change in human organizations. Indicators of organizational development may include effective communication, a sound group morale, administrative efficiency, and productivity. Outcomes such as these equip the organization for performing its core functions and reaching its goals and are usually achieved through adult education and action research programs that are codesigned and guided by a change agent or team.

Organizations come in many forms, from family to workplaces, charitable and religious organizations, government agencies, sports teams, social clubs, labor unions, and so on. These organizations form the social structures within and through which human development may be achieved; they should ideally be understood using local worldviews and indigenous knowledge systems as points of departure (e.g., Broodryk, 2005; Nabudere, 2011). The major focus of organizational development is the total system and its interdependent parts, such as work groups, task teams, committees, departments, or individuals. Occupational therapists are trained to perform service-related managerial tasks and organizational maintenance functions. They are able to draw on these competencies to design in-service training for human resources, such as community health workers; facilitate the organizational efficiency of community-led action groups; and assist grassroots organizations with project design, implementation, and monitoring.

Community Development

Community development is a discipline in itself, with a body of theory, standards of practice, and professional associations. It involves "the facilitation of growing awareness and consciousness such that people are able to take control of their own lives and circumstances, and exert responsibility and purpose with respect to their future" (Kaplan, 1999, p. 12). Community development creates the conditions for community well-being (economic, social, environmental, and cultural) through collective empowerment emerging from reliance on a community's initiative and active participation (Swanepoel & de Beer, 2011). Discussing the foundations of community development from a social justice perspective, Ife (2002, p. 61) suggested that empowerment increases the power of structurally disadvantaged groups over personal choices, chances, needs definition, ideas, institutions, resources, economic activity, and reproduction. This is achieved through policy and planning, social and political action, and education. Structurally disadvantaged groups may be identified by class (women), race/ethnicity (indigenous people, minorities), age (children, the elderly), ability (people with disabilities), sexual orientation (LGBT communities), and location (slum dwellers, people living in geographically isolated areas or on garbage dumps).

Communities are groups of people of any size who share a physical and geographic location, common cultural heritage, language and beliefs, or shared interests. Individuals usually belong to more than one community at the same time, based on different relationships, needs, and goals. For example, an individual can be part of a neighborhood, a religious community, and a sporting community. To speak of "the community" presumes that it exists as a single, uniform, and undifferentiated unit with anthropomorphic characteristics that can be steered, influenced, and empowered. This is not the case. Community is the product of the complex interactions between human beings. It is a living entity but not an actor in its own right; at most, it is the context within which humans act (Theron, 2008). Relationships and development processes are therefore messy, complicated, contested, and invisible (Kaplan, 2002). Some communities are inchoate and unready or incapable of making a sustainable contribution to their collective development, some lack interest in coalescing efforts to change their circumstances, and others may feel too hopeless and marginalized to try. In some settings, the elite dominate, are corrupt, and even threaten those who seek to change the status quo. It cannot be assumed that a community has the capacity or interest to effect change, that its members are ready to donate their energy and time for the benefit of the community, or that they are democratic in their collective decision making (Theron, 2008). Effective community development balances competing interests among subgroups, promotes responsible execution of negotiated goals, and fosters the capacity of people to address their shared concerns. Against this backdrop, community development is a long, slow, fluid, multilayered, volatile but ultimately rewarding process of change that is fraught with multiple personal, structural, and sociopolitical challenges. A growing body of social occupational therapy literature supports the profession's role in community development (Lauckner, Krupa, & Paterson, 2011; Lauckner, Pentland, & Paterson, 2007).

Social Development

Social development addresses welfare issues such as social and food security, housing, law enforcement, roads and transport, and disaster risk management. It targets the structural elements that are necessary for the development of an inclusive, cohesive, and accountable society—one in which people treat each other (more) fairly in their daily lives, whether in the family, workplace, or public office (Davis, 2004). Social development seeks to advance democracy, social justice, equity, and human rights through efficient and effective local governance. It puts people at the center of development by supporting the capacity for self-determination of formal and informal social structures and institutions, including families, civic associations, and local government bodies. Box 12-3 reviews some indices of social development (Institute for Social Studies, n.d.), all of which have an occupational dimension.

The egalitarian assumptions of social development must be critiqued at this point. Bond (2007) mapped five international ideological currents that influence how social justice is understood, the distribution of wealth and poverty may be conceptualized, and development targeted. Ideological currents range from socialism and anarchism on the left, through capitalism, social democracy, and neoliberalism in the center left and right, to neoconservativism on the right. Global justice movements, supporting socialism in the fight against poverty and inequality, argue for deglobalization of capital (not people), antiracism, women's liberation, decommodified state services, and radical participatory democracy. Third world nationalism, supporting national capitalism, argues for fairer global integration, expanded market access, reformed global governance, third world unity, and anti-imperialism. The Post Washington consensus movement, supporting social democracy, opposes US unilateralism and militarism and advocates for sustainable development via United Nations and similar global state-building frameworks. The Washington Consensus lobby, supporting neoliberalism, argues for the inclusion of emerging markets under the umbrella of a US-led empire. The main agenda of neoconservatists is the defense of particular right-wing ideologies, including religious extremism, patriarchy, unilateral petro-military imperialism, and globalization of people via racism and xenophobia. It is beyond the scope of this chapter to review these ideological currents, the philosophical tenets on which they are based and their role in creating, perpetuating, or alleviating poverty. Suffice to acknowledge that the conceptual and theoretical terrain of social development is complex and contested among the proponents of different political positions. The gestalt (configuration, pattern, form) of occupational therapy and its contributions to social development are determined by the ideological and political context within which the profession is located (Frank & Zemke, 2009). It cannot be assumed that a focus on occupational justice as a rationale for the profession's contribution to social development is in fact feasible or even considered desirable in some contexts. Practitioners may not have the sociopolitical freedoms necessary to promote occupational therapy practices that advance social justice. Care therefore needs to be taken in discerning the potential for theoretical imperialism in occupational therapy social development discourse (Whalley Hammel, 2010).

Box 12-3. Indices of Social Development

- **Civic activism:** extent of citizen involvement in public policies and decisions. For example, occupations of citizenship may be linked to the activities of civic associations addressing the social concerns of minority groups through lobbying the media and staging petitions.

- **Clubs and associations:** extent to which people are part of social networks and potentially supported by community ties. Examples of occupations may include engagement in informal saving clubs, women's groups, religious organizations, sports clubs, and special interest groups, or time spent socializing in and working for voluntary associations.

- **Intergroup cohesion:** extent of cooperation and respect between groups in a society. The potential for conflict exists where social cooperation breaks down due to ideological differences (e.g., ethnicity and religion) or when access to resources becomes constrained (e.g., through land and job distribution among urban citizens and rural migrants) or between local citizens, foreign nationals, and refugees. Intergroup conflict finds expression in occupations associated with looting, public riots, and gang violence.

- **Interpersonal safety and trust:** level of trust and confidence between people who may or may not know each other personally. This index is concerned with the likelihood, rates, and types of criminal activities and interpersonal violence that occur in different pockets of society. Forms of trust violation include white- and blue-collar crime; gender-based, domestic, and sexual violence; child and other forms of abuse; racial intolerance; and xenophobia. Violations of interpersonal safety have a negative impact on the occupational human, whether as victim or perpetrator, affecting his or her developmental structure, mental and physical health and well-being, occupational performance, and patterns of occupational engagement.

- **Gender inequality and inclusion of minorities:** monitors discrimination against and exploitation of women in the labor market, education, health care, and home. The indices of social development also monitor equality in other intersectional dimensions of human identity, such as age, race, class, sexual orientation, and ability/disability (Duncan & Creek, 2014). The inequality, poverty, and exploitation of marginalized people are a result, primarily, of unequal economic and power relations rather than social exclusion. Marginalized people are, in fact, socially included but on adverse terms, and adverse incorporation places constraints on people's occupational choices and opportunities. Indeed, total exclusion on any dimension is rare, and so adverse incorporation might be a preferable term to social exclusion for some situations where inequality exists (Hickey & du Toit, 2007).

Adapted from the Institute for Social Studies. (n.d.). *Indices for social development*. International Institute for Social Studies in the Hague, Erasmus University, Rotterdam, Netherlands. Available online: http://www.ind-socdev.org/home.html

Rural Development

Rural development targets spatial inequality. It is a strategy for enabling people in remote geographic areas to gain for themselves and their children more of what they want and need to live meaningful lives (Chambers, 2005; Kanbur & Venables, 2005). Approximately three quarters of the world's poorest people live in rural areas, including small-scale farmers, tenants, and the landless. Inclusive development argues for careful attention to be paid to the needs of women, children, and people with disabilities in rural areas (Chervin & Geiser, 2012). The primary aim of rural development is the improvement of sustainable livelihoods through investment in basic infrastructure and social services, skills training, and ensuring the safety and security of the rural population.

Seasonal population influxes to cities in developing countries are often made up of rural people in search of work, education, health care, and social security. Most of the poorest among them are forced to live in urban slums, exposed to health-compromising living conditions. Seeking to secure a future for themselves and their households, they send financial remittances and other assets to their homesteads in rural areas. Migration to cities leads to loss of labor in agrarian communities, where women, children, and the elderly tend to remain carrying the brunt of working the land to secure a livelihood (Bishop-Sanbrook, 2014). The oscillation of people between their urban and rural households creates a poverty trap, a spiraling mechanism that forces people to remain poor (Bowles, Durlauf, & Hoff, 2006; Moore, Grant, Hulme, & Shepherd, 2008). Rural development is therefore an important poverty reduction strategy. Enhancing living standards, income generation opportunities, and access to land, education, and basic health care, including rehabilitation, in rural areas can curtail depopulation and the erosion of human and other forms of capital (Chambers, 2005).

Occupational therapists are a scarce human resource. The reach of occupational therapy into rural communities hinges, among other factors, on a country's health, rehabilitation, and disability service models and on the profession's commitment to addressing rurality as a social determinant of health and well-being. *Rurality* refers to the structure and quality of life of people living in sparsely settled and underdeveloped places that are significant distances away from resourced urban centers. Bishop-Sanbrook, writing about women's time poverty in sub-Saharan Africa, calls for

> more visibility in policy dialogue to promote public infrastructure investments that reduce rural workloads. We need to make greater use of proven methodologies that are available to create a supportive environment for positive behaviour change and equitable workload balance, such as community conversations, community listeners' clubs and household methodologies. (2014, p. 1)

Occupational therapists, by virtue of their skills in occupational performance-enhancing methods, are equipped to address time and other forms of poverty that erode the quality of life of persons with disabilities in rural areas (Watson & Duncan, 2010).

LEVELS OF DEVELOPMENT AND MODES OF THINKING

This section outlines the essential features of macro- and microdevelopment and associated modes of thinking. Macrodevelopment involves transnational, national, and regional economic and political strategizing to secure a country or region's future. Microdevelopment is local, people-centered, and concerned with intrapersonal and interpersonal processes of social change that lead to some form of growth in humans and their social institutions.

Macrodevelopment

Macrodevelopment is a prerequisite for all forms of development because it links the economic and political systems of a country—the production, distribution, and regulation of commodities—to human lives. Macrodevelopment is a precursor of socioeconomic progress which, in turn, determines the health, well-being, and potential of a country's people to thrive. The increase in material welfare (e.g., having access to the resources needed for a decent life, such as food, clothing, shelter, education) and infrastructure (e.g., having access to transport, electricity, markets) brought about through macrodevelopment opens up opportunities for microdevelopment, through which people can become more than they are.

Although occupational therapy is not a role-player in macrodevelopment, the profession is directly affected by it in two ways: first, in terms of the recognition given to the profession by a government as an essential health service provider and, second, in terms of the influence that macrodevelopment has on the various contexts in which the profession is practiced. Occupational therapy has an established record as an essential health service profession in developed countries. Supported by the WFOT, as well as by regional and national occupational therapy associations, the profession is gaining recognition in developing and transitioning countries for its contribution to national health (e.g., the Occupational Therapy Africa Regional Group). It could be argued that the visibility and utility of the profession may be enhanced by championing its contribution to nation building in the different facets of development discussed in the previous section. A country's level of macrodevelopment creates the backdrop to the resources, infrastructure, and opportunities available to its citizens. As such, it plays a significant role in human occupation. Development-orientated occupational therapists use macromode thinking to inform their understanding of the complex dynamics operating in a society that influence people's occupations, health, and well-being. Two meta-theoretical streams that inform macromode thinking are considered here: modernization theory and dependency theory.

Macromode Thinking

Modernization theory has its roots in structuralist functionalist social theory. Structuralism theorizes the relationships between the various social institutions and systems that make up a particular society (Cotterrell, 2010). Functionalism addresses society as a whole in terms of the function of its constituent elements, such as norms, customs, traditions, and institutions (Parsons, 1975). A combination of structuralism and functionalism offers contemporary social theorists the tools for thinking about the social transitions associated with an increasingly globalized and technologically sophisticated world. Modernization theory attempts to explain how a society becomes progressively more modernized and developed through interdependent networking between its various institutions (Joshi, 2005). Social institutions (e.g., government, law, social care, education, religion, and sports) and systems (e.g., clans and family units) carry out collective activities to ensure that the needs of society (such as survival, cohesion, and progress) are fulfilled. Modernization theory insists that the third world is underdeveloped and remains in such a state because of the existence of counterproductive traditions and social practices, as well as a historical failure to industrialize and modernize with technology (Davids et al., 2009).

Dependency theory is opposed to the assessments and solutions offered by modernization theory (Joshi, 2005). It argues that development is a form of imperialism and exploitation that deliberately creates donor dependency. Dependency theory offers resistance to the subversive intentions of economic and knowledge colonization (e.g., wealthy nations actively perpetuate a state of dependence by the manipulation of banking and financial systems, media control, politics, education, culture, and sport) (Joshi, 2005). In exchange for development donor funding, poor nations provide for developed nations the markets, natural resources, cheap labor, and destinations for obsolete technology without which the latter could not have the standard of living they enjoy. In summary, macromode thinking makes use of grand social theories, including the two examples briefly introduced here. These and other macrodevelopment theories are of relevance to occupational therapists who want to understand the socioeconomic contexts that shape people's occupational opportunities, choices, and engagement at individual, group, and collective levels.

Microdevelopment

Contemporary development experts acknowledge that the deeper microdimensions of development are subtle, often invisible and complex (Kaplan, 2002). Selected aspects of microdevelopment are reviewed here to illustrate the range of factors that occupational therapists as change agents have to think about in terms of principles, methods, and evaluation.

Microdevelopment: Principles

The most commonly identified microdevelopment principle is participation (Davids et al., 2009, p. 161). Participation is made possible through equity, sustainability, empowerment, freedom, capacity, and self-esteem. These principles are briefly summarized in Box 12-4.

An understanding of the structural constraints of the society within which people live, and the sociocultural frameworks that shape their life-worlds, is needed to inform the developmental direction that people wish to pursue. Finding appropriate development paths in collaboration with a specific group of people hinges on an intimate knowledge of their history, culture, and current structural and social concerns. This suggests that occupational therapists should ideally be cultural insiders or, if this is not possible, should make concerted efforts to acquire social and anthropological understanding of the contexts in which they work. More important, individuals matter. Microdevelopment primarily involves going the extra mile to build and maintain trustworthy and inclusive relationships.

Microdevelopment: Methodologies

Microdevelopment is achieved through social research methodologies such as participatory learning and action research, participatory rural appraisal, and participatory action research. These methodologies are considered in the occupational therapy literature (e.g., Letts, 2003; Townsend, Cockburn, Letts, Thibeault, & Trentham, 2007) and addressed in the social research and development literature (e.g., Bless, Higson-Smith, & Kagee, 2006; Chambers, 2005; Chevalier & Buckles, 2013a, 2013b; Davids et al., 2009; Kaplan, 1999, 2002; Theron, 2008). Each of these participatory research methodologies is a combination of investigation and social change. It investigates the forms of and ways that knowledge is produced by being clear about who the knowledge is for. Participatory research works prefiguratively (i.e., it anticipates a better society in the very process of struggling for it). The broader political patterns of power and resistance operating in a particular social space are uncovered, revealed, and described while they are being enacted through the participatory research process. The task of the researcher as change agent or the change agent as researcher is not to measure microdevelopment but to ignite and understand it in partnership with development beneficiaries. Theron and Wetmore (2008, p. 203) pointed out that this form of research has "a cardinal role to play in enabling communities to assess their own needs and resources, to assess and share ideas, or to design and/or develop particular feasible development intervention."

Microdevelopment: Methods

Participatory data gathering and change-precipitating methods include, among others, arts-based inquiry (culturally appropriate storytelling, drama, art, games, photographs as codes for group work discussion), mapping, rapid rural appraisals, and surveys. They allow data (information) to surface while simultaneously facilitating social learning through three dynamic, iterative processes or research stages: analysis, action, and reflection. These processes unfold in communal spaces through occupation, defined here as the different activities, tasks, and roles that people assume when engaging with a participatory research method and process. Participatory research as occupation facilitates change over time by bringing people together and setting them firmly in their meaning-giving context during research events (Cockburn & Trentham, 2002).

To facilitate something is to make it easier. Inclusive development facilitation is therefore a process through which a change agent makes it easier for people to discover their strengths, acquire competencies for self-reliance, and develop dormant capabilities. It involves "creating something new that is rooted but latent in the ecology of ideas with agent and community as co-creators" (Theron, 2008, p. x). It may be argued that some participatory research methods can be considered as collective occupations of citizenship (Ramugondo & Kronenberg, 2015). Citizenship refers to the qualities that a person is expected to have as a responsible member of a community. Community-orientated microdevelopment methods provide the means through which the qualities of responsible civic engagement (knowledge, skills, and attitudes) can evolve.

BOX 12-4. MICRODEVELOPMENT PRINCIPLES

- **Participation:** "participation is an essential part of human growth i.e. the development of self-confidence, pride, initiative, responsibility, and cooperation. Without development *within* [italics added] people themselves, all efforts to alleviate their poverty will be immensely more difficult, if not impossible. This process, whereby people take charge of their own lives and solve their own problems, is the essence of development" (Burkey, 1993, p. 56). Participation facilitates the will to create a meaningful life. In development, meaning refers to people's experience of subjective reality within their life-worlds. Life-world refers to the micro-social reality between individuals; the world of shared, ongoing experience from which they constitute objects and abstract ideas. The personal and social growth that flows from participation in a development project does not necessarily imply improvement in material welfare. It does, however, imply the potential for shifts in the way people feel about themselves and what they believe they are capable of achieving through their own efforts. The problem is that although people may desire to take charge of their lives, they are prevented from doing so by their positioning in society. For example, in the disability literature, the concept of participation highlights the structural and systemic barriers people with disabilities encounter in accessing their opportunities for social inclusion (WHO, 2001). In occupational therapy literature, participation is theorized as occupational engagement (e.g., Stav, Hallenen, Lane, & Arbesman, 2012).

- **Equity:** the equity principle ensures that historical and current disparities in resources and access to opportunities are redressed. Equity features in recent occupational therapy literature (e.g., Belagamage & Jull, 2012).

- **Freedom:** the freedom from servitude releases people's ability to make choices that will influence or determine their future. Occupational therapists have an established and expanding body of literature that addresses social justice (Whalley Hammell & Iwama, 2012; Whiteford & Townsend, 2011).

- **Capacity:** capacity is the ability to produce something. Development paradoxically and simultaneously requires and develops a fundamental set of abilities. Capacity building is creating the building blocks required to produce change. Community practice in occupational therapy considers the need for capacity building through occupation (Meyers, 2010).

- **Self-esteem:** the ability to experience a sense of worth, dignity, and respect for self enables people to hold the same attitude toward others. Occupational therapists are trained to assess the psychological and psychodynamic factors that influence people's self-esteem (Bryant, Fieldhouse, & Bannigan, 2014).

- **Sustainability:** meeting the needs of the present without compromising the ability of future generations to meet their own needs (Sachs, 2012; United Nations Development Programme, 2013, 2014).

- **Empowerment:** the process by which disadvantaged people work together to take control of the factors that determine their development, such as education, health care services, livelihoods, governance, and safety. By definition, one cannot empower someone else: empowerment is something that people do for themselves. However, health workers as development facilitators can sometimes help open the way for people to empower themselves. De Sardan (2005, p. 168) saw empowerment as "knowledge transfer in both directions," a mutually beneficial social learning process and task shifting partnership in which the change agent acts as a mediator of different types of knowledge systems. Chambers's (2005, pp. 191-192) famous development injunctions are a helpful guide for empowerment: "Ask them, Be kind to people, Do not rush, Embrace error, Hand over the stick, Have fun."

Adapted from Davids, I., Theron, F., & Maphunye, K. J. (2009). *Participatory development in South Africa. A development management perspective.* Pretoria, South Africa: van Schaik.

Box 12-5. Evaluating Development

Max-Neef (1991), in his seminal book on human-scale development (HSD), pointed out that people are not simply human *havings* or human *doings*, they have to be valued as *interacting* human *beings*. He argued that the evaluation of development (i.e., describing the economic and social outcomes of development projects and programs) should not be reduced to numerical indices. To objectify and measure shifts in human needs and assets for the purposes of documenting developmental progress is to reduce humanity to an abstract concept, sanitized of the spiritual and ethical complexities that give meaning to being human. Max-Neef proposed that HSD could be plotted on a matrix, by participating stakeholders, throughout the development engagement. The Y-axis of the HSD matrix represents human needs according to nine axiological categories: subsistence, protection, affection, understanding, participation, idleness, creation, identity, and freedom. The X-axis of the HSD matrix represents human needs according to four existential categories: being, having, doing, and interacting. The HSD matrix can be used as a tool for identifying and monitoring qualitative and quantitative indicators of human well-being and social change (Cruz, Stahel, & Max-Neef, 2009).

Microdevelopment: Evaluation

Development unfolds tacitly in the midst of a fragmented, ever-changing reality (Kaplan, 2002). The meaning-giving processes and interactions that lead to substantive change, stability, or even stagnation and regression, emerge at different times and in different places between parts of the whole (individual, organization, community, society). It is therefore methodologically impossible to determine causal relationships among mutually interacting variables. No linear relationship can be established between the impact of a change agent's influence and the resulting response from or benefit to individuals or community groups who are the beneficiaries of microdevelopment. While some forms of structural change can be measured (e.g., number of schools built, roads repaired, jobs created, or patients treated), the evaluation of microdevelopment requires qualitatively descriptive shifts in meeting people's fundamental human needs. Human-scale development (Max-Neef, 1991) provides one such evaluative framework. Box 12-5 reviews the essential features of human scale development, indicating its close alignment with the values of occupational therapy (WFOT, 2009).

How do occupational therapists measure or evaluate the impact of their development-orientated practice? How may the personal growth of individuals and groups through occupational engagement be evaluated? In what ways can evidence for social change through occupational justice be monitored? These are challenging questions because the evaluation of microdevelopment requires a nonclinical approach. Occupational therapists in clinical practice settings are expected to record and evaluate their treatment sessions. Making use of standardized and nonstandardized tools, they have to provide measured evidence that their interventions have made a difference, added value, or resulted in functional improvement. Evaluation of microdevelopment is the joint monitoring and evaluation responsibility of all stakeholders rather than solely the responsibility of the occupational therapist. It entails oral and written documentation of democratically identified objectives and indicators of change over a designated time period and the submission of outcomes for external auditing. Practice-based evidence of individual and social change can be captured in vignettes, memorandums, and reports of events, using indicators that hold meaning for the people concerned, for example, success stories of children with disabilities enrolled in a local crèche or thriving disabled women entrepreneurs.

Micromode Thinking

The focus of micromode, people-centered development thinking is threefold: first, to understand the needs and meaning-giving contexts of development beneficiaries; second, to engage the personal and social capital that they possess; and third, to understand and manage the complexities of the intersecting participatory spaces that arise among beneficiaries as members of a particular community and between beneficiaries and change agents/service providers (Coetzee, 2001). The reasoning task of the development practitioner is to create synergies between his or her professionally informed thinking (e.g., clinical and professional reasoning in the case of the occupational therapist) and the various structures of thinking in a community, social system, or organization. The change agent's reasoning should identify the latent potential in the individual, community, social system, or organization and, in the process of interacting with the people concerned, link with their ways of thinking so that there is increasing emphasis on their capacity for self-determination (Theron, 2008). However, acquiring and exercising agency and self-reliance are easier said than done. Thinking is deeply personal and shaped by experience. It may reveal internalized oppression, compliance with entrenched patriarchal attitudes, or alignment with hegemonic practices (e.g., the dominance of Whiteness and privilege), all of which make it difficult for people to find their voice or, alternatively, to refrain from imposing power. In the next section, I consider three forms of reasoning that may assist the change agent to understand and deal with the complexities of microdevelopment practice: sociological imagination, public reasoning, and axiological reasoning.

FORMS OF DEVELOPMENT REASONING

Sociological imagination serves as a resource for the change agent, a tool for clarifying the rationale for microdevelopment in a particular context at a particular time. Public reasoning serves as a resource for development beneficiaries, a tool for collective thinking that may or may not lead to gradual liberation of individual and collective agency. Axiological reasoning guides the participatory spaces between change agents and development beneficiaries. It is a resource for ensuring mutual accountability during the messy and slow process of microdevelopment, albeit at individual, group, or community levels.

Sociological Imagination

C. Wright Mills, a pioneer sociologist during the Cold War era in the United States, wrote a seminal introductory text for sociology in 1959 on sociological imagination. He described sociological imagination as an intellectual quality, the understanding and acquisition of which forms the basis for social change. It is a way of thinking that makes links between the taken-for-granted lived experiences of individuals (the particular) and the social forces that shape these experiences (the universal). Sociological imagination as a form of reasoning enables its user to understand the impact of the larger historical scene on the inner life of individuals and the external lives that they are able to pursue in different social strata or classes. It guides the user to take account of how individuals in the "welter of their daily experience become falsely conscious of their social positions" (Mills, 1959, p. 9). Sociological imagination traces the complex ways through which individuals and groups develop over time a belief that they belong to a particular social stratification or class. The belief systems that people hold about their social class may be mirrored in their cultural practices and the patterns of consumption that they pursue. They come to believe that life is what it is because it has always been that way, and then they act accordingly.

Mills described how society shapes individuals and how individuals contribute to shaping society. Every society, with its structures, values, and history, affects the individuals who live in it in specific ways, including their occupational choices and opportunities. An essential tool of sociological imagination is to differentiate between personal troubles of milieu and public issues of social structure. A trouble is a private matter; it is concerned with the self and those areas of social life of which the person is directly aware. An issue is a public matter that exists in a particular social structure at a particular historical moment. Some individual troubles are precipitated or exacerbated by social issues. The larger structure of the social and historical life of society is formed by the ways in which different issues and various milieus overlap and interpenetrate (Mills, 1959, p. 8). For example, becoming unemployed or disabled is more than an individual or personal experience; it is also something collective, or common to a class. When an ordinary man becomes unemployed, it is seen as his trouble or problem, but when it involves thousands of people, it becomes a public issue or concern. In short, the framework of society formulates the psychologies and behaviors of people both individually and collectively. Sociological imagination illuminates this framework by being "the most fruitful form of . . . self-consciousness" (Mills, 1959, p. 12).

Mills argued that although many social scientists rightly condemn the state of affairs within the capitalist context (e.g., class stratification), they are unable to break with the rhetoric of domination and engage in real social change. When individuals begin to understand the intersections between biography and history, they are able to grasp what is going on in their world and understand what is happening within them. Sociological imagination leads them to "adequate summations, cohesive assessments and comprehensive orientations" of the dialogical (mutually reinforcing) relationship between personal troubles and public issues. "By such means the personal uneasiness of individuals is focused upon explicit troubles and the indifference of publics is transformed into involvement with public issues" (Mills, 1959, p. 12). Sociological imagination plays a role in people-centered development, first as a way of helping change agents and beneficiaries think about themselves in relation to society and, second, as a means of mobilizing structural change. Box 12-6 provides examples of triggers for using sociological imagination as a form of development reasoning.

In summary, sociological imagination reveals the dynamic relationship among the nature, needs, and aspirations of individuals; the milieus that shape their personal (and occupational) troubles; and the collective public issues prevailing in the social (and occupational) structures within which their daily lives are situated. Sociological imagination provides insights into the social determinants of individual and collective occupational engagement. It is relevant to development-orientated occupational therapy because it offers a way of thinking about the broader contextual forces that influence human occupation in personal and communal environments. Ramugondo (2012) proposed that social change can be effected if people become occupationally conscious, entailing an ongoing awareness of the dynamics of hegemony, an appreciation of the role of personal and collective occupations of daily life in perpetuating hegemonic practices, and an appraisal of resultant consequences for individual and collective well-being. A combination of sociological imagination and occupational consciousness can bolster the reasoning skills of development-orientated occupational therapists.

Public Reasoning

Public reasoning is a way of thinking out what appropriate justice would entail for people situated in less than fully just social circumstances. In social and political forums where issues of collective concern are debated and actions decided, public reasoning forms the basis of group thinking. People and their actions change when they reason together and when they are helped, through skilled group conductors, to talk about, analyze, and critique their thinking and actions (Rohr, 2011). Amartya Sen (2009, p. 18), writing about the idea of justice, described reason as the "ultimate arbitrator of ethical beliefs." He described public reason as any system that allows

---

BOX 12-6. TRIGGERS FOR SOCIOLOGICAL IMAGINATION

Mills (1959, p. 15) suggested that social scientists ask three basic questions to foster socio-logical imagination:

1. **What is the structure of this society as a whole?** Think about its essential components, how they are related to each other, and what the meaning of any particular feature is for its continuance and change.

2. **Where does this society stand in human history?** Think about the mechanisms through which it is changing, the historical period within which it moves, its place within and meaning for the development of humanity as a whole.

3. **What varieties of men and women prevail now in this society and period?** Think about the ways they are coming to prevail; the ways they are selected, formed, liberated, repressed, blunted, or made sensitive; the kinds of human nature that are revealed in the conduct and character observed in this society at this period; and the meaning for human nature of each feature of society being imagined.

From an occupational consciousness perspective, it could be asked how the structure, history, and varieties of people in this society create or obstruct their opportunities to engage in occupations of choice. Galvaan (2012) identified occupational choice as involv-ing the application of choice to participation in occupations, manifesting as both a process where the choice is made and as an outcome of a decision to participate; this occurs implic-itly and explicitly when agency is applied to occupational engagement.

---

people to talk without getting punished by someone. If democracy is a subideal of social justice, then public reason and freedom of speech are important because they contribute to justice and, hence, to democracy (Sen, 2009). However, public reason is not necessarily rational or inclusive. It does not mean that everyone in a community or group is committed to the idea of social justice or that they have an equal and fair chance to participate in deliberations about desired social change. Rawls (1997) suggested that public reasoning, in the context of democracy, occurs at multiple levels in society through consultative hierarchies that allow people to express their views, even though there may be no institutional mechanisms (egalitarian or otherwise) for registering them. Consultative hierarchies are open forums where public reasoning and social learning occur. They are social structures that represent different levels of authority in public and communal affairs, ranging from parliamentary and other governance structures, such as traditional leader forums, to local street committees, health clinic committees, parent–teacher associations, and informal women's groups. The change agent and stakeholders have to make connections between the public reasoning occurring in different public spaces. Occupational therapists as change agents must therefore be informed about and, where possible, actively participate in a wide range of public dialogue spaces. Box 12-7 briefly explains how structural coupling may make these connections possible.

Axiological Reasoning

Axiological (values-based) reasoning considers the intrinsic (personal), extrinsic (communal/societal), procedural (methodological), and regulatory (systemic) values by which people live and according to which change agents may precipitate microdevelopment. It endeavors to create alignment between these four sets of values during participatory events, especially when relationships flounder or projects derail. Axiological reasoning enables change agents to make the ethical dimension of their work explicit to themselves and to those they work with. It requires reflexive

---

BOX 12-7. STRUCTURAL COUPLING: MAKING SENSE OF PUBLIC REASONING

The term *structural coupling* denotes the structure determined and structure determining engagement of a given system or unity (e.g., an individual, a group, a project, a service) with its environment or with another system or unity (Maturana & Varela, 1987). It is a process through which structurally determined transformations in two or more systemic unities induce for each a trajectory of reciprocally triggered change. Maturana and Varela (1987, p. 75) proposed that "recurrent engagement and interaction leads to the structural congruence between two or more systems." Structural coupling has connotations of reciprocal influence, coordination and co-evolution among structures, systems, and unities within a given environment. At a practical level this means that public reasoning (e.g., disabled women's rights and time poverty) that is structured in one forum will resonate with structured public reasoning in another forum (e.g., time burden of mothers of children with disabilities). The task of development reasoning is to discern the congruencies and disjunctions between public reasoning taking place within and between different forums. The change agent identifies helpful linkages between different structures (e.g., services across public sectors in a particular district) and finds ways to enable or support recurrent interforum engagement. During structural coupling, each participating system is, with respect to the other(s), a source (and a target) of perturbations (conflict, disruption, agitation) or compatibility (harmony, good match). The participating systems reciprocally serve as sources of perturbations or compatibility for each other and, in so doing, precipitate actions that gradually contribute to desired social change.

---

engagement with critical incidents and a willingness to give and receive feedback when assumptions and actions contradict or potentially dehumanize, dominate, or violate people's beliefs, cultural practices, and value systems (Chan, 2014).

The processes of microdevelopment can be difficult and discomforting for everyone concerned. Participatory action approaches are used precisely because they allow different perspectives and interests to surface: It is better to focus on points of difference than to pretend they can be smoothed over. Processing difference can be emotionally taxing and therefore requires regular time-out for self-nurturing and reflection. Theron (2008) suggested that

> before change agents can change others they have to change themselves and their consciousness. They have to constantly try to shed their own contradictions, weaknesses, prejudices . . . it is essential to have regular sessions of criticism and self-criticism. Only through such sessions can a genuine understanding of each other and of the work one is doing emerge. (p. 20)

Axiological reasoning can be used as a values-based cognitive tool to guide the development work that unfolds in the participatory spaces between change agent and beneficiaries. Boxes 12-8 through 12-11 summarize how to do axiological reasoning by considering each of the four value domains: intrinsic, extrinsic, procedural, and regulatory.

Box 12-8. Axiological Reasoning and Intrinsic Values

Chambers (2005) identified the following five mutually reinforcing impediments to the development process, all of which are connected to the power and dominance of intrinsic (personal) values and attitudes of the people involved.

1. **Conditioning:** We jealously defend our own thinking and attach value to our training and/or worldview, and we expect people to respect this. If we do not reflect on what we know and on how we think and view the world, it becomes easy to colonize (transplant our knowledge and understanding onto) the lives and intentions of others. Axiological reasoning encourages respect for and integration of different regimes of thinking, doing, and constructing knowledge.

2. **Dominance:** Dominance (use of authority and power) is conveyed through speech, behavior, accessories, and associates.

   - *Speech:* becoming culturally literate, learning the local language, and using easily understood words goes a long way toward shifting power imbalances.

   - *Behavior:* dominance can be conveyed through body language (e.g., where one stands and sits, wagging a finger, looking at a watch, or clapping hands to speed up proceedings). A willingness to listen, keep quiet, and let people do things for themselves is indicated.

   - *Accessories:* ways of dressing, carrying a briefcase, using tape recorders, and even arriving in a car can be symbolic expressions of dominance. The impression of superiority can be counteracted by attending community events, visiting homes, and contributing labor to a communal project.

   - *Associates:* initial contact for community entry and decision making is usually made via the local elite. Dominance is perpetuated if the association with the community stays at that level. Change agents demonstrate the values of humility and inclusivity by creating both vertical and horizontal social relationships.

3. **Isolation:** Development projects may run in isolated areas away from professional accountability and support structures. Change agents may work long hours with limited resources, travel far distances, and struggle to communicate due to language and cultural differences. Isolation may require the development practitioner to dig deep, ethically and emotionally, to sustain personal well-being and professional standards. Seeking regular supervision, debriefing, and in-service training will go some way toward alleviating a sense of isolation.

4. **Denial:** Change agents may react to difficulties by discrediting the motives of others and by becoming intolerant of different opinions and insensitive to local values and customs. Values clarification can help to reduce projections, denial, and rejection.

5. **Blaming:** When a development project fails or derails, the most common defense is to blame the beneficiaries. Blame shifting shuts down self-criticism and becomes part of the disciplinary apparatus through which change agents try to control the people with whom they work. It is necessary to hold the process lightly, trust the people, and not step into rescue or fix-it mode. People will carry on helping themselves long after the change agent has left.

Box 12-9. Axiological Reasoning and Extrinsic Values

Change agents may be outsiders who do not understand the extrinsic (communal, cultural) values of development beneficiaries. They are unlikely to appreciate or understand the meanings and purposes that people attribute to life events when they do not share the same history, socialization, or language. There is always a danger of the change agent essentializing people's experiences and worldviews (i.e., reducing them to uniform, unchanging, and inescapable ways of being in the world). Sillitoe, Dixon, and Barr (2005, pp. 12-18) proposed that understanding indigenous knowledge systems, including traditional beliefs, values, and practices, has mutually reinforcing benefits for change agents and development beneficiaries.

The change agent who respects indigenous knowledge systems does the following:
- Uses ethnographic immersion to gain some appreciation of local worldviews and cultural practices
- Uses informed diplomacy to facilitate uptake of externally introduced information
- Refrains from judgment and interpretation and is willing to acknowledge mistakes

Box 12-10. Axiological Reasoning and Procedural Values

Theron (2008, pp. 7-9) suggested the following five values to guide change agents in thinking about the procedures they follow and the methods they use in microdevelopment.

1. **People can be more than they are:** Social change is possible because people have the potential and ability to create a better life for themselves.

2. **Meaning:** People experience their social reality in a particular meaning-giving context. They progress when their will to lead a meaningful life is supported by social reconstruction (e.g., policies and programs that reduce poverty and inequality) and access to development opportunities (e.g., infrastructure, education, and training).

3. **Emphasis on the experience of the life-world:** People attribute meaning to their life circumstances based on their experiences within a microsocial reality. The impact of a development initiative or project is enhanced when it legitimizes and incorporates the sociocultural meaning-making context of the people involved.

4. **Desirable direction:** The focus and trajectory of development must be identified by the people themselves, drawing on their experience of their reality and including their needs and aspirations. Development strategies should incorporate indigenous knowledge systems and locally appropriate and culturally relevant technologies.

5. **Consciousness:** People know what they need and what is at stake in their lives. People have the right to make their own decisions about how to use themselves and their environment to meet their needs and those of others. The participatory occupational justice framework (Whiteford & Townsend, 2011) could pave the way for occupational therapy to enact procedural values.

Box 12-11. Axiological Reasoning and Regulatory Values

Change agents, besides being accountable to development beneficiaries, funders, and other stakeholders, are bound in one way or another to the rules, regulations, and ethical guidelines of employers, professional organizations, and a range of contractual or legal entities. The agreement may be formal or informal.

- **Formal project protocol:** Participatory research requires that the terms and conditions of the collaborative process be submitted to a recognized research ethics approval body, such as those available in government departments or universities.
- **Informal project agreement:** Entry into a community must be contracted with community representatives, such as the tribal authority, using customary approaches. Subject to ongoing negotiations, the project plan should ideally be co-constructed with the people involved.

Participatory methodology is always a step into the unknown, raising new questions and creating new risks over time. The norms of ethical conduct and their implications have to be revisited as the project unfolds to ensure that potential risks are identified timeously and that the welfare of all concerned is protected (Chevalier & Buckles, 2013a, 2013b; Duncan & Watson, 2012). For example, empowerment through being recognized and heard may be deemed more important than anonymity, confidentiality, or privacy. Terms of reference and indicators of progress should therefore:

- Explicitly acknowledge shared values, collective rights, interests, and mutual obligations. Consent forms may be replaced with consenting processes in which the participatory project is ratified by witnesses. If used, they must be available in the local language and be regularly revisited and revised through inclusive discussions between the parties involved.
- Value people's dignity more than the progress or change that is being reported. People may agree to the public or academic dissemination of the project processes and outcomes without realizing the implications of their consent. Ways of equalizing knowledge generation and ownership include proper quoting, acknowledgments, coauthorship, protecting the identity of people in photographs, and granting intellectual property rights.

Case Study

The next section presents a case study of a participatory research project to illustrate some of the features of development reasoning in community practice.

The Research Context

The Mount Frere subdistrict in the Alfred Nzo district of the Eastern Cape Province of South Africa consists of a cluster of villages with populations ranging between 1,500 and 5,000 people. This remote rural region is home to the Baça and Xhosa people, traditional pastoralists who have reared livestock and worked the fields for many generations. Alfred Nzo is one of the poorest districts in South Africa. Residents in some areas do not yet have access to electricity, potable water, sanitation services, or regular, affordable public transport. An estimated 78% of the population are unemployed and subsist on informal trade, social security grants (such as old age pensions, child care grants, and disability grants), and remittances from employed relatives who reside elsewhere.

Box 12-12. Imagining the Social

Occupational therapists, rendering services in collaboration with other stakeholders to individuals and/or the community as a whole, need to think about (imagine) the fabric of society in the region. Doing so will sensitize the therapist to the factors influencing occupational performance and engagement, hence ensuring reasoned responsiveness to prevailing challenges. For example, current South African social, health, and poverty literature repeatedly asks, "Where are the men?" This question confirms what we have observed about the challenges facing men and male youth in the context of rurality and rapid modernization. The redistribution of land, the demands of an industrializing South African economy, and the political duress that Black people suffered during apartheid have contributed to the perceived loss of authority by traditional leaders. Tribal elders have expressed concern about the erosion of traditional values. Alongside high unemployment, they have reported increase of domestic violence, rape, serious substance abuse (some children as young as 9 years of age), vandalism, theft, and substance-induced psychosis. A number of the men among our research informants were disabled due to violence-related trauma, some sustained in fights during manhood initiation processes. Hospital-based health interventions, including medical and substance abuse rehabilitation, are clearly not sufficient to address the bigger picture of the context within which these men live. What else may be offered by occupational therapists in collaboration with other role-players at village level to address the crises facing males?

The structural underdevelopment of the Eastern Cape Province is a legacy of the apartheid history of South Africa (du Toit & Neves, 2007). For more than 40 years, the systematic process of racial segregation meant that Black people were marginalized in the least developed areas of the country, called *homelands*. Alfred Nzo forms part of the former homeland called the Transkei. Despite the intention of the apartheid government to promote separate development in the homelands, the Transkei offered Black people fewer social and economic opportunities and less access to basic public services, such as health care and education. It is against this historic backdrop of racially motivated disadvantage that the postapartheid democratic dispensation in South Africa started redressing past inequalities in public service delivery in 1994. Disadvantage is compounded for people with disabilities in the region because they are subject to institutional, environmental, and attitudinal exclusion, all of which are relative to the structural underdevelopment and multidimensional poverty in the Eastern Cape (Chakwizira, Nhemachena, Dube, & Maponya, 2010). Box 12-12 illustrates ways of *imagining the social* from a gender perspective in this particular region.

The South African government is a signatory to the CRPD (United Nations, 2006). The CRPD undertakes to "promote, protect and ensure the full and equal enjoyment of all human rights and fundamental freedoms by all persons with disabilities, and to promote respect for their inherent dignity" (Article 1). The government is also committed to the United Nations Millennium Development Goals (United Nations, 2000), thus raising "the prospect for the poor and poorest to be seriously considered in policy analysis and to become actors in policy making" (Moore et al., 2008, p. 19). Concrete evidence of disability policy implementation is, however, dismally slow. In a constitutional democracy such as South Africa, citizens with disabilities should be key figures in shaping and translating policy into real change in their everyday lives, but national policies are not always known, accessible, or useful to those for whom they are intended. For example, social security and primary health care policies are intended to make the disability grant and rehabilitation available at primary levels of care, but public service officials and people with disabilities themselves are often uninformed about disability and the benefits of rehabilitation, making it difficult for their citizen rights to be realized (Booi, 2012).

Research Project 1: Poverty, Disability, and Occupation

Two research projects were run in the Mpoza subdistrict between 2006 and 2013.[1] The first project investigated the dynamics between poverty, disability, and occupation (PDO) in rural households. It replicated a study carried out in urban informal human settlements in Cape Town (2004–2006) that confirmed some of the ways in which rural–urban migratory patterns within households shaped their livelihood occupations (Duncan, Swartz, & Kathard, 2011a, 2011b). The PDO survey of 102 households in 15 rural villages, between 2006 and 2009, revealed the extent to which people with disabilities, their households, and their communities were marginalized by poorly coordinated and erratic public service delivery in health, education, and social development (Watson, 2013; Watson & Duncan, 2010).

The researchers (occupational therapists) were guided throughout their time in the area by a local resident, who acted as research assistant and cultural broker, and by a community-appointed research advisory group (see Acknowledgments). They worked closely with community health workers, nurses at local primary care health clinics, and rehabilitation professionals at the district hospital to ensure that appropriate referrals, arising from needs identified during the survey, were made and followed up. Besides documenting and responding when possible to the impairment and disability-related needs of research informants, the researchers also initiated occupation-based informal income generation opportunities for members with disabilities in some destitute households by sourcing equipment and material such as hand sewing machines, woodwork and gardening tools, and by coupling the entrepreneurs with public sector training resources in the area. Drawing on anthropological, sociological, economic, and political literature sources, and dialogue with local residents, the researchers spent much time learning about the history, cultural practices, and worldviews of local residents, including sociopolitical dynamics such as land owner- ship, gender roles, and clan rivalries. The researchers also studied the occupations being pursued in the context of chronic and structural poverty, rurality, and disability. In the spirit of reciprocal learning, they followed through, where possible, on the basics of social inquiry, such as seeking and giving regular feedback and making occupational therapy–informed recommendations and referrals when indicated.

Research Project 2: People Informing Policy— Power and Progress

From the PDO study, it became clear that more needed to be known and done about the social inclusion of people with disabilities, especially in light of the South African social and rural devel- opment agenda. Building on established relationships and following the principles and methods of participatory research methodology, the second project, called People informing Policy: Power and Progress (PPP&P), was launched in 2009 and terminated in 2013. A participatory process was followed at the start of the PPP&P project, involving multiple stakeholders concerned with dis- ability (people with disabilities, caregivers of people with disabilities, public sector service provid- ers responsible for the implementation of disability policies) to clarify the methodology, identify outcome indicators, and negotiate roles (Roseveare & Longshaw, 2006). The purpose of the project was to inform how citizen engagement with disability-related matters could strengthen policy- aligned access to health, education, and social development. These public sectors were identified by participants as the most critical in the short term to the service-related needs of persons with disabilities in the Mpoza subdistrict.

The aim of the PPP&P project was to promote disability-inclusive activism in one case study village by strengthening disability policy literacy and collaboration among community members and service providers. Lessons learned in one village would then be disseminated to other villages

[1] The two projects described in this section were funded by the South African Netherlands Partnership in Development.

organically through information sharing among villagers, community workers, and service providers. Village X (not named to protect anonymity) was selected as the research site through community decision-making processes that were ratified by the tribal chief, the headmen of the Mpoza subdistrict villages, and other representatives (collectively called the *imbizo*). Criteria for inclusion were the presence of a school and a health clinic within walking distance of most residents, engaged village health and social development workers, traditional healers and midwives, an active imbizo (tribal authority), an operational local chapter of Disabled People South Africa, and a range of community interest groups such as women's groups, religious organizations, savings scheme groups, and youth sports clubs. Participation in the PPP&P project was open to everyone in the case study village, including people with disabilities and their households, as well as anyone from the surrounding villages who wished to learn more about disability. Headmen from other villages travelled for 2 to 3 hours by horseback to participate in project-related events, taking what they had learned back to their constituencies.

The project unfolded in collaboration with community stakeholders, as well as local government officials and, where possible, public sector staff (e.g., nurses, teachers, social workers, therapists, police, agriculturalists, and labor advisors). The involvement of public sector employees was sporadic and problematic due to time, resource, and policy constraints (e.g., lack of transport, heavy workloads, and not being granted permission by managers to participate in community-led projects, despite primary health care policy mandates). The research team visited the area for 5 to 7 days every 3 to 4 months between 2006 and 2013. Although this longitudinal relationship promoted the gradual development of credibility and some trust between the people involved, the project initiators remained outsiders, with limited appreciation of the tacit sociocultural processes at play. They could not speak isiXhosa, and some research assistants who could speak the language were unfamiliar with the Baça dialect spoken in the area. The team relied heavily on the practical assistance, cultural brokerage, and strategic guidance of a locally trusted resident, who acted as translator, mediator, and driver, to deal with these and other community entry challenges. Box 12-13 describes some of the challenges of enabling public reasoning when using participatory research methods.

Axiological reasoning proved to be a personally challenging and humbling process of learning through many mistakes (Duncan & Watson, 2010; Richardson & Duncan, 2013), one of which is described in Box 12-14. Despite good intentions, the researchers often failed to understand what was actually happening in the community. They felt overwhelmed by the harsh conditions that people faced and powerless to effect any change. Smith (1999, p. 44), in discussing colonizing forms of development-orientated research, suggested that researchers ask the following questions: "Whose research is it? Who owns it? Whose interests does it serve? Who will benefit from it? Who has designed its questions and framed its scope? Who will carry it out? Who will write it up? How will its results be disseminated?" Although these questions sound politically correct, the most desirable answers can still be judged ethically incorrect because they are, according to Smith (1999, p. 10), not part of a larger set of judgments such as: "Is her spirit clear? Does he have a good heart? What other baggage are they carrying? Are they useful to us? Can they fix our generator? Can they actually do anything?" A critical component of axiological reasoning was to think about ways of demonstrating respect and care during the seemingly incidental, everyday exchanges with the people we met. Although our ethical commitment was to align the research methodologies with the historical and cultural traditions of indigenous people, we did not always get this right (Chilisa, 2011).

Microlevel Change Through Participatory Research

The outcome indicators set at the PPP&P planning workshop in 2009 gradually emerged during the life span of the project, the sustainability of which remained uncertain. Examples of gradual social change that emerged include the following:

Box 12-13. Enabling Public Reasoning

Taking fluctuating attendance into consideration, a group of approximately 150 to 180 people was exposed to some of the participatory learning processes associated with the PPP&P project over 4 years. Q methodology (McKeown & Thomas, 1988) was used as an outcome measure at the start and end of the project to ascertain shifts, if any, in perceptions about disability among community members and service providers. Participatory research methods, such as workshops, role-plays, and codes to stimulate discussion (e.g., drawings, photos, and stories of disability experiences by local residents) were used. The workshops covered topics such as definitions of disability, disability policies and rights, promoting mental health, coping with mental illness, inclusive education, and employment equity. Learning occurred through rudimentary exploration of policy entitlements and mismatches, taking local needs and disability experiences into consideration.

The PPP&P research events (workshops) provided a structure that allowed people to think and talk about disability-related issues. Did public reasoning happen and, if so, how effective was it? The short answer is that this is not known. Participation was fraught with logistical challenges, fluid social dynamics, and cultural ambiguities. Dissemination of information and emergent actions were made more difficult by the geographic isolation and dispersion of people and the time lapses between research visits. Communication between the researchers and community representatives and among community members themselves was organic and nondirective. It happened by word of mouth, cell phone calls (if owned), posters, newspapers, and handout notes (in accessible English and isiXhosa), and by discussion items on the agenda of *imbizo* (tribal authority structure) and other community meetings. Being cultural and language outsiders, the researchers missed a great deal of what was happening and had to rely on verbal feedback from stakeholders about emergent changes in the lives of people with disabilities, none of which could be directly attributed to the PPP&P project.

- A mother who had previously hidden her child with disability at home started bringing him into public spaces.
- A teacher and a few parents with children with disabilities started looking at ways to enroll children with disabilities at the village junior school.
- Village health workers and nurses at the clinic reported being more confident in mobilizing resources for residents with disabilities, including those with mental illness.
- An educator who became aware of disability prevention arranged for an audiologist to do screening hearing tests on children at local schools.
- The tribal elders responsible for allocating piece (ad hoc) jobs in an extended public works program reported greater awareness of including persons with disabilities.
- A few people with disabilities were able to increase their income, using hand sewing machines, woodwork, and shoe repair tools that were distributed by the researchers.
- The *imbizo* called a meeting with the police to discuss the prevalence of substance abuse and management of violence in the community.
- Two community health workers who attended an in-service training workshop in the village on mental health screening shared their knowledge at a regional community health worker gathering.
- Rehabilitation professionals at the district hospital were motivated to work toward disability inclusion through outreach trips to primary health care clinics.

BOX 12-14. AXIOLOGICAL REASONING: DISCERNING BENEFICENT OPPORTUNITIES

A number of valuable lessons about active citizenship unfolded during the research project, one being that the capacity of community members for, and interest in, self-representation cannot be assumed. The researchers informed the research advisory group about a national conference on community engagement, indicating that they were willing to support community-led efforts to attend. The advisory group agreed with the suggestion. Acting on behalf of the advisory group, because they did not have access to electronic communication with the conference organizers, the researchers secured funding for two members to attend the conference and present a paper on a topic of their choice. Capacity-building opportunities were created to prepare the elected individuals for participation at the conference, including discussions on how to write and read a paper. The researchers were clear that they would not present or speak on behalf of the community and that attendance hinged on the group taking ownership of the project. Some members of the group struggled to conceptualize what was involved, never having been exposed to a conference or to the idea of presenting a paper. Others were concerned that only those fluent in English stood a chance of being elected by the advisory group to attend, and others said people were only interested in the event because they would get free food. The impasse remained unresolved, resulting in the opportunity being abandoned. The timing of the researchers' suggestion and their understanding of the dynamics at play were flawed. They learned that engaged citizenship is a complex competency in its own right, one that requires the development and pooling of different literacies before action can ensue. Ethically, they had to refrain from blaming, dominating, rescuing, and judging.

- Eighteen months after the project was terminated, the tribal chief, local headmen, and the research advisory group arranged a community gathering to address the needs of people with disabilities, without any involvement of the researchers. They invited key service providers from the police, health, social development, labor, and agriculture public sectors concerned with disability policy implementation to give an account of their responsibilities to the people of Mpoza.

- Two years after the project ended, the regional department of social development reported cognizance of active citizenship in Mpoza subdistrict. Officials requested the partnership of the Mpoza research advisory group to implement new development projects.

CONCLUSION

This chapter located occupational therapy as a potential agent of social change through inclusive development practice using participatory research methodologies. It argued that the profession is equipped to apply different forms of reasoning to address the social determinants of health and human well-being from an occupational perspective. Occupational therapy is eminently positioned as a development change agent, by virtue of its philosophical roots in holism, humanism, and pragmatism, its biopsychosocial and occupational knowledge base, and its unique reasoning and skills set. However, the dominance of modernist thinking tends to prevail in occupational therapy services and structures. The preferred fallback position is traditional, individualized treatment or rehabilitative, project-driven interventions based on biomedical, therapeutic, and clinically orientated thinking. While the therapeutic roots of occupational therapy indicate a crucial contribution to public health, there is much more that the profession has to offer society. A holistic, developmental approach would position occupational therapy as a change agent within and across various parts of the social whole—that is, at individual, clan, family, household, community, and public systems. A combination of clinical and development reasoning is therefore indicated because it will enable occupational therapists to think about the parts of society as they pertain to individual human action in health and disability, while simultaneously considering and addressing the needs of the population.

ACKNOWLEDGMENTS

This chapter is dedicated to the memory of occupational therapist and emeritus professor Ruth Watson, who passed away in 2014. She provided occupational therapy leadership in South Africa throughout her career and, after retirement, served the people of Mpoza with her heart and soul.

We acknowledge the contribution of the following people to the Mpoza studies described in this chapter: Dr. Hanneke van Bruggen (exENOTHE) and Dr. Mayke Kaag (Centre for African Studies, Leiden University), who were appointed by South African Netherlands Partnership in Development as research consultants; Kate Sherry (occupational therapist and PhD Public Health researcher), Mpilo Booi (audiologist and MPhil Disability Studies researcher), Xakathile Dabula (research assistant), and the Mpoza Research Advisory Group (Chief Ndutyana, Mr. Ndutyana, Mr. Nonjeke, Mr. Lungongolo, Mrs. Nozihewu, Mr. Mpiti, and Mrs. Ngabase).

REFERENCES

Ampim, A. (2003). The five major African initiation rites. *Africana Studies*. Retrieved from http://www.manuampim .com/AfricanInitiationRites.htm

Belagamage, L., & Jull, J. E. (2012). Considering health inequities to enhance conference presentations. *Occupational Therapy Now*, 16, 16-17.

Bishop-Sanbrook, C. (2014). *The time poverty trap: Rural women's poverty of time is one of the biggest challenges facing smallholder development in sub-Saharan Africa*. Retrieved from http://ifad-un.blogspot.com/2014/10/the-time -poverty-trap-rural-womens.html

Bless, C., Higson-Smith, C., & Kagee, A. (2006). *Fundamentals of social research methods: An African perspective*. Cape Town, South Africa: Juta.

Bond, P. (2007). *Five international ideological currents*. G8 Club Governance, Perils of elite pacting: Appendix (pp. 50-51). Durban, South Africa: Centre for Civil Society, University of KwaZulu-Natal.

Booi, M. (2012). *Disability and service delivery: Perspectives of service users in a rural community in the Eastern Cape Province, South Africa*. Unpublished master's thesis, Division of Disability Studies, Faculty of Health Sciences, University of Cape Town, South Africa.

Bowles, S., Durlauf, S., & Hoff, K. (2006). *Poverty traps*. Princeton, NJ: Princeton University Press.

Boyt Schell, B. A., & Schell, J. W. (2008). *Clinical and professional reasoning in occupational therapy*. Philadelphia, PA: Lippincott Williams & Wilkins.

Broodryk, J. (2005). *Ubuntu management philosophy: Exploring ancient African wisdom into the global world*. Randburg, South Africa: Knowres.

Bryant, W., Fieldhouse, J., & Bannigan, K. (2014). *Creek's occupational therapy and mental health*. Edinburgh, Scotland: Churchill Livingstone.

Burkey, S. (1993). *People first: A guide to self-reliant participatory rural development*. London, England: Zed Books.

Canadian Association of Occupational Therapists. (2006). Position statement: Occupational therapy and primary health care. *Canadian Journal of Occupational Therapy*, 73, 122-124.

Chakwizira, J., Nhemachena, C., Dube, S., & Maponya, G. (2010). *Rural travel and disability in Leroro and Moremela Villages, South Africa*. Paper delivered at The 12th International Conference on Mobility and Transport for Elderly and Disabled Persons (TRANSED), Hong Kong, June 2-4, 2010.

Chambers, R. (2005). *Ideas for development*. London, England: Earthscan.

Chan, S. (2014). Can there be mercy without the merciful? A meditation on Martha Nussbaum's questions. *Third World Quarterly*, 35, 1728-1747.

Chervin, P., & Geiser, P. (2012). *Disability and development.* Handicap International. Retrieved from http://www .hiproweb.org/fileadmin/cdroms/Handicap_Developpement/www/index_en.html

Chevalier, J. M., & Buckles, D. J. (2013a). *Handbook for participatory action research, planning and evaluation.* Retrieved from http://www.participatoryactionresearch.net/sites/default/files/sites/all/files/manager/Toolkit_En_ March7_2013-S.pdf

Chevalier, J. M., & Buckles, D. J. (2013b). *Participatory action research: Theory and methods for engaged enquiry.* London, England: Routledge.

Chilisa, B. (2011). *Indigenous research methodologies.* Thousand Oaks, CA: Sage Publications.

Cockburn, L., & Trentham, B. (2002). Participatory action research: Integrating community occupational therapy practice and research. *Canadian Journal of Occupational Therapy.* Retrieved from http://www.caot.ca/CJOT_pdfs/ CJOT69/Cockburn69%281%2920-30.pdf

Coetzee, J. K. (2001). A micro foundation for development thinking. In J. K. Coetzee & J. Graaf (Eds.), *Development theory, policy and practice* (pp. 118-139). Cape Town, South Africa: Oxford University Press.

Connell, R. (2007). *Southern theory.* Cambridge, United Kingdom: Polity Press.

Cotterrell, R. (Ed.). (2010). *Emile Durkheim: Justice, morality and politics* (Queen Mary School of Law Legal Studies Research Paper No. 57/2010). Surrey, England: Ashgate. Retrieved from http://ssm.com/abstract=1620127

Creek, J. (2010). *The core concepts of occupational therapy: A dynamic framework for practice.* London, England: Jessica Kingsley.

Cutchin, M. P., Aldrich, R. M., Baillard, A. L. & Coppola, S. (2008). Action theories for occupational science: The contributions of Dewey and Bourdieu. *Journal of Occupational Science, 15,* 157-164.

Cutchin, M. P., & Dickie, V. A. (2013). *Transactional perspectives on occupation.* London, England: Springer.

Cruz, I., Stahel, A., & Max-Neef, M. (2009). Towards a systemic development approach: Building on the human-scale development paradigm. *Ecological Economics, 68,* 2021-2030.

Davids, I., Theron, F., & Maphunye, K. J. (2009). *Participatory development in South Africa. A development management perspective.* Pretoria, South Africa: van Schaik

Davis, G. (2004, March). *A history of the Social Development Network in the World Bank* (Social Development, Paper No. 56). Washington DC: The World Bank.

de Sardan, J. P. (2005). *Anthropology and development: Understanding contemporary social change.* London, England: Zed Books.

Duncan, M., & Creek, J. (2014). Working on the margins: Occupational therapy and social inclusion. In W. Bryant et al. (Eds.), *Creek's occupational therapy and mental health* (pp. 457-473). Edinburgh, Scotland: Churchill Livingstone.

Duncan, M., Swartz, L., & Kathard, H. (2011a). The burden of psychiatric disability on chronically poor households: Part 1 (costs). *The South African Journal of Occupational Therapy, 41,* 55-63.

Duncan, M., Swartz, L., & Kathard, H. (2011b). The burden of psychiatric disability on chronically poor households: Part 2 (coping strategies). *The South African Journal of Occupational Therapy, 41,* 64-70.

Duncan, M., & Watson, R. (2010). Taking a stance: Socially responsible ethics and informed consent. In M. Saven-Baden & C. Taylor (Eds.), *New approaches in qualitative research: Wisdom and uncertainty.* London, England: Taylor & Francis.

du Toit, A., & Neves, D. (2007). In search of South Africa's Second Economy: Chronic poverty, economic marginalisation and adverse incorporation in Mt Frere and Khayelitsha. *Chronic Poverty Research Centre Working Paper, 107.* Programme for Land and Agrarian Studies, School of Governance: University of Western Cape.

Escobar, A. (1995). *Encountering development: The making and unmaking of the Third World.* Princeton, NJ: Princeton University Press.

Frank, G., & Zemke, R. (2009). Occupational therapy foundations for political engagement and social reformation. In N. Pollard, D. Sakellariou, & F. Kronenberg (Eds.), A political practice of occupational therapy (pp. 126-136). Edinburgh, Scotland: Elsevier Ltd.

Freire, P. (2005). *Pedagogy of the oppressed* (30th anniversary ed.; Trans. Myra Bergman). New York, NY: Continuum.

Fukuda-Parr, S. (2003). The human development paradigm: Operationalizing Sen's ideas on capabilities. *Feminist Economics, 9*(2-3), 301-317.

Galheigo, S. M. (2011). What needs to be done? Occupational therapy responsibilities and challenges regarding human rights. *Australian Occupational Therapy Journal, 58,* 60-66.

Galvaan, R. (2012). Occupational choice: The significance of socio-economic and political factors. In G. E. Whiteford & C. Hocking (Eds.), *Occupational science: Society, inclusion, participation* (pp. 152-162). Oxford, England: Wiley-Blackwell.

Gibson, N. (2011). *Living Fanon: Global perspectives.* New York, NY: Palgrave Macmillan.

Hickey, S., & du Toit, A. (2007). *Adverse incorporation, social exclusion and chronic poverty* (CPRC Working Paper 81). Institute for Development Policy and Management School of Environment and Development, University of Manchester, and the Programme for Land and Agrarian Studies School of Government, University of the Western Cape.

Ife, J. (2002). *Community development: Community-based alternatives in an age of globalisation.* Frenches Forest, Australia: Pearson Education.

Institute for Social Studies. (n.d.). *Indices for social development.* International Institute for Social Studies in the Hague, Erasmus University, Rotterdam, Netherlands. Available online: http://www.indsocdev.org/home.html

Joshi, S. (2005). *Theories of development: Modernisation vs dependency*. Retrieved from http://infochangeindia.org/defining-development/theories-of-development-modernisation-vs-dependency.html

Kanbur, R., & Venables, A. J. (Eds.). (2005). *Spatial inequality and development*. Oxford, England: Oxford University Press.

Kaplan, A. (1999). *The development of capacity* (10th Occasional Paper, United Nations Non-Governmental Liaison Service). Geneva, Switzerland: United Nations

Kaplan, A. (2002). *Development practitioners and social process: Artists of the invisible*. London, England: Pluto Press.

Kothari, U. (Ed.). (2005). *A radical history of development studies: Individuals, institutions and ideologies*. London, England: Zed Books.

Kronenberg, F., Pollard, N., & Sakellariou, D. (Eds.). (2011). *Occupational therapy without borders* (Vol. 2). Edinburgh, Scotland: Elsevier/Churchill Livingstone.

Lauckner, H. M., Krupa, T. M., & Paterson, M. L. (2011). Conceptualizing community development: Occupational therapy practice at the intersection of health services and community. *Canadian Journal of Occupational Therapy, 78*, 260-268.

Lauckner, H., Pentland, W., & Paterson, M. (2007). Exploring occupational therapists' understanding of and experiences in community development. *Canadian Journal of Occupational Therapy, 74*, 314-325.

Leclair, L. L. (2010). Re-examining concepts of occupation and occupation-based models: Occupational therapy and community development. *Canadian Journal of Occupational Therapy, 77*, 15-21.

Letts, L. (2003). Occupational therapy and participatory research: A partnership worth pursuing. *American Journal of Occupational Therapy, 57*, 77-87.

Levasseur, M., & Carrier, A. (2012). Integrating health literacy into occupational therapy: Findings from a scoping review. *Scandinavian Journal Occupational Therapy, 19*, 305-314. Retrieved from http://www.ncbi.nlm.nih.gov/pmc/articles/PMC3586251

Macionis, J. J., & Plummer, K. (2008). *Sociology: A global introduction* (4th ed.). Harlow, England: Pearson Education Limited.

Mandela, N. (2005, February 3). *Make poverty history*. Speech given in Trafalgar Square, London, England. Retrieved from http://www.makepovertyhistory.org/extras/mandela.shtml

Maturana, H., & Varela, F. (1987). *The tree of knowledge*. Boston, MA: Shambhala.

Max-Neef, M. (1991). *Human scale development: Conception, application and further reflections*. New York, NY: Apex Press.

McKeown, B., & Thomas, D. (1988). *Q methodology*. Newbury Park, CA: Sage.

McLean, G. N. (2005). *Organization development principles, processes, performance*. San Francisco, CA: Berrett-Koehler.

Meyers, S. K. (2010). *Community practice in occupational therapy: A guide to serving the community*. Sudbury, MA: Jones & Bartlett.

Mills, C. W. (1959). *Sociological imagination*. New York, NY: Oxford University Press.

Mloka, E. (Ed.). (2004). *Africa's development thinking since independence—A reader*. Pretoria, South Africa: Africa Institute of South Africa (AISA), Human Sciences Research Council.

Moore, K., Grant, U., Hulme, D., & Shepherd, A. (2008). *Very poor, for a long time in many ways. Defining the poorest for policy makers* (Chronic Poverty Research Centre Working Paper No. 124). Manchester, England: Brooks World Poverty Institute.

Nabudere, D. W. (2011). *Afrikology, philosophy and wholeness: An epistemology*. Pretoria, South Africa: Africa Institute of South Africa.

Narayan, D. (1999). Can anyone hear us? Voices from 47 countries. *Voices of the Poor* (Vol. 1). Poverty Group, PREM, World Bank.

Naz, F. (2006). Arturo Escobar and the development discourse: An overview. *Asian Affairs, 28*, 64-84.

Nussbaum, M. (2011). *Creating capabilities: The human development approach*. Cambridge, MA: Belknap Press of Harvard University Press.

Parsons, T. (1975). The present status of "structural-functional" theory in sociology. In T. Parsons (Ed.), *Social systems and the evolution of action theory*. New York, NY: The Free Press.

Pollard, N., Sakellariou, D., & Kronenberg, F. (2008). *A political practice of occupational therapy*. Edinburgh, Scotland: Elsevier/Churchill Livingstone.

Ramugondo, E. (2012). Intergenerational play within family: The case for occupational consciousness. *Journal of Occupational Science, 19*, 326-340.

Ramugondo, E., & Kronenberg, F. (2015). Explaining collective occupations from a human relations perspective: Bridging the individual-collective dichotomy. *Journal of Occupational Science, 22*, 3-16.

Rawls, J. (1997). The idea of public reason revisited. *The University of Chicago Law Review, 64*, 765-807.

Richardson, P., & Duncan, M. (2013). A context for mental health research in occupational therapy. In E. Cara & A. MacRae (Eds.), *Psychosocial occupational therapy: An evolving practice* (pp. 61-90). New York, NY: Delmar/Cengage Learning.

Robertson, L. (2012). *Clinical reasoning in occupational therapy: Controversies in practice*. Chichester, England: Blackwell.

Rohr, E. (2011). *From conflict to recognition: Cultural transformation through group supervision in Guatemala*. Keynote address at the 2011 Symposium of the Group Analytic Society International. Retrieved from http://vimeo.com /28624238

Roseveare, C., & Longshaw, M. (2006). *The opportunities and feasibility of addressing disability as a cross cutting research issue*. A report for the Department of International Development, DFID Central Research Department.

Sachs, J. D. (2012). From millennium development goals to sustainable development goals. *Lancet, 379*, 2206-2211.

Said, E. (1994). *Culture and imperialism*. London, England: Vintage.

Sen, A. (2009). *The idea of justice*. London, England: Penguin Books.

Sen, A. (2011). *Development as freedom*. London, England: Knopf Doubleday.

Sillitoe, P., Dixon, P., & Barr, J. (2005). *Indigenous knowledge inquiries: A methodologies manual for development*. Warwickshire, England: Practical Action.

Smith, L. T. (1999). *Decolonising methodologies: research and indigenous peoples*. London, England: Zed Books.

Stav, W. B., Hallenen, T., Lane, J., & Arbesman, M. (2012). Systematic review of occupational engagement and health outcomes amongst community-dwelling older adults. *American Journal of Occupational Therapy, 66*, 301-310.

Sullivan, A., & Sheffrin, S. M. (2003). *Economics: Principles in action*. Upper Saddle River, NJ: Pearson Prentice Hall.

Swanepoel, H., & de Beer, F. (2011). *Community development: breaking the cycle of poverty*. Lansdowne, South Africa: Juta.

Theron, F. (2008). *The development change agent: A micro-level approach to development*. Pretoria, South Africa: van Schaik.

Theron, F., & Wetmore, S. (2008). Action research methodology—alternative options for grassroots research and community participation. In F. Theron (Ed.), *The development change agent: A micro-level approach to development*. Pretoria, South Africa: van Schaik.

Townsend, E. A. (2012). Boundaries and bridges to adult mental health: Critical occupational and capabilities perspectives of justice. *Journal of Occupational Science, 19*, 8-24.

Townsend, E. A., Cockburn, L., Letts, L., Thibeault, R., & Trentham, B. (2007). Enabling social change. In E. A. Townsend & H. J. Polatajko (Eds.), *Enabling occupation 11: Advancing an occupational therapy for health, well being, and justice through occupation*. Ottawa, Canada: CAOT Publications.

United Nations. (2000). *Millennium development goals*. New York, NY: Author.

United Nations. (2006). *Convention on the rights of persons with disabilities*. New York, NY: Author.

United Nations Development Programme. (2013). *The rise of the South: Human progress in a diverse world*. Retrieved from http://hdr.undp.org/en/2013-report

United Nations Development Programme. (2014). *Human development report 2014: Sustaining human progress: reducing vulnerabilities and building resilience*. New York, NY: Author. Retrieved from http://hdr.undp.org/en/2014-report

van Bruggen, H. (2009). *Competencies for poverty reduction (CAPORE)*. Copenhagen, Denmark: European Network of Occupational Therapists in Higher Education. Retrieved from www.enothe.eu

Venkatopuram, S. (2011). *Health justice: An argument from the capabilities approach*. Cambridge, England: Polity Press.

Watson, R. (2013). A population approach to occupational therapy. *South African Journal of Occupational Therapy, 43*, 35-39.

Watson, R., & Duncan, E. M. (2010). The right to occupational participation in the presence of chronic poverty. *WFOT Bulletin, 62*(1), 26-32.

Wells, T. R. (2013). *Reasoning about development: Essays on Amartya Sen's capability approach*. Doctoral dissertation, Erasmus University, Rotterdam, the Netherlands. Retrieved from http://www. repub.eur.nl/pub/40509/thesis

Whalley Hammel, K. R. (2010). Resisting theoretical imperialism in the disciplines of occupational science and occupational therapy. *British Journal of Occupational Therapy, 74*(1), 27-33.

Whalley Hammell, K. R., & Iwama, M. K. (2012). Well-being and occupational rights: An imperative for critical occupational therapy. *Scandinavian Journal of Occupational Therapy, 19*, 385-394.

Whiteford, G., & Hocking, C. (2012). *Occupational science: Society, inclusion, participation*. Oxford, England: Wiley-Blackwell.

Whiteford, G., & Townsend, E. (2011). Participatory occupational justice framework (POJF 2010). In F. Kronenberg, N. Pollard, & D. Sakellariou (Eds.), *Occupational therapies without borders: Towards an ecology of occupation-based practices* (Vol. 2). Edinburgh, Scotland: Elsevier/Churchill Livingstone.

Wilcock, A. A., & Townsend, E. A. (2009). Occupational justice. In E. B. Crepeau, E. S. Cohn, & B. A. B. Schell (Eds.), *Willard & Spackman's occupational therapy* (11th ed.). Philadelphia, PA: Lippincott Williams & Wilkins.

Wilkinson, R. G., & Pickett, K. (2010). *The spirit level: Why equality is better for everyone*. London, England: Penguin Books.

World Bank. (2013). *Gini index*. Retrieved from http://data.worldbank.org/indicator/SI.POV.GINI

World Federation of Occupational Therapists. (2006). *Position paper: Human rights*. Retrieved from http://www.wfot.org/ResourceCentre.aspx

World Federation of Occupational Therapists. (2009). *Guiding principles on diversity and culture*. Available at: http://www.wfot.org/ResourceCentre.aspx

World Federation of Occupational Therapists. (2014). *Draft international guidelines for the education of occupational therapists—2014*. The Council of the World Federation of Occupational Therapists, Forrestfield, Australia.

World Health Organization. (2001). *International classification of functioning, disability and health* (ICF). Retrieved from http://www.who.int/classifications/icf/en

World Health Organization. (2007). *Interim statement of the commission on social determinants of health.* Retrieved from http://www.who.int/social_determinants/thecommission/interimstatement/en/index.html

World Health Organization. (2010). *Community-based rehabilitation guidelines.* Retrieved from http://www.who.int/disabilities/cbr/guidelines/en

Glossary

agency: the conscious capacity to exercise control over the nature and quality of one's life (Chapter 9).

borrowed story: a narrative that draws from figures in popular cultural mythology, such as action figures, idols, or superheroes (Mattingly, 2010).

butterfly effect: two states differing by imperceptible amounts may eventually evolve into two considerably different states (Chapter 11).

clinical reasoning: the modes of thinking that the therapist uses when trying to understand people's needs and what to do about them, such as defining problems and making judgments (Schell & Schell, 2008; Sinclair, 2007).

collaboration: working in partnership with others, whether with other professionals, the client–therapist relationship, or therapists within services collaborating with other organizations to achieve mutual goals (Chapter 4).

community: a group of any size of people who share a physical and geographic location, common cultural heritage, language and beliefs, or shared interests. Individuals usually belong to more than one community at the same time, based on different relationships, needs, and interests (Chapter 12).

community-based rehabilitation (CBR): a strategy within community development for education, vocational, and social services (International Labour Organization, 2004). CBR is not a service in itself but an approach that benefits everyone in a community because it promotes and emphasizes the inherent values of human development (World Health Organization, 2010).

complexity: some systems, such as social groups and neural networks, are made up of multiple components that interact both with each other and with the environment (Creek, 2010). "Complexity results from the interaction between the components of a system [and] is manifested at the level of the system itself" (Cilliers, 1998, pp. 2-3). Nonlinear relationships between components that are history dependent have fuzzy boundaries and the presence of amplifying or damping feedback loops. Behavior reorganizes in unexpected ways giving rise to increased complex patterns over time (Lazzarini, 2004).

Cole, M. B., & Creek, J. (Eds.).
Global Perspectives in Professional Reasoning (pp. 239-246).
© 2016 Taylor & Francis Group.

conscientization: a process in which individuals and communities become critically aware of their potential to initiate and manage positive change; emphasizes the values of autonomy and self-determination (Freire, 2005).

control parameters: variables that lead the system through the variety of possible patterns or states but do not prescribe or contain the code for emerging patterns (Freeman, 1988a, 1988b; Kay, Lancaster, & Freeman, 1996; Kelso, 1999).

coupling: pairing, linking, or joining things together (*Shorter Oxford English Dictionary*, 2002).

> **coupling, body–environment:** the activity or occupation and the body are tightly linked to the environment so that thinking cannot easily be isolated from the immediate task at hand for fear of an accident or poor performance (Chapter 11).

> **coupling, mind–environment:** the person is completely engrossed in an occupation for its own sake and oblivious to her or his body position or exposure (Chapter 11).

> **coupling, structural:** the structure determined and structure determining engagement of a given system or unity with either its environment or another system or unity (Maturana & Varela, 1987). It is a process through which structurally determined transformations in two or more systemic unities induce for each a trajectory of reciprocally triggered change (Chapter 12).

creativity: a combination of three components: area of expertise, creative thinking skills, and motivation (Chapter 10).

cultural brokerage: "the act of bridging, linking or mediating between groups or persons of differing cultural backgrounds for the purpose of reducing conflict or producing change" (Jezewski & Sotnik, 2001).

decision making: evaluating information, predicting the outcomes of alternative courses of action, planning interventions, setting priorities, and justifying actions taken (Sinclair, 2007).

development: the advancement of human well-being through the "constant elimination of situations of dehumanization at all levels of society" (Davids, Theron, & Maphunye, 2009, p. 133). The gradual unfolding or bringing out of latent potential in people, their environments, or social systems; growth, maturation, and advancement to a more organized and preferred state of being (Chapter 12).

> **development, community:** "the facilitation of growing awareness and consciousness such that people are able to take control of their own lives and circumstances, and exert responsibility and purpose with respect to their future" (Kaplan, 1999, p. 12).

> **development, health:** the active participation of people in promoting and caring for their own health. It involves a participatory process by which individuals and families assume responsibility for their own health and welfare and for those of the community, and develop the capacity to contribute to their and the community's development (Chapter 12).

> **development, human:** improving people's lives and capabilities by expanding their choices, freedoms, and dignity (Chapter 12).

> **development, individual:** the biopsychosocial, behavioral, and other changes in human attributes and abilities that occur at each age and stage of the life span and are considered normative in a particular society, culture, or historical period. There is no universally applicable understanding of individual development because people across the world interpret the human life cycle differently (Chapter 12).

> **development, macro-:** structurally orientated and system-centered development involving transnational, national, and regional economic strategizing; social and environmental reconstruction; and political transition to address issues of universal concern such as the reduction of extreme poverty, hunger, and (gender) inequality (Chapter 12).

> **development, micro-:** people-centered development that is concerned with processes of social change that lead to some form of growth in humans and their social institutions (Chapter 12).

development, occupation-based: focuses on human occupation to advance an occupational therapy vision of health, well-being, and social justice for individuals, groups, and communities (Chapter 12).

development, organizational: developing the values, attitudes, norms, and management practices that will enable the organization and its members to grow (Chapter 12).

development practice: involves local people playing an integral part in decision-making processes related to any projects that are identified and implemented in their community so that development is more likely to be sustainable (Chapter 6).

development studies: a multidisciplinary branch of social science and a discipline in its own right (Chapter 12).

dualism: assumption that there is an essential division between mind and body (Block, 1980).

empathy: the ability to "feel, detect, imitate and express emotions and to communicate verbal and nonverbal signals to understand each other" (Abreu, 2011, p. 624). In the emotional intelligence literature, empathy is viewed both as the identification of the other's emotional experience and as the ability to communicate that understanding, as well as the capacity to solve problems and react with an appropriate therapeutic response (Salovey & Mayer, 1990).

emplotment: creating plots or story lines in the "therapeutic encounters with patients, that is, [helping to] create a therapeutic story that becomes a meaningful short story in the larger life story of the patient" (Mattingly, 1991, p. 998).

evidence discovery: the mode of reasoning the therapist uses when gathering data, carrying out assessments, identifying potential problems, recognizing relevant clinical cues, and defining the problems to be addressed during intervention (Sinclair, 2007).

expertise: "includes a rich, integrated knowledge base, qualitatively different strategies, automaticity in problem solving, and the ability to reflect on problem solving when necessary" (Carr & Shotwell, 2008, p. 52).

film as metaphor: a film may be used to represent concepts that go beyond its literal meaning and to present comparisons between ideas and/or things that constitute analogies applicable to the film's subject matter or to life in general outside the parameters of the film (Chapter 8).

Foundation Trust: a corporation responsible to a board of governors that typically provides hospital, mental health, or ambulance services within a local area of the United Kingdom (Chapter 4).

functionalism: defines mind as set of mechanisms that can perform functions independently of the physical platform on which it is implanted (Block, 1980).

generative themes: bring together a group's thinking and feelings on a current topic that is of concern to them, reflecting the ideas, hopes, doubts, frustrations, and challenges that they face in everyday life (Chapter 7).

illness experience: a phenomenon related to the impact of a disease on the process of living with the ongoing consequences of that condition. It encompasses the way a disease affects a person's life and their response (as well as their family's reaction) to living with an illness in their unique social, economic, and cultural context (Helman, 2007).

intentional leadership: a conscious choice of action that draws the ideals of collaboration, proactivity, and transformation into a focused, purposeful direction (Chapter 7).

judgment: the ability to use evidence in drawing inferences and conclusions, to weigh arguments, to determine the best course of action, to recognize the ramifications of decisions taken, and to take responsibility for them. Good judgments take into account the weight of evidence, the context, the potential utility of solutions, and the pragmatic need for action (Sinclair, 2007).

language: "a system of human communication using words, written and spoken, and particular ways of combining them" (*Shorter Oxford English Dictionary*, 2002).

meaning: "experienced as a total life orientation including a person's global beliefs, spiritual beliefs and a motivation to meaning" (Lethborg, Aranda, & Kissane, 2008, p. 68).

Millennium Development Goals: developed by the United Nations to focus attention and mobilize resources to address the major gaps in human development and poverty reduction (Chapter 6).

narrative: storytelling as a form of communication that people use in relating events, including the process of describing life experiences of special significance (Bruner, 1986, 1990). "The realization of self as a narrative in process serves to gather together what one has been, in order to imagine what one will be, and to judge whether that is what one wants to become" (Polkinghorne, 1988, p. 154).

narrative, chaos: description of an unrelenting, painful course of illness with loss of control or hope of recovery (Schell & Schell, 2008).

narrative, illness: the stories that patients tell about their illness; the plot related to their stage and perception of their illness and the path that is traveled. Frank (1995, 2013) described three types of plot: restitution narrative, chaos narrative, and quest narrative.

narrative, occupational: a narrative that reveals "the overall meaning of life events, signifying their place in a plot that integrates past, present and future" (Goldstein, Kielhofner, & Ward, 2004, p. 119). This narrative reflects the client or patient's response to the illness or limitations as they affect occupational performance; their description of meaningful occupations as they have evolved over time for the individual and the relationship of these to sense of health, well-being, and community participation; and how one may revise their occupational identity in response to the condition/limitations (Schell & Schell, 2008).

narrative, quest: way of describing an experience with illness in which there is an archetypal journey manifesting the ability to withstand or adapt to illness and develop greater self-awareness (Schell & Schell, 2008).

narrative, restitution: way of describing a quest for victory over the illness and return to health, often viewed as a victory of the biomedical processes over the medical condition (Frank, 2013; Schell & Schell, 2008).

occupational genesis: the process through which creativity enables humans to engage in a series of evolving occupations, throughout individual lifetimes and throughout the millennia (Chapter 10).

occupational therapy: "a client-centered health profession concerned with promoting health and well-being through occupation" (World Federation of Occupational Therapists, 2012).

offline cognition: cognitive operations are decoupled from real time and the world environment (Chapter 11).

online cognition: situated cognition, where all cognitive operations occur in real time are environmentally embedded and demand immediate action (Varela, Thompson, & Rosch, 1991).

participation: a multidimensional process that contributes to human growth in such areas as self-confidence, initiative, cooperation, self-reliance, pride, and responsibility. These, and other forms of change within people, liberate them to enact their personal values, take charge of their lives, and solve their own problems (Burkey, 1993).

pattern: an arrangement or order discernible in objects, actions, ideas, situations, etc. (*Shorter Oxford English Dictionary*, 2002).

pattern, formation: the brain's basic means of storing information (Chapter 11).

pattern, recognition: the brain's basic means of sharing information (Chapter 11).

pedagogy of suffering: what the ill have to teach about suffering (Frank, 1995). Suffering is literally embodied in an individual "and when the body's vulnerability and pain are kept in the foreground, a new social ethic is required" (p. 146), encompassing not just medical perspectives but restoring "agency to ill people [whose] testimony is given equal place alongside professional expertise" (p. 145).

power: possession of control, authority, or influence over others (*Merriam-Webster Dictionary*, 2015).

reasoning: the action of thinking in a logical or connected manner; the arguments involved in arriving at a conclusion or judgment (*Shorter Oxford English Dictionary*, 2002).

reasoning, axiological: considers the intrinsic (personal), extrinsic (communal/societal), procedural (methodological), and regulatory (systemic) values by which people live and according to which change agents practice. When relationships flounder or projects derail, axiological reasoning endeavors to create alignment between these four sets of values (Chapter 12).

reasoning, ethical: the process of thinking through the moral dimensions of a situation to reach the best decision (Chapter 2).

reasoning, narrative: the therapist's thinking related to understanding the story of the client's illness, the impact on occupational performance and his or her lifestyle, and working with the client and family to engage them in treatment supporting their values, spirituality, and goals (Chapter 8).

reasoning, professional: the full range of thinking skills and "cognitive processes used to guide professional actions" (Schell & Schell, 2008, p. 447). Professional reasoning includes the types of thinking used when working with clients, teaching students, establishing new services, developing existing services, negotiating with funders, managing staff, and so on (Chapter 2).

reasoning, public: a form of thinking out what appropriate justice entails for people situated in less than fully just circumstances. It forms the basis of group thinking in social and political forums where issues of collective concern are debated and actions decided (Chapter 12).

reasoning, social: thinking about occupations from a social perspective, including social contexts, expectations, sources of support, and considering the social groups and/or significant relationships within which occupational choices are made and performed (Chapter 9).

reasoning, strategic: a thinking process through which occupational therapists work out the best course of action to take in a complex situation or how to position themselves in a constantly changing world (Chapter 3).

self-efficacy: belief in one's own abilities (Chapter 9).

self-organization: the spontaneous, self-generated occurrence of some kind of pattern; the brain's ability to demonstrate pattern formation and change under nonparametric conditions (Kelso, 1999).

self-regulation: people's capacity to modify the extent of their motivation and expectations of themselves, based on the extent to which they believe they possess the prerequisite abilities and can control their own functioning (Chapter 9).

social identity: "the sense of self that people derive from their membership in social groups (e.g., family, work, community)" (Jetten, Haslam, & Haslam, 2012, p. 4).

social inclusion: a process through which efforts are made to ensure equal opportunities for all, regardless of their background, so that they can achieve full potential in life: the process of improving the terms for individuals and groups to take part in society (World Bank, 2013).

social learning: the thinking process that occurs when people watch the behaviors of others, leading to an appreciation of their own abilities and the way other people think and feel about them (Chapter 9).

social network: the people with whom one has relationships through frequent interactions, trusting connections, and/or shared group membership; not necessarily related to Internet group participation (Christakis & Fowler, 2010).

sociological imagination: an intellectual quality, the understanding and acquisition of which forms the basis for revolutionary social change. It is a way of thinking that makes links between the taken-for-granted lived experiences of individuals (the particular) and the social forces that shape these experiences (the universal) (Mills, 1959).

spirituality: the "aspect of humanity that refers to the way individuals seek and express meaning and purpose and the way they experience their connectedness to the moment, to self, to others, to nature, and to the significant or sacred" (Puchalski et al., 2009, p. 887).

story making: the therapist's effort to make the patient's illness a narrative, unfolding a chapter related to their ongoing story in the course of clinical treatment. The process of reconstructing the client's narrative, drawing on influences of personal contexts (family, culture, occupational profile) and their current condition, and positioning the therapist to develop with the client a positive and engaging vision of occupational performance in the future to reaffirm occupational identity and function (Mattingly, 1991).

storytelling: the engagement of therapists in developing descriptions of their perspective of the patient's and family members' participation in therapy as an unfolding story with emotional challenges, reflecting the patient's unique experiences with his or her illness (Mattingly, 1991).

strategic planning: working out how to realize and support strategies developed through strategic thinking and integrate these back into the association, network, etc. (Chapter 3).

strategy: the art or skill of careful planning toward a desired end (*Shorter Oxford English Dictionary*, 2002).

suffering: paying honor to the "pedagogy of suffering" speaks to a social ethic of recognizing the vulnerability of the person and stories that are told "through a wounded body" (Frank, 2013, p. 2).

system: a way of looking at the world, a theoretical construct that simplifies nature (Chapter 11).

system, nonlinear dynamic: a system that changes over time and is characterized by complexity, randomness, and nonlinearity (Kelso, 1999; Thelen & Smith, 1994).

system, open: a system that can interact with the environment, exchanging information, energy, and matter (Chapter 11).

therapeutic interactive encounter: therapists' engagement in directing "complex action and interaction as they (1) used verbal behaviors, (2) used nonverbal behaviors, and (3) interacted with co-participants within the given settings and contexts of the evaluation" (Burke, 2010, p. 859).

therapeutic use of self: using "one's personality, insights, perceptions, and judgments, as part of the therapeutic process" (American Occupational Therapy Association [AOTA], 2008, p. 653). This skill "allows occupational therapy practitioners to develop and manage their therapeutic relationships with clients by using narrative and clinical reasoning; empathy; and a client-centered, collaborative approach to service delivery" (AOTA, 2014, p. S12; Taylor & van Puymbroeck, 2013).

thinking: consists of both processes and skills and "includes such mental actions as applying rules, choosing, conceptualizing, evaluating, judging, justifying, knowing, perceiving and understanding" (Creek, 2007, p. 9).

thinking, strategic: an integrative process that crosses interorganizational boundaries and spans multiple levels of analysis as a way of thinking built on the foundation of a systems perspective from which a problem or opportunity is seen as a part of the whole situation or system (Bonn, 2005; Liedtka, 1998).

thinking, systems: a way of thinking that enables the identification and clarification of patterns and supports effective change, thereby increasing creativity. It consists of the key elements of systems thinking, creativity, and vision (Chapter 3).

third sector organizations: not-for-profit organizations that are typically charities or community organizations, each one established to help tackle a particular issue, such as supporting people with a health condition, addressing a local community problem, or raising funds for research (Chapter 4).

values: the principles or moral standards of a person or social group; the generally accepted or personally held judgments of what is valuable and important in life (*Shorter Oxford English Dictionary*, 2002).

REFERENCES

Abreu, B. (2011). Accentuate the positive: Reflections on empathic interpersonal interactions. Eleanor Clarke Slagle Lecture. *American Journal of Occupational Therapy, 65*, 623-634. doi:10.5014/ajot.2011.656002

American Occupational Therapy Association. (2008). Occupational therapy practice framework: Domain and process (2nd ed.). *American Journal of Occupational Therapy, 62*, 625-683.

American Occupational Therapy Association. (2014). Occupational therapy practice framework: Domain and process (3rd ed.). *American Journal of Occupational Therapy, March/April, 68*(Suppl. 1), S1-S41. doi:10.5014/ajot.2014.682006

Block, N. (Ed.). (1980). What is functionalism? In *Readings in Philosophy of Psychology* (Vol. 1). Cambridge, MA: Harvard University Press.

Bonn, I. (2005). Improving strategic thinking: A multilevel approach. *Leadership and Organization Development Journal, 26*, 336-354.

Bruner, J. (1986). *Actual minds, possible worlds*. Cambridge, MA: Harvard University Press.

Bruner, J. (1990). *Acts of meaning*. Cambridge, MA: Harvard University Press.

Burke, J. P. (2010). What's going on here: Deconstructing the interactive encounter. Eleanor Clarke Slagle Lecture. *American Journal of Occupational Therapy, 64*, 855-868. doi:10.5014/ajot.2010.64604

Burkey, S. (1993). *People first: A guide to self-reliant participatory rural development*. London, England: Zed Books.

Carr, M., & Shotwell, M. (2008). Information processing theory and professional reasoning. In B. A. B. Schell & K. W. Schell (Eds.), *Clinical and professional reasoning in occupational therapy* (pp. 36-68). Philadelphia, PA: Lippincott Williams & Wilkins.

Christakis, N., & Fowler, J. (2009). *Connected: The surprising power of our social networks and how they shape our lives*. New York, NY: Little, Brown, & Co.

Cilliers, P. (1998). *Complexity and postmodernism: Understanding complex systems*. London, England: Routledge.

Creek, J. (2007). The thinking therapist. In J. Creek & A. Lawson-Porter (Eds.), *Contemporary issues in occupational therapy: reasoning and reflection* (pp. 1-21). Chichester, England: Wiley.

Creek, J. (2010). *The core concepts of occupational therapy: A dynamic framework for practice*. London, England: Jessica Kingsley.

Davids, I., Theron, F., & Maphunye, K. J. (2009). *Participatory development in South Africa. A development management perspective*. Pretoria, South Africa: van Schaik.

Frank, A. W. (1995). *The wounded storyteller: Body, illness and ethics*. Chicago, IL: University of Chicago Press.

Frank, A. W. (2013). *The wounded storyteller: Body, illness and ethics* (2nd ed.). Chicago, IL: University of Chicago Press.

Freeman, W. J. (1988a). Nonlinear neural dynamics in olfaction as a model for cognition. In E. Basar (Ed.), *Dynamics of sensory and cognitive processing by the brain* (pp. 19-29). Berlin, Germany: Springer.

Freeman, W. J. (1988b). Strange attractors that govern mammalian brain dynamics as shown by trajectories of electroencephalographic (EEG) potential. *IEEE Transactions on Circuits and Systems, 35*, 781-783.

Freire, P. (2005). *Pedagogy of the oppressed* (30th anniversary ed.; Trans. Myra Bergman). New York, NY: Continuum.

Goldstein, K., Kielhofner, G., & Ward, A. (2004). Occupational narratives and the therapeutic process. *Australian Occupational Therapy Journal, 51*, 119-124. doi:10.1111/j.1440-1630.2004.00443.x

Helman, C. G. (2007). *Culture, health and illness* (5th ed.). New York, NY: Taylor & Francis.

International Labour Organization. (2004). *Community based rehabilitation joint position paper* (ILO, UNESCO, & WHO). Geneva, Switzerland: World Health Organization.

Jetten, J., Haslam, S. A. & Haslam, C. (2012). The case for a social identity analysis of health and well-being. In J. Jetten, C. Haslam, & S. A. Haslam (Eds.), *The social cure: Identity, health, & well-being* (pp. 3-21). New York, NY: Psychology Press.

Jezewski, M. A., & Sotnik, P. (2001). *The rehabilitation service provider as culture broker: Providing culturally competent services to foreign born persons*. Buffalo, NY: Center for International Rehabilitation Research Information and Exchange.

Kaplan, A. (1999). *Organizational capacity*. Cape Town, South Africa: Community Development Resource Association. Available: http://www.cdra.org.za

Kay, L. M., Lancaster, L., & Freeman, W. J. (1996). Reafference and attractors in the olfactory system during odor recognition. *International Journal of Neural Systems, 7*, 489-496.

Kelso, S. J. A. (1999). *Dynamic patterns: The self-organization of brain and behavior*. Cambridge, MA: MIT Press.

Lazzarini, I. (2004). Neuro-occupation: The nonlinear dynamics of intention, meaning and perception. *British Journal of Occupational Therapy, 67*, 1-11.

Lethborg, C., Aranda, S., & Kissane, D. (2008). Meaning and adjustment to cancer: A model of care. *Palliative and Supportive Care, 6*, 61-70. doi:10.1017/S1478951508000096

Liedtka, J. (1998). Strategic thinking: Can it be taught? *Long Range Planning, 31*, 120-129.

Mattingly, C. (1991). The narrative nature of clinical reasoning. *American Journal of Occupational Therapy, 45*, 998-1005.

Mattingly, C. (2010). *The paradox of hope: Journey through a cultural borderland.* Berkeley, CA: University of California Press.

Maturana, H., & Varela, F. (1987). *The tree of knowledge.* Boston, MA: Shambhala.

Merriam-Webster Dictionary. (2015). http://www.merriam-webster.com/dictionary

Mills, C. W. (1959) *Sociological imagination.* New York, NY: Oxford University Press.

Polkinghorne, D. E. (1988). Transformative narratives: From victim to agentic life plots. *American Journal of Occupational Therapy, 50,* 299-305.

Puchalski, C., Ferrell, B., Virani, R., Otis-Green, S., Baird, P., Bull, J., et al. (2009). Improving the quality of spiritual care as a dimension of palliative care: The report of the consensus conference. *Journal of Palliative Medicine, 12,* 885-904. doi:10.1089/jpm.2009.0142

Salovey, P., & Mayer, J. D. (1990). Emotional intelligence. *Imagination, cognition and personality, 9,* 185-211. doi:0.2190/DUGG-P24E-52WK-6CDG

Schell, B., & Schell, J. (2008). *Clinical and professional reasoning in occupational therapy.* Philadelphia, PA: Wolters Kluwer/Lippincott Williams & Wilkins.

Shorter Oxford English Dictionary. (2002). Oxford, England: Oxford University Press.

Sinclair, K. (2007). Exploring the facets of clinical reasoning. In J. Creek & A. Lawson-Porter (Eds.), *Contemporary issues in occupational therapy: Reasoning and reflection* (143-160). Chichester, England: Wiley.

Taylor, R. R., & van Puymbroeck, L. (2013). Therapeutic use of self: Applying the intentional relationship model in group therapy. In J. C. O'Brien & J. W. Solomon (Eds.), *Occupational analysis and group process* (pp. 36-52). St. Louis, MO: Elsevier.

Thelen, E., & Smith, L. B. (1994). *A dynamic approach to the development of cognition and action.* Cambridge, MA: MIT Press.

Varela, F., Thompson, E., & Rosch, E. (1991). *The embodied mind: Cognitive science and human experience.* Cambridge, MA: MIT Press.

World Bank. (2013). *Social development brief: Social inclusion.* Retrieved from http://www.worldbank.org/en/topic/socialdevelopment/brief/social-inclusion

World Federation of Occupational Therapists. (2012). *Definition of occupational therapy.* Retrieved from www.wfot.org

World Health Organization. (2010). *Community-based rehabilitation guidelines.* Geneva, Switzerland: Author.

Financial Disclosures

Dr. Angela Birleson has no financial or proprietary interest in the materials presented herein.

Dr. Estelle B. Breines has no financial or proprietary interest in the materials presented herein.

Marilyn B. Cole has no financial or proprietary interest in the materials presented herein.

Dr. Jennifer Creek has no financial or proprietary interest in the materials presented herein.

Dr. E. Madeleine Duncan has no financial or proprietary interest in the materials presented herein.

Dr. Ivelisse Lazzarini has no financial or proprietary interest in the materials presented herein.

Dr. Theresa Lorenzo has no financial or proprietary interest in the materials presented herein.

Sílvia Martins has no financial or proprietary interest in the materials presented herein.

Dr. Anne Hiller Scott has no financial or proprietary interest in the materials presented herein.

Richard Scott has no financial or proprietary interest in the materials presented herein.

Dr. Kit Sinclair has no financial or proprietary interest in the materials presented herein.

Dr. Hanneke van Bruggen has no financial or proprietary interest in the materials presented herein.

Index

Printed in the United States
by Baker & Taylor Publisher Services